PROSTATE CANCER - LEADING-EDGE DIAGNOSTIC PROCEDURES AND TREATMENTS

Edited by **Ravinder Mohan**

Prostate Cancer - Leading-edge Diagnostic Procedures and Treatments
http://dx.doi.org/10.5772/61619
Edited by Ravinder Mohan

Contributors

Hojjat Ahmadzadehfar; Md, MSc, Yasemin Parlak, Weranja Ranasinghe, Raj Persad, Meral Huri, Burcu Semin Akel, Sedef Şahin, Naoki Sakai, Sunao Shoji, Jeremy Teoh, Ming-Kwong Yiu, Miltiadis Paliouras, Mark Trifiro, Carlos Alvarado, Sanjay Gupta, Eswar Shankar, Mario Candamo, Gregory MacLennan, Goran Brajuskovic, Appu Rathinavelu, Arkene Levy, Yasuyoshi Miyata, Jue Wang, John W. Davis

Published by InTech

Janeza Trdine 9, 51000 Rijeka, Croatia

Publishing Process Manager Andrea Koric

Technical Editor SPi Global

Cover InTech Design team

First published September, 2016

Printed in Croatia

Additional hard copies can be obtained from orders@intechopen.com

Prostate Cancer - Leading-edge Diagnostic Procedures and Treatments, Edited by Ravinder Mohan

p. cm.

Print ISBN 978-953-51-2644-7

Online ISBN 978-953-51-2645-4

For EU product safety concerns:
IN TECH d.o.o., Prolaz Marije Krucifikse Kozulić 3, 51000 Rijeka, Croatia,
info@intechopen.com or visit our website at intechopen.com.

Meet the editor

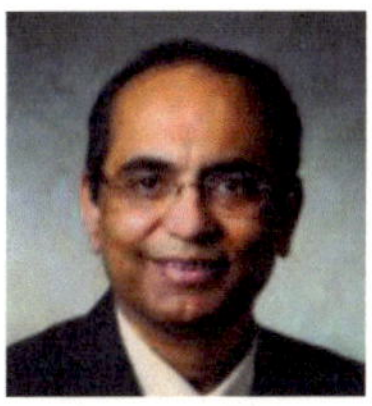

Ravinder Mohan, MD, PhD, teaches and practices family medicine in Virginia and also works as a hospitalist physician. He became interested in research on health-related quality of life in Belgium, where he studied outcomes of cardiac surgery. He did similar research in the United States in survivorship of patients newly diagnosed with localized prostate cancer. This is his third book as editor on clinical outcomes in cancer.

Contents

Preface

Prostate cancer is a common cancer that is usually slow growing and may be mistakenly perceived as harmless. In nonsmoking American men, it is the commonest cause of cancer death. In the past two decades, the norm was to screen for this cancer actively in any man over 50, find it, and treat it with surgery or radiotherapy. Many patients then suffered erectile dysfunction and urinary incontinence, and large studies questioned whether their survival had been prolonged even slightly. In the last five years, the pendulum has swung extremely to the opposite side; national recommendations have declared that screening for this cancer is harmful, and screening for the cancer has almost halted—at times even in African-American men who have the cancer more commonly and die due to it more commonly. Whether this approach will lead to a large increase in prostate cancer mortality remains to be seen.

At such a time, we have to again review the usefulness of newer screening protocols and biomarkers that can help in identifying cancers that we should treat before they spread rapidly and also be ready to treat more advanced cancers with newer, more effective, and safer methods of hormone therapy, chemotherapy, and radiotherapy. In this book, some of the best investigators in the world present their cutting-edge research, clinical practice, and discussions in both of these aspects.

Prof. Ravinder Mohan
Associate Professor,
Eastern Virginia Medical School,
Norfolk, Virginia, USA

Chapter 1

Prostate-Specific Antigen-Based Prostate Cancer Screening

Naoki Sakai

Additional information is available at the end of the chapter

http://dx.doi.org/10.5772/63751

Abstract

Serum prostate-specific antigen (PSA) testing is a simple and effective method for diagnosing prostate cancer. The widespread PSA screening resulted in increased diagnosis of early-staged, localized prostate cancer and marked reduction in advanced, metastatic cancer, which contributed to subsequent reduction in prostate cancer mortality. Most patients with localized prostate cancer, especially low-grade cancer, have an indolent clinical course. In addition, the rate of death from prostate cancer itself is very low. Therefore, early diagnosis of prostate cancer can lead to overdiagnosis and overtreatment. There has been a controversy regarding the effect of PSA screening on prostate cancer mortality. Results of the two largest randomized trials concerning PSA screening were totally contrary. European countries-based trial showed a significant prostate cancer mortality reduction, whereas the USA-based trial showed no benefit in reducing prostate cancer mortality. In 2013, based on these arguments, the American Urological Association updated a guideline regarding PSA screening, which did not recommend routine PSA screening but a selective screening, according to patient's age, coexisting medical condition, and risks, such as family history. The guideline also emphasized shared decision making.

However, older patients have been shown to be more likely to have high-risk prostate cancer at diagnosis. Older patients more often have other medical conditions and are more likely to die from causes other than prostate cancer. Prostate cancer is more often diagnosed with older patients. These facts bring PSA-based screening for prostate cancer more and more complex. In this chapter, problems concerning PSA screening are presented.

Keywords: prostate-specific antigen, prostate cancer, screening, mortality, evidence

1. Introduction

Prostate cancer is the most common cancer, accounting for up to 29% of all incident cases and is the second most common cause of cancer death among men in the United States in 2012 [1]. The lifetime probability of being diagnosed as prostate cancer is approximately 16% [1]. Serum prostate-specific antigen (PSA) measurement is an extremely effective tool for identifying men with prostate cancer. Today, almost all prostate cancer patients are being diagnosed with an elevated PSA. It is well known that PSA screening has increased the incidence of prostate cancer but decreased a rate of advanced, metastatic prostate cancer and resulted in a subsequent drastic reduction in prostate cancer mortality.

In the United States, following the introduction of widespread PSA screening in the late 1980s, there was a 70% increase in prostate cancer incidence. In 1992, there was a peak of incidence, as if it can be called the prostate cancer incidence surge. Several years after the introduction of PSA testing, from around 1994, mortality rate began to fall [1].

In European countries, PSA screening decreased the absolute risk of being diagnosed with advanced prostate cancer [2]. A population-based, prospective, randomized, controlled screening study for prostate cancer, with biennial PSA testing group and control group, showed that after a follow-up of 10 year, the diagnosis of prostate cancer increased by 1.8-fold; however, the risk of being diagnosed with metastatic prostate cancer was reduced by 48.9% ($p = 0.0084$) [2].

The incidence of prostate cancer in Japan rapidly increased between 2000 and 2003, while the mortality rate started to decrease in 2004, immediately after the increase in incidence [3]. The proportion of localized prostate cancer rapidly increased between 1997 and 2003, from 40 to 60% or higher. These facts are explained by early diagnosis using serum PSA measurement [3].

The primary aim of PSA-based prostate cancer screening should be the early detection of asymptomatic patients with potentially fatal cancers resulting in reduction of cancer-specific mortality [4]. However, early diagnosis of the prostate cancer due to widespread PSA screening has also led to increased diagnosis of clinically indolent cancers. Almost all localized cancers, especially low-grade disease, rarely progress to advanced disease and even fewer have a fatal clinical course [5, 6]. Prostate biopsy as well as any treatment has some adverse events and harms. Thus, PSA screening itself is associated with overdiagnosis and overtreatment. PSA screening in asymptomatic individuals involves a trade-off of benefit and harm.

Randomized trial is the most valuable study design for making evidence in medical fields. To address whether there is a mortality benefit in PSA screening, several randomized trials were performed. However, results of the two largest randomized trials were extremely confusing. The USA-based, the prostate component of the Prostate, Lung, Colorectal, and Ovarian Cancer Screening Trial (PLCO trial) showed no benefit in reducing mortality rate [7]; however, the European-based, the European Randomized study of Screening for Prostate Cancer (ERSPC trial) showed a significant mortality reduction [8].

The United States Preventive Health Services Task Force (USPSTF) has regarded harms associated PSA screening more important and has recommended against PSA screening in asymptomatic men regardless of age [9]. The USPSTF stated that current empiric evidence is insufficient to assess the risks and benefits of prostate cancer screening. Potential harms from screening and treatment are much more significant and clinicians should recommend against PSA screening for prostate cancer [9].

In 2013, based on these arguments, the American Urological Association (AUA) updated clinical guideline for PSA screening, "Early detection of Prostate cancer", which recommended against an organized PSA screening but for a selective PSA screening according to age, comorbidities, and risks such as family history [10]. In addition, the AUA strongly recommended shared decision making, a thorough discussion between physician and patient regarding the risks and benefits of PSA-based screening [10].

In general, the rate of prostate cancer incidence increases with age [1, 11]. Compared with younger men, older men are more frequently diagnosed with high grade and high risk prostate cancer [12]. In addition, coexisting medical conditions are also more prevalent in older patients. These facts bring PSA screening much more confusing.

As an alternative data source, a population level data, cohort study, concerning PSA screening is presented. Although cohort study is considered a lower level of evidence compared to the randomized study, it has some merit in reflecting "real world" clinical data.

2. Conflicting two large randomized trials concerning PSA screening

In 2009, totally conflicting two large randomized trials addressing the effect of PSA screening on the prostate cancer-specific mortality rate were published at the same time in the same journal, and consecutively [7, 8]. The USA-based, the prostate component of the Prostate, Lung, Colorectal, and Ovarian Cancer Screening Trial (the PLCO trial), showed no benefit in reducing mortality rate, after 7–10 years of follow-up (rate ratio (RR) 1.13; 95% confidence interval (CI) 0.75–1.70) [7]. In contrast, European countries-based trial, the European Randomized study of Screening for Prostate Cancer (the ERSPC trial), showed a benefit of PSA screening in reducing prostate cancer mortality [8]. The ERSPC trial reported that during a median follow-up of 9 years, the rate ratio for death from prostate cancer in the screening group, as compared with the control group, was 0.80 (95% CI, 0.65–0.98; adjusted $p = 0.04$) [8].

The prostate component of the Prostate, Lung, Colorectal, and Ovarian Cancer Screening Trial (PLCO trial) is a multicenter, randomized trial designed to evaluate the effect of PSA screening for prostate cancer-specific mortality. A total of 76,685 men, aged 55–74 years, were randomly assigned to the intervention arm (offered annual PSA testing for 6 years and annual digital rectal examination for 4 years) and to the control arm (usual, opportunistic PSA examination) at 10 centers in the United States between 1993 and 2001. A PSA cutoff 4.0 ng/ml was used for prostate biopsy. The PLCO trial extended follow-up period to 13 years and concluded that there was also no evidence of a mortality benefit for organized annual screening compared with opportunistic screening (RR, 1.09; 95% CI, 0.87–1.36) [13].

On the other hand, the European Randomized study of Screening for Prostate Cancer (ERSPC trial) is also a randomized multicenter trial with core age group (55–69 years) evaluating the benefit of screening for prostate cancer with serum PSA in eight European countries, including the Netherlands, Belgium, Sweden, Finland, Italy, Spain, Switzerland, and France. Briefly, a total of 162,388 aged 55–69 men were randomly assigned as an intervention arm (invited to PSA screening once every 4 years in seven countries and once every 2 years in Sweden) or a control arm with no PSA testing offered. A PSA cutoff 3.0 ng/ml was used for prostate biopsy. The ERSPC group also extended follow-up to 11–13 years and reported that the rate ratio (RR) of prostate cancer incidence between the intervention and control arms was 1.91, 1.66, and 1.57 after 9, 11, and 13 years, respectively, and the RR of prostate cancer mortality was 0.85, 0.78, and 0.79 at 9, 11, and 13 years, respectively (95% confidence interval 13 years 0.69–0.91, p = 0.001), corresponding to a relative risk reduction of 21% at 13 years [14, 15]. The updated ERSPC study concluded a substantial prostate cancer mortality reduction due to PSA testing. In the ERSPC trial, a significant decrease in metastatic disease at diagnosis was demonstrated. The rate of advanced group (M1 and/or PSA > 100 ng/ml) was 3.4 and 9.6%, in the intervention and control arm, respectively.

The reasons why the results of these two trials were totally different might be due to differences in study design: screening protocol and PSA cutoff value. For example, the ERSPC trial compared screening group to no screening group, while the PLCO trial compared annual PSA screening to opportunistic PSA testing in the control arm [16].

Randomized trial has some unavoidable limitations: compliance in the intervention arm, nonparticipation in the screening arm, and PSA contamination, opportunistic PSA testing in the control arm. Because investigated individuals have the will, PSA contamination cannot be excluded completely. The contamination rates were 20–25% in the ERSPC trial and 40% in the first year and increased to 52% in the sixth years in the PLCO trial [7, 8]. Increased exposure to opportunistic PSA testing in the control arm reduces the reliability of the randomized study. The Rotterdam section of the ERSPC trial demonstrated that after correction for both nonattendance in the screening arm and PSA contamination in the control arm, PSA-based screening conducted in the Dutch center reduced the risk of dying from prostate cancer up to 51% (RR of 0.49; 95% CI, 0.27–0.87) in men who undergo organized screening at a median follow-up of 13 years [17].

In addition, randomized trial has another limitation. The primary end point of the trial is prostate cancer-specific mortality. Therefore, randomized trials would require a considerably long time to withdraw some conclusions. These trials randomly registered asymptomatic, healthy men and had followed until assigned men developed prostatic cancer and, further, died from prostate cancer or other causes. When a result is provided, the diagnostic method that is prostate biopsy method as well as treatment methods usually have progressed.

In addition, the rate of the death from prostate cancer is very low and there is a difficulty in assessing the effect of PSA screening on the prostate cancer-specific mortality. For example, the PLCO trial reported that after 7–10 years of follow-up, the incidence of death per 10,000 person-years was only 2.0 (50 deaths) in the screening group and 1.7 (44 deaths) in the control group (rate ratio, 1.13; 95% CI, 0.75–1.70) [7].

3. Localized, low-grade prostate cancer most often has an indolent character

The majority of prostate cancer patients with early, localized, low-grade cancer with proper treatments most often have an indolent clinical course. An analysis of 828 case records of men treated conservatively (with observation and delayed hormone therapy) for clinically localized prostate cancer showed that 10 years after diagnosis, disease-specific survival was 87% for men with grade 1 or 2 tumors and 34% for those with grade 3 tumors [5]. Most early-stage (T0-T2 NX M0 classification), initially untreated prostate cancer, had an indolent course during the first 10–15 years [6].

4. Patients with some coexisting conditions are more likely to die from causes other than prostate cancer

Patients with some comorbidities were more likely to die from causes other than prostate cancer [18]. The Surveillance, Epidemiology, and End Results (SEER) group conducted a 10-year competing risk analysis of men 66 years age and older with localized prostate cancer and received no surgery and radiation within 180 days of diagnosis and found that relatively few men died as a result of prostate cancer within 10 years of diagnosis [19]. Patients were more likely to die from comorbid causes other than prostate cancer during the first 10 years after diagnosis. Depending on patient age, Gleason score, and number of coexisting conditions, 10-year overall mortality rates increased from 28.8% (95% CI, 25.3–32.6%) to 94.3% (95% CI, 87.4–100%), in contrast, prostate cancer-specific mortality rates varied from 2.0% (95% CI, 0.0–5.3%) to 27.5% (95% CI, 21.5–36.5%). The group reported that most patients with localized prostate cancer older than 65 years would not die from prostate cancer within 10 years of diagnosis. Most prostate cancer patients with either no or one comorbidity would survive at least 10 years; in contrast, those with two or more comorbid conditions would have a substantial risk of dying from a coexisting disease within this time period [19]. Another randomized study demonstrated a similar result. After 10-year follow-up of 76,693 men with prostate cancer, a significant decrease in the risk of prostate cancer-specific mortality was observed in patients with no or minimal comorbidity (adjusted hazard ratio (HR), 0.56; 95% CI, 0.33–0.95; $p = 0.03$); however, no reduction of that was observed in patients with at least one significant comorbidity (adjusted hazard ratio, 1.43; 95% CI, 0.96–2.11; $p = 0.08$). The group concluded that selective use of PSA screening for men in good health appeared to reduce the risk of prostate cancer-specific mortality [20].

5. The AUA updated a guideline concerning early detection of prostate cancer

In 2013, the American Urological Association (AUA) updated clinical guideline regarding PSA screening, "Early detection of Prostate cancer", which recommended a selective PSA screening, for example, according to age, coexisting medical conditions, or risks such as family history [10]. In addition, the AUA guideline strongly recommended "shared-decision making", which is a thorough discussion between clinicians and patients concerning the risks and benefits of PSA screening and treatment.

Above-mentioned arguments were the main reasons why the AUA recommended against routine PSA screening but for a selected screening and emphasized "shared-decision making". For example, the AUA guideline did not recommend routine PSA screening in 70 years of age or older men.

However, we must pay attention to the fact that the AUA guideline does not address diagnosis of symptomatic patients, where symptoms imply those that could be related to locally advanced or metastatic disease, but detection of disease at an early, pre-symptomatic stage when a man would have no reason to seek medical care.

6. Prostate cancer incidence increases with age

The rate of prostate cancer incidence increases with age. The incidence rate of prostate cancer increases, especially older than 70 years. In the United States, probability of developing prostate cancer for 60–69 years of age, 70 and older, and birth to death were 6.84, 12.54, and 16.48%, respectively [1]. As for in Japan, the Japan Cancer Surveillance Research Group reported that the prostate cancer incidence rate of all ages, crude rate, was 63.1 per 100,000 population in 2004; however, age-adjusted incidence rate increased from 32.2 in the 55- to 59-year-old group to 401.2 in the 80- to 84-year-old group [11].

7. Older men are more likely to be presented with high-risk prostate cancer

Older men are more likely to be presented with high-risk prostate cancer and to have lower cancer-specific survival [12]. A study from the Cancer of the Prostate Strategic Urologic Research Endeavor (CaPSURE) demonstrated that 26% of men above 75 years of age presented with high-risk prostate cancer and older men were less likely to receive curative treatment, partially explaining the higher prostate cancer-specific mortality rate [12]. Furthermore, post PSA screening follow-up study showed that compared with cancers detected during the screening period for men up to 69 year of age, cancers diagnosed after screening for men beyond 69 year of age were shifted toward more advanced, high-risk cancers with a low rate of low-risk cancers [21]. In addition, an extended follow-up study revealed that even patients with initially low risk tumors showed local progression and distant metastasis and eventually resulted in lethal outcome. A comparative study of early-staged prostate cancer patients between the first 15 years and the next 15–20 years demonstrated a substantial decrease in progression-free survival, from 45.0 to 36.0%; survival without metastases, from 76.9 to 51.2%; and prostate cancer-specific survival, from 78.7 to 54.4% [6]. In addition, the prostate cancer-specific mortality rate increased from 15 per 1000 person-years (95% CI, 10–21) during the first

http://dx.doi.org/10.5772/63751

15 years to 44 per 1000 person-years (95% CI, 22–88) following the first 15 years ($p = 0.01$) [6]. After 32 years of follow-up of this series, 90 (41.4%) cases showed local progression and 41 (18.4%) exhibited progression to distant metastasis [22]. These facts imply that localized prostate cancer most often has an indolent course; however, local progression and distant metastasis could develop over the long term, even among patients considered as low-risk disease at diagnosis.

8. Population-based cohort study reflects the real -world clinical outcome

Population-based cohort study is the second best study design for evidenced-based decision making in medicine. Randomized study searches for an idealized world data, while cohort study uses a real-world clinical data. Different from the randomized trials, the cohort study targets the patients with prostate cancer from the beginning.

Authors conducted a population-based cohort study of pathologically diagnosed prostate cancer patients in Yokosuka City, Japan, between 2001 and 2010 and compared their clinical outcomes until 2013. Prostate cancer patients were divided into two groups: 524 detected by PSA-based screening in Yokosuka City (screening, S group) versus 1044 those detected by opportunistic PSA examinations (non-screening, NS group) [23]. Median age at diagnosis in the S group was significantly lower than that in the NS group: 71 and 73 years of age, respectively ($p < 0.001$). The rate of Gleason score (GS) 8–10 in the S group was significantly lower than that in the NS group: 9.7 and 16.7%, respectively ($p < 0.001$). The rate of patients with metastasis or PSA 100 ng/ml or more in the S group was also significantly lower than that in the NS group: 7.8 and 23.0%, respectively ($p < 0.001$). The group reported 8 (1.5%) prostate cancer deaths in the S group, whereas 70 (6.7 %) deaths in the NS group during the follow-up period. There were 42 (8.0%) deaths from other causes in the S group and 119 (11.4%) such deaths in the NS group. In the study, the group found a significantly higher 10-year cancer-specific survival rate in the S group than in the NS group: 97 and 86%, respectively ($p < 0.001$). The 10-year overall survival rate in the S group was also significantly higher than the NS group, 77 and 64%, respectively ($p < 0.001$). Multivariate Cox regression analysis showed that GS 8–10 was significantly associated with cancer-specific survival rate (HR, 4.808; 95% CI, 1.044–22.14; $p = 0.044$). The significantly lower prevalence of advanced prostate cancer, especially lower prevalence of GS 8–10 in the S group, was considered to be associated with higher cancer-specific survival. Older patients are more likely to have high-risk prostate cancer at diagnosis [12, 21]. The difference in the median age between the two groups was only 2 years; however, this difference might be responsible for the significantly lower prevalence of GS 8–10 prostate cancer in the S group.

Prostate cancer patients are in general more likely to die from coexisting diseases other than prostate cancer [18–20]. This study also demonstrated that overall 5.0% of patients died from prostate cancer, whereas 10.3% died from other causes. However, we must pay attention to the fact that in patients with advanced disease group, metastasis positive, or PSA 100 ng/ml or more, especially in the NS group, the incidence of death from prostate cancer was higher than those from other causes, 22.5 and 13.8%, respectively.

The ERSPC trial demonstrated similar overall survival rates between the intervention and the control arms [8]. In contrast, this real-world analysis revealed a significantly higher 10-year overall survival rate in the S group. The higher cancer-specific survival rate in the S group and the 2 years difference in median age between the two groups might be partly responsible for the higher overall survival rate. In addition, a plausible reason for this difference is considered as follows: the S group might consist of health-conscious men, who are willing to seek PSA screening at their own will, in other words, who are eager to be in good health. PSA screening itself is not a national duty. In fact, the group noticed a significantly lower Charlson comorbidity score in the S group than in the NS group, 0.5 and 1.3, respectively ($p < 0.001$). These factors might be associated with a higher overall survival rate in the S group [23]. PSA-based population screening in Yokosuka City could contribute to reduce the rate of advanced prostate cancer and might help to reduce prostate cancer mortality rate.

Cancer statistical analysis reported that among men, prostate cancer was the most common cancer, accounting for up to 29% of all incident cases and was the second most common (9%) cause of cancer death in the United States in 2012 [1]. While lung and bronchus cancer was the second most common (14%) estimated new cases and the most common (29%) cause of cancer death among men in the United States in 2012 [1]. These figures suggest that at least prostate cancer, totally, is less aggressive than lung and bronchus cancer. In this statistical analysis, disease duration was not clearly shown; however, prostate cancer patients would seem to survive much longer than lung and bronchus patients. Prostate cancer is a highly heterogeneous cancer, ranging from low-grade, slow-growing, and indolent tumors to high grade, rapidly growing, and fatal carcinomas associated with significant morbidity [24].

An ideal tumor marker should be such that it could mainly detect asymptomatic patients with potentially fatal cancers; however, in fact, this would be rather impossible for PSA screening. Because PSA screening is an extremely sensitive examination, it inevitably detects indolent tumors as well as fatal carcinomas. Rather, if PSA screening could not detect a variety of prostate cancers, PSA would have no value as a screening marker for prostate cancer.

Prostate cancer is an extremely heterogeneous cancer, from low-grade, slow-growing, and indolent tumors to high-grade, rapidly growing, and fatal carcinomas. Prostate cancer incidence increases with age. Older men are more likely to be presented with high-grade prostate cancer. Older men are more likely to have comorbid medical conditions, such as diabetes, cardiovascular diseases, and cerebrovascular diseases. Health-conscious men would seek PSA screening. According to these facts, prostate cancer management should be tailored based on an individual patient's health status, coexisting medical conditions, life expectancy, and tumor characteristics [25]. One man argued as follows: the time has come from a "one size fits all" approach to a tailored approach based on an individual patient's health condition [26]. Physicians should be aware of these facts and should use PSA screening to offer the most appropriate approach to prostate cancer management for each patient.

http://dx.doi.org/10.5772/63751

Author details

Naoki Sakai

Address all correspondence to: sakai@wakakusa.saiseikai.or.jp

Department of Urology, Saiseikai Wakakusa Hospital, Yokohama, Kanagawa, Japan

References

[1] Siegel R, Naishadham D and Jemal A. Cancer statics, 2012. CA Cancer J Clin. 2012: 62: 10–29.

[2] Aus G, Bergdahl S, Lodding P, et al. Prostate cancer screening decreases the absolute risk of being diagnosed advanced prostate cancer-results from a prospective, population-based randomised control trial. Eur Urol. 2007; 51: 659–664.

[3] Katanoda K, Matsuda T, Matsuda A, et al. An updated report of the trends in cancer incidence and mortality in Japan. Jpn J Clin Oncol. 2013; 43: 492–507.

[4] Gomella LG, Liu XS, Trabulsi EJ, et al. Screening for prostate cancer: the current evidence and guidelines controversy. Can J Urol. 2011; 18: 5875–5883.

[5] Chodak GW, Thisted RA, Gerber GS, et al. Results of conservative management of clinically localized prostate cancer. N Engl J Med. 1994; 330: 242–248.

[6] Johansson JE, Andrén O, Andersson SO, et al. Natural history of early, localized prostate cancer. JAMA. 2004; 291: 2713–2719.

[7] Andriole GL, Crawford ED, Grubb IIIRL, et al. Mortality results from a randomized prostate-cancer screening trial. N Engl J Med. 2009; 360: 1310–1319.

[8] Schroder FH, Hugosson J, Roobol MJ, et al. Screening and prostate-cancer mortality in a randomised European study. N Engl J Med. 2009; 360: 1320–1328.

[9] Melnikow J, LeFevre M, Wilt TJ, et al. Counterpoint: randomized trials provide the strongest evidence for clinical guidelines: the US Preventive Services Task Force and prostate cancer screening. Med Care. 2013; 51: 301–303.

[10] Carter HB, Albertsen PC, Barry MJ, et al. Early detection of prostate cancer AUA guideline. J Urol. 2013; 190: 1134–1137.

[11] Matsuda T, Marugame T, Kamo K, et al. Cancer incidence and incidence rates in Japan in 2004: based on data from 14 population-based cancer registries in the monitoring of cancer incidence in Japan (MCIJ) project. Jpn J Clin Oncol. 2010; 40: 1192–1200.

[12] Bechis SK, Carroll PR and Cooperberg MR. Impact of age at diagnosis on prostate cancer treatment and survival. J. Clin Oncol. 2011; 29: 235–241.

[13] Andriole GL, Crawford ED, Grubb IIIRL, et al. Prostate cancer screening in the randomized prostate, lung, colorectal, and ovarian cancer screening trial: mortality results after 13 years of follow-up. J Natl Cancer Inst. 2012; 104: 125–132.

[14] Schroder FH, Hugosson J, Roobol MJ, et al. Prostate-cancer mortality at 11 years of follow-up. N Engl J Med. 2012; 366: 981–990.

[15] Schroder FH, Hugosson J, Roobol MJ, et al. The European randomized study of screening for prostate cancer-prostate cancer mortality at 13 years of follow-up. Lancet. 2014; 384: 2027–2035.

[16] Kim EH and Andriole GL. Prostate-specific antigen-based screening: controversy and guidelines. BMC Med. 2015; 13: 61–64.

[17] Bokhorst LP, Bangma CH, van Leederd GJLH, et al. Prostate-specific antigen–based prostate cancer screening: reduction of prostate cancer mortality after correction for nonattendance and contamination in the Rotterdam section of the European randomized study of screening for prostate cancer. Eur Urol. 2014; 65: 329–336.

[18] Lu-Yao GL, Albertson PC, Moore DF, et al. Outcomes of localized prostate cancer following conservative management. JAMA. 2009; 302: 1202–1209.

[19] Albertsen PC, Moore DF, Shih W, et al. Impact of comorbidity on survival among men with localized prostate cancer. J Clin Oncol. 2011; 29: 1335–1341.

[20] Crawford ED, Grubb III R, Black A, et al. Comorbidity and mortality results from a randomized prostate cancer screening trial. J Clin Oncol. 2011; 29: 355–361.

[21] Bergdahl AG, Holmberg E, Moss S, et al. Incidence of prostate cancer after termination of screening in a population-based randomised trial. Eur Urol. 2013; 64: 703–709.

[22] Popiolek M, Rider JR, Andrén O, et al. Natural history of early, localized prostate cancer: a final report from three decades of follow-up. Eur Urol. 2013; 63: 423–435.

[23] Sakai N, Taguri M, Kobayashi K, et al. Clinical outcomes of prostate cancer patients in Yokosuka City, Japan: a comparative study between cases detected by prostate-specific antigen-based screening in Yokosuka and those detected by other means. Int J Urol. 2015; 22: 747–753.

[24] Roobol MJ and Carlsson SV. Risk stratification in prostate cancer screening. Nat Urol Rev. 2013; 10: 38–48.

[25] Hoffman KE. Management of older men with clinically localized prostate cancer: the significance of advanced age and comorbidity. Semin Radiat Oncol. 2012; 22: 284–294.

[26] McNaughton MF and Barry MJ. One man at a time-resolving the PSA controversy. N Engl J Med. 2011; 365: 1951–1953.

Chapter 2

Advances in Prostate Cancer Diagnosis: Triggers for Prostate Biopsy

John W. Davis and Chinedu Mmeje

Additional information is available at the end of the chapter

http://dx.doi.org/10.5772/64402

Abstract

In the early years of screening for prostate cancer with serum PSA, absolute cutoffs were typically utilized such as greater than 4.0 ng/mL or even 2.5 ng/mL. A biopsy of the prostate would commonly be recommended in a man with greater than 10-year life expectancy who had a confirmed elevation above such a threshold or in the presence of an abnormal digital rectal examination. The unmet need, however, is to be more selective in recommending a prostate biopsy, due to the risk of complications and the high rate of false-positive PSAs. More recently, various clinical nomograms can be used to refine selection. In addition, clinicians can now utilize various advanced serum biomarkers that have enhanced specificity—especially for the patient with a rising PSA with prior negative biopsy. In this chapter, we will focus on the biomarkers PCA3, Prostate Health Index, and 4 K score to illustrate key concepts in biomarker development and clinical utility.

Keywords: prostate cancer, prostate biopsy, PCA3, urine, Prostate Health Index, serum, 4 K score, serum

1. Introduction—a narrative on contemporary management of prostate cancer risk with ordinary clinical tools

The male disease process "prostate cancer" is a heterogeneous entity at multiple subtopics including epidemiology, screening, diagnosis, treatment options, side effects, and cancer control results. It is common to introduce a peer-reviewed article or text chapter focused on any aspect of prostate cancer with the observation that the disease is common but a much smaller subset result in a disease-specific mortality—almost to the point of useless repetition. The heterogeneity of prostate cancer extends well beyond population statistics, and in this chapter, we will focus on one aspect of heterogeneity—diagnosis. The key paradigm in contemporary practice is a male screened for prostate cancer with serum prostate specific antigen (PSA) and digital rectal examination (DRE). The alternate/related paradigm is the male with lower urinary tract or other pelvic symptoms who is evaluated for prostate cancer with serum PSA/DRE as a differential diagnosis. Performing a biopsy and subsequent treatment has certainly altered key statistics in prostate cancer compared to pure clinical detection. The incidence has increased as well as treatment numbers. Recently, Welch et al. demonstrated with SEER/Medicare data that the incidence of metastatic disease at diagnosis significantly declined with the introduction of PSA, compared with the relatively flat effect of mammography screening to breast cancer staging [1].

The problem faced from this paradigm is that the results of a prostate biopsy are frustrating for a growing list of reasons:

1. Too many negative or indeterminate biopsies.
2. Too many negative or indeterminate biopsies that are found to be falsely negative with future evaluations.
3. Too many positive biopsies for low grade disease—leads to overtreatment.
4. Too many positive biopsies for low grade disease that with future radical prostatectomy or repeat biopsies are found to have missed higher grade disease.
5. Cost, discomfort, and an occasional septic infection as the side effects of this effort to make the *correct* diagnosis for a patient.

The concepts can be illustrated in the following case vignettes:

- A patient with Gleason Score 3+3 on biopsy has a radical prostatectomy, and the final pathology showed Gleason 4+4.
- A patient with three negative biopsies has a continuous rising PSA—should he have a 4th biopsy or accept the cause as benign?
- A patient with a negative biopsy and stable PSA—should he continue screening? What age to stop?
- An elderly patient with Gleason 7 prostate cancer is unsure of overall longevity—does he need curative therapy or just watchful waiting based on symptoms?

Physicians managing patients at risk for prostate cancer can certainly use clinical features to frame many questions. In the asymptomatic patient who might have clinically localized disease, a life expectancy of less than 10 years would be treated differently than a life expectancy greater than 10 years. Family history of prostate cancer (father, brothers, uncles) and African American race are well-known adverse risk features for prostate cancer. The PSA has its statistical problems with specificity (related to false positives), but does have sensitivity (related to true positives) related to its value—higher PSAs have more risk of cancer, but hard to determine a clear line to draw where you call the test clearly normal versus abnormal. Translating these narrated elements into summary numerical estimates (noncited as widely available):

- For the common case with elevated PSA between 2.5 and 6.0, and leading to a prostate biopsy, the overall cancer detection rate can be 30%, ±10% depending upon region. Of all positive biopsies, 10–25% may have high grade elements. This means that the majority of prostate biopsies are free of cancer, and an even higher number are free of clinically significant cancer.
- For men with a previous negative biopsy, a repeat biopsy for continued rise is often positive in 10–20%. Subsequent repeat biopsies lower the rate further but not to something approaching zero.
- For men placed on active surveillance for low grade cancer, approximately 30% will be upgraded at some point with repeat testing.

Moving forward, the unmet needs in prostate cancer evaluation are to increase the detection of clinically significant disease when it is present, and to effectively rule out significant disease when it is not present, such that subsequent monitoring can be reduced or eliminated. *To emphasize—both of these needs are critical and equal: the need to diagnose cancer that is present and potentially lethal, and the need to eliminate diagnostic attempts when cancer is absent or nonlethal.*

2. Prostate biopsy triggers—mild improvement from mathematics and clinical trials

In a state-of-the-art lecture at the 2015 American Urological Association Annual Meeting, Stacy Loeb (New York, USA) made the key analogy that the first 10 or more years of use of PSA was analogous to a pregnancy test—in search of when to call the test positive or negative. The initial cut-point was 4.0, and many labs still flag a result in red at >4.0, and subsequent proposals were for >2.5. Clinical experience clearly showed the fallacy of this version of laboratory medicine—a man's risk of prostate cancer does not go from zero at PSA 3.9 to 100% at PSA of 4.1. The point was well illustrated by a follow-up report from the Prostate Cancer Prevention Trial that showed the biopsy results of men with different PSA cut-points who were all biopsied and on a placebo medication—sample size of 2950 participants and 449 cancers [2].**Table 1** shows a sample of their report. Note that the pregnancy illustration was carried forward in this trial, as men with a PSA > 4.0 were biopsied "for cause" and the data represent the men followed for the 7-year duration of the trial who were considered clinically "normal range". Prior to this publication, there was very limited data available on the results of a prostate biopsy in men with a normal DRE and PSA < 4.0.

With this data, you can certainly counsel a man on the concept of a relative range of prostate cancer risk rather than oversimplify it to a positive/negative result. This same dataset was refined further into an online calculator tool where you can input multiple clinical variables and receive an estimate on overall cancer detection and high grade (Gleason 7 or higher) cancer. The web link is: http://deb.uthscsa.edu/URORiskCalc/Pages/uroriskcalc.jsp.

Here are two example cases:

1. Race Caucasian, age 59, PSA 2.1, no family history, abnormal DRE, no prior biopsy. Result: 3% high-grade cancer, 14%, low-grade cancer, and 83% negative biopsy.

2. Race African American, age 59, PSA 9.8, positive family history for prostate cancer, DRE abnormal, no prior biopsy. Result: 35% high-grade cancer, 20% low-grade cancer, 45% negative biopsy.

PSA level	Percentage positive biopsy	Percentage of positive biopsies with high grade
≤0.5	6.6	12.5
0.6–1.0	10.1	10.0
1.1–2.0	17.0	11.8
2.1–3.0	23.9	19.1
3.1–4.0	26.9	25.0

Table 1. Data from the Prostate Cancer Prevention Trial [2]. This cohort of men were biopsied as part of the trial design and were on a placebo. Men with a PSA > 4.0 would have been biopsied earlier "for cause".

The results also remind you that regardless of the biopsy result, there may be a 2–4% chance of an infection requiring hospitalization. Thus, the absolute risks of cancer and side effects can be discussed and a personalized choice made. We should not forget why we are considering these efforts. The third update to the Bill-Axelson trial of radical prostatectomy versus watchful waiting reminds us that the treatment arm had a 12.7% absolute difference in overall mortality, with a relative risk of 0.71 in favor of surgery and number needed to treat to avoid a death of 1:8 [3]. Additional benefits were observed in palliation, metastatic progression, and androgen deprivation utilization.

3. Biomarkers in prostate cancer—highlights of evaluation and early improvement of specificity

As established thus far, PSA is the gold standard for prostate cancer detection. Many experts have voiced the opinion that this might change in the next generation [4]. First, we should review key biomarker nomenclature recognized by the FDA—whether a biomarker is serum, urine, or tissue base. **Table 2** shows four key distinctions and a biomarker such as PSA has elements of all four.

Data on biomarkers is a separate and vast topic and we will not review it. But the key headings would be whether a study is in preclinical exploratory trials, assay development, assay validation, retrospective use/repositories, prospective screening, or randomized controlled.

Biomarkers can be described based on their validity with a number of statistical expression and eventually need to be described based upon clinical utility, i.e., strength of ability to alter key clinical decisions and add value to health care.

Biomarker type	When	Indications
Prognostic	Prior to treatment	Risk of a specific outcome
Predictive	Prior to treatment	Identify which patients benefit from a treatment
Response indicator	During or after treatment	Response to treatment (pharmacology, physiology)
Efficacy-response (surrogate)	After treatment	Early/accurate prediction of a clinical endpoint

Table 2. FDA biomarker classification based on context of use.

As stated, there are many statistical advantages to PSA screening compared to using prostatic acid phosphatase (PAP) [5], or clinical exam [6]. However, there is significant room to improve accuracy and especially specificity. Early efforts to make progress were numerous such as adding the percent-free PSA to PSA ratio [7], age adjustment [8], PSA velocity of ≥0.75 ng/mL/year [9], and PSA density of 0.15 [10]. These methods all made incremental practice, but perhaps the most significant is in making decisions about a repeat biopsy versus a primary biopsy. Another useful contribution to PSA screening interval questions came from Lilja et al., who showed that a single PSA before age 50 could be predictive of lifetime prostate cancer incidence [11].

4. A focus on novel diagnostic biomarkers: prostate Health Index and 4 K score

Similar themes in advancing future prostate cancer screening have come from focusing on "isomers" or molecular variants of the PSA molecule. Another variant of PSA is called Pro-PSA and can be more prevalent in the free-fraction within cancer versus noncancer [12]. In a validation study of Pro-PSA versus percent-free PSA, the area under the curve (AUC) was 0.68 for %ProPSA and 0.567 for %free PSA. At sensitivity of 75%, the %ProPSA would eliminate 59% of negative biopsies versus 33% with %fPSA [13]. Catalona et al. [14] also did a serum bank study on biopsied patients with elevated PSA and found the %proPSA can eliminate 19–33% of biopsies while holding 90% sensitivity.

The next iteration came from the discovery of an isoform p2PSA, and the concept of combining the information with free PSA and total PSA into an equation: ([−2]pPSA/fPSA)/√(tPSA). This is now the Prostate Health Index and licensed by Beckman Coulter laboratories. Jansen et al. [15] reported a multisite study showing that prostate cancer patients had higher PHI levels and %p2PSA. A U.S. validation study of 829 patients holding sensitivity at 95% had specificity of 16% for PHI and 8.5% for %fPSA [16]. Relevant to our case vignettes in the introductory narrative, the higher PHI values were also correlating with *a higher risk of Gleason score ≥7.*

A PHI score is currently reported in four "brackets" of results: 0–24.9, 25.0–34.9, 35.0–54.9, and >55. The PHI, as stated will include a total PSA, the free PSA, and the Pro-PSA. The PHI result is then translated into a percentage risk of prostate cancer. The source reference [16] includes the high grade numbers, but an actual test result for some reason does not. **Table 3** shows a commercial report range. The study listed ranges for Gleason ≥7 were PHI 0–24.9 = 26.1%, PHI 25.0–34.9 of 28.2%, PHI 35.0–54.9 of 30.1%, and PHI >55.0 of 42.1%. Thus, the trends are strongest comparing the lowest versus highest PHI brackets.

Biomarker	Sample result	Reference interval			
Total PSA	7.8	Normal < 2.0 At risk ≥ 2.0			
Free PSA	1.16	See below			
Pro2PSA	20.78	See PHI			
%free PSA	15	% Free PSA prostate cancer probability by age			
		%Free PSA	**<60**	**60–70**	**>70**
		<7	85%	95%	96%
		7–15	25%	50%	60%
		16–25	11%	27%	35%
		>25	2%	6%	10%
PHI	49.9	**PHI**	**Cancer probability**		
		0–24.9	11.0%		
		25.0–34.9	18.1%		
		35.0–54.9	32.7%		
		>55.0	52.1%		

Table 3. PHI result reporting as of 2015.

A European cohort was published by Lazzeri et al. [17] and showed an AUC of 0.67 for PHI as well as %proPSA—both superior to total PSA and %free PSA. At a PHI cutoff of 27.6, biopsies could have been avoided in 15.5%. The Gleason ≥7 trend was also observed in their statistical analyses.

Another research direction developing in parallel has been human glandular kallikrein 2—hK2. It is also part of the serine protease family along with PSA. Nam et al. [18], for example, looked at hK2 and hK2 to %free PSA ratios could find trends elevated in PCa. Vickers et al. then expanded the concept as a panel of Kallikrein markers: total PSA, free PSA, intact PSA, and hK2. This coined the phrase 4 K score [19]. The process developed a nomogram that includes the four markers, age, DRE, and determines a probability of cancer. The model adds to a clinical base model and increases prediction for high grade prostate cancer. The AUC for the full model was 0.832 and high-grade cancer was 0.870, and a decision curve analysis is presented to propose a threshold value of 20% as a biopsy trigger that would spare a significant number of biopsies and only miss 3% high-grade cancers. Parekh et al. [20] then published a U.S. prospective trial that used the PCPT risk calculator above as a control. Again, the full model had an AUC of 0.821 and higher AUC for Gleason ≥7, as well as decision curve benefit. As an illustration, a 4 K score cutoff of 9% led to 43% of biopsies avoided and 2.4% risk of delay in Gleason ≥7 diagnosis.

For the clinician, the question then becomes which test to use? PHI had a slight advantage in being earlier in regulatory approval. Nordstrom et al. presented a comparison study of PHI versus 4 K [21]. The PHI and 4 K both had improved prediction for overall and high grade prostate cancer. The AUC for 4 K was 0.69 and for PHI was 0.704, and for high-grade prostate cancer was 0.718 and 0.711, respectively. Comparable metrics were observed with a 4 K cutoff of 10% and PHI of 39.

	PHI	4K	PCA3
Components	Serum ([−2]pPSA/fPSA)/√(tPSA)	Serum tPSA, fPSA, intact PSA, hk2, age Clinical model (add DRE results)	Urine; (mRNA PCA3/ mRNA PSA) × 1000
Patient population	>50 y/o, PSA 4–10 ng/mL, normal DRE	Any patient referred for TRUS Bx	>50 y/o; prior negative Bx
FDA approval	2012	n/a	2012
Outcome measure	PCa	High risk PCa (GS ≥ 7)	PCa
Cutoff	0–29 = low risk; 8.7% risk PCa 21–39.9 = mod risk; 20.6% risk PCa >40 = high risk; 43.8% risk PCa	≥9%, eliminates 43% of unnecessary Bx, w/2.4% risk of delayed dx of HG PCa	>35 sensitivity = 58%, and specificity = 72% for PCa
Disadvantages		Not currently covered by private insurances/Medicaid/ Medicare	Requires prostate message
Comparisons	Comparable diagnostic accuracy to both 4 K and PCA3, and both their recommended indications	No comparison to PCA3; comparable accuracy and utility to 4 K	No comparison to 4 K; comparable diagnostic accuracy to PCA3 for initial & repeat Bx
Cost	$71–80	$395	$385

Table 4. Comparison of serum biomarkers PHI, 4K, and urine biomarker PCA3.

Another biomarker with a little more clinical experience and validation data is the PCA3 score —different in being a urinary marker rather than serum as for PHI and 4 K. The assay uses a ratio of messenger RNA for the PCA3 molecule with a PSA ratio built in. The AUCs for PCA3 are generally in the 0.0.68–75 range [22]. In the validation study for repeat biopsy patients, Marks et al. showed an AUC of 0.68 for PCA3 versus 0.52 for PSA [23]. The cutoffs recommended are in the 25–35 range. In the Marks study, a PCA3 cutoff of 35 showed 58% sensitivity and 72% specificity. A particular advantage of PCA3 has been that it is not affected by prostate volume and performed well across multiple PSA levels [24].

Back to comparative studies, Ferro et al. compared PCA3 to PHI in a prospective observational study [25]. The diagnostic accuracy was similar at 90% sensitivity: PHI specificity of 40% and PCA3 of 40% with 31.6 and 22 cutoffs, respectively. In a decision curve analysis, PHI had slightly higher benefit at probability of 25%. The Scattoni study [26] looked at these markers in initial and repeat biopsy populations and found a slight benefit to PHI but not significant. A comparison of AUC for initial biopsy showed PSA of 0.54, %fPSA of 0.67, PCA3 of 0.57, and PHI of 0.69. In repeat biopsy, it showed PSA of 0.60, %fPSA of 0.52, PCA3 of 0.63, and PHI of 0.72.

In **Table 4**, we consolidate these statistics into a final comparison with existing data.

The cost comparison certainly favors PHI, although the PCA3 test has more clinical experience and strong metrics in repeat biopsy decisions. It remains to be determined whether the 4 K cost is justified; however, when this test is up and running and through regulation, it may give a more objective reporting of specific high grade prostate cancer risk that clinicians may prefer.

5. Moving forward—similar themes in imaging, biopsy techniques, and tissue biomarkers

In this chapter, we have outlined the PSA problem with emphasis on triggers for a biopsy. A separate but related topic is the technique of biopsy. The gold standard for all of these biomarker studies has been the 10–12 core transrectal ultrasound-guided biopsy. Emerging data, however, demonstrate that a transperineal template biopsy may sample the apex and anterior zones better. Other areas of research are looking at improvements in multiparametric MRI staging, and commercial software platforms that fuse the images such that an ultrasound biopsy now has a more accurate target to sample rather than random sampling by anatomic region. The endpoints are the same—ability to improve Gleason score ≥7 and the ability to trust that a negative test is actually negative. For diagnosed patients, commercial genetic profiling products can then look at specific grades of prostate cancer and offer additional prognostic information such as risk of upgrading/upstaging at surgery, mortality rates untreated, biochemical relapse after surgery, or metastatic relapse after surgery [27]. These topics can be separate chapters, but the themes are consistent—solving heterogeneity in prostate cancer diagnosis such that the downstream monitoring and treatment decisions are optimized.

http://dx.doi.org/10.5772/64402

Author details

John W. Davis* and Chinedu Mmeje

*Address all correspondence to: johndavis@mdanderson.org

University of Texas MD Anderson Cancer Center, Houston, Texas, USA

References

[1] Welch HG, Gorski DH, Albertsen PC. Trends in metastatic breast and prostate cancer —lesson in cancer dynamics. N Engl J Med 2016; 374: 596.

[2] Thompson IM, Pauler DK, Goodman PJ, et al. Prevalence of prostate cancer among men with a prostate-specific antigen level ≤ 4.0 ng per milliliter. N Engl J Med 2004; 350: 2239–2246.

[3] Bill-Axelson A, Holmberg L, Garmo H, et al. Radical prostatectomy or watchful waiting in early prostate cancer. N Engl J Med 2014; 370: 10.

[4] Loeb S. Time to replace prostate-specific antigen (PSA) with the Prostate Health Index (PHI)? Yet more evidence that the PHI consistently performs PSA across diverse populations. BJU Int 2015; 115: 500.

[5] Seamonds B, Yang N, Anderson K, et al. Evaluation of prostate-specific antigen and prostatic acid phosphatase as prostate cancer markers. Urology 1986; 28: 472–479.

[6] Catalona WJ, Smith DS, Ratliff TL, et al. Measurement of prostate-specific antigen in serum as a screening test for prostate cancer. N Engl J Med 1991; 324: 1156–1161.

[7] Catalona WJ, Smith DS, Eolfert RL, et al. Evaluation of percentage of free serum prostate-specific antigen to improve specificity of prostate cancer screening. JAMA 1995; 274: 1214–1220.

[8] Oesterling JE, Jacobsen SJ, Chute CG, et al. Serum prostate-specific antigen in a community-based population of healthy men. Establishment of age-specific reference ranges. JAMA 1993; 270: 860–864.

[9] Smith DS, Catalona WJ. Rate of change in serum prostate specific antigen levels as a method for prostate cancer detection. J Urol 1994; 152: 1163–1167.

[10] Benson MC, Whang IS, Pantuck A, et al. Prostate specific antigen density: a means of distinguishing benign prostatic hypertrophy and prostate cancer. J Urol 1992; 147: 815–816.

[11] Lilja H, Cronin AM, Dahlin A, et al. Prediction of significant prostate cancer diagnosed 20 to 30 years later with a single measure of prostate-specific antigen at or before age 50. Cancer 2011; 117: 1210–1219.

[12] Mikolajczyk SD, Millar LS, Wang TJ, et al. A precursor form of prostate-specific antigen is more highly elevated in prostate cancer compared with benign transition zone prostate tissue. Cancer Res 2000; 60: 756–759.

[13] Sokioll LJ, Chan DW, Mikolajczyk SD, et al. Proenzyme psa for the early detection of prostate cancer in the 2.5-4.0 ng/ml total psa range: preliminary analysis. Urology 2003; 61: 274–276.

[14] Catalona WJ , Bartsch G, Rittenhouse HG, et al. Serum pro prostate specific antigen improves cancer detection compared to free and complexed prostate specific antigen in men with prostate specific antigen 2 to 4 nl/ml. J Urol 2003; 170: 2181–2185.

[15] Jansen FH, van Schaik RH, Kurstjens J, et al. Prostate-spcirfic antigen (PSA) isoform p2PSA in combination with total PSA and free PSA improves diagnostic accuracy in prostate cancer detection. Eur Urol 2010; 57: 921–927.

[16] Le BV, Griffin CR, Loeb S, et al. [−2]Proenzyme prostate specific antigen is more accurate than total and free prostate specific antigen in differentiating prostate cancer from benign disease in a prospective prostate cancer screening study. J Urol 2010; 183: 1355–1359.

[17] Lazzeri M, Haese A, de la Taille A, et al. Serum isoform [−2] proPSA derivatives significantly improve prediction of prostate cancer at initial biopsy in a total PSA range of 2–10 ng/ml: a multicentric European study. Eur Urol 2013; 63: 986–994.

[18] Nam RK, Diamandis EP, Toi A, et al. Serum human glandular kallikrien-2 protease levels predict the presence of prostate cancer among men with elevated prostate-specific antigen. J Clin Oncol 2000; 18: 1036–1042.

[19] Vickers AJJ, Cronin AM, Aus G, et al. A panel of kallikrein markers can reduce unnecessary biopsy for prostate cancer: data from the European Randomized Study of Prostate Cancer Screening on Goteborg, Sweden. BMC Med 2008; 6: 19.

[20] Parekh DJ, Punnen S, Sjoberg D, et al. A multi-institutional prospective trial in the USA confirms that the 4 K score accurately identifies men with high grade prostate cancer. Eur Urol 2015; 68: 464–470.

[21] Nordstrom T, Vickers A, Assel M, et al. Comparison between the four-kallikrein panel and the prostate health index for predicting prostate cancer. Eur Urol 2015; 68: 139–146.

[22] Groskopf J, Aubin SM, Deras IL, et al. APTIMA PCA3 molecular urine test: development of a method to aid in the diagnosis of prostate cancer. Clin Chem 2006; 52: 1089–1095.

[23] Marks LS, Fradet Y, Deras IL, et al. PCA3 molecular urine assay for prostate cancer in men undergoing repeat biopsy. Urology 2007; 69: 532–535.

[24] Deras IL, Aubin SM, Blase A, et al. PCA3: a molecular urine assay for predicting prostate biopsy outcome. J Urol 2008; 179: 1587–1592.

[25] Ferro M, Bruzzese D, Perdona S, et al. Prostate health indiex (PHI) and prostate cancer antigen3 (PCA3) significantly improve prostate cancer detection at initial biopsy in a total PSA range of 2–10 ng/ml. Plos One 2013; 8.

[26] Scattoni V, Lazzeri M, Lughezzani G, et al. Head-to-head comparison of prostate health index and urinary PCA3 for predicting cancer at initial or repeat biopsy. J Urol 2013; 190: 496–501.

[27] Davis JW. Novel commercially available genomic tests for prostate cancer: a roadmap to understanding their clinical impact. BJU Int 2014; 112: 531–532.

Chapter 3

The Role of Prostate-Specific Antigen (PSA) and PSA Kinetics in the Management of Advanced Prostate Cancer

Jeremy Teoh and Ming-Kwong Yiu

Additional information is available at the end of the chapter

http://dx.doi.org/10.5772/64180

Abstract

Prostate-specific antigen (PSA) plays an important role in the diagnosis and management of prostate cancer. The utility of PSA has been extended to a number of parameters which may guide clinical decision-making in subsequent treatment. This book chapter systematically reviewed the current evidence of PSA and PSA kinetics in the management of advanced prostate cancer. Results showed that the prognostic significance of pre-treatment PSA level is uncertain. PSA nadir predicts survival outcomes but may be confounded by the pre-treatment PSA level, and the PSA nadir may only be known after there is a PSA rise in subsequent follow-up. Time to PSA nadir has some prognostic significance but is limited by the potential immortal bias. Evidence on the use of PSA doubling time is limited and the different calculation methodologies render difficulties in generalization of such parameter. PSA progression is the best surrogate marker of survival and can be considered as the primary endpoint in future clinical trials. PSA response predicts survival but has not been shown prospectively to be a surrogate of clinical benefit. PSA and its kinetics should play an important role in the management of advanced prostate cancer and should be utilized in a more standardized manner.

Keywords: prostate cancer, prostate-specific antigen, prostate-specific antigen nadir, time to prostate-specific antigen nadir, prostatic-specific antigen doubling time, prostate-specific antigen progression, prostate-specific antigen response

1. Introduction

The first study investigating tissue-specific antibodies in the human prostate can be traced back to 1969 by Ablin et al. [1]. Nadji et al. [2] later characterized prostate-specific antigen (PSA) as a potential immunohistologic marker for prostatic neoplasms. The landmark article by Stamey et al. [3] showed that serum PSA has a much better performance than prostatic acid phosphatase in the detection of prostate cancer, and appeared to be useful in detecting residual or early recurrence of tumour, and in monitoring response to primary treatment. It has led to extensive researches in this area, and the discovery of PSA has revolutionized the management of prostate cancer, from early detection to definitive treatment and monitoring of the disease. The utility of PSA has been extended to a number of parameters that may have prognostic significance in prostate cancer and hence has gained wide interest in the past two decades.

2. Objectives

In this chapter, we systemically reviewed and appraised the current role of PSA and PSA kinetics in the management of advanced prostate cancer. We further discussed the potential benefits and controversies of the different PSA-related parameters.

3. Methods

A systematic search was conducted in the PubMed database through November 2015 using the following terms: 'prostate cancer', 'prostate-specific antigen', 'prostate-specific antigen nadir', 'time to prostate-specific antigen nadir', 'prostatic-specific antigen doubling time', 'prostate-specific antigen progression' and 'prostate-specific antigen response'. Only original full research articles published in English with full-length text available were reviewed. A manual search using the Web-based search engine Google Scholar was also performed. Reference lists of the retrieved articles were reviewed for other relevant studies.

4. Results

4.1. Pre-treatment PSA level

To a certain extent, the pre-treatment PSA level may reflect the volume of cancer cells, and hence, it is a parameter of interest in predicting disease prognosis. However, it does not reflect the sensitivity of cancer cells in response to subsequent therapy, in particular hormonal therapy in the context of metastatic disease. The prognostic significance of pre-treatment PSA level is uncertain. Some studies showed that higher pre-treatment PSA level was associated with disease progression, cancer-specific mortality and all-cause mortality [4–14], while other studies either showed no association or failed to demonstrate statistical significance upon multivariate analyses [15–32]. The wide range of pre-treatment PSA level in metastatic disease also limited its clinical application.

4.2. PSA nadir

PSA nadir was defined as the lowest PSA level achieved after the initiation of treatment. An undetectable PSA nadir level reflects that most if not all of the prostate cancer cells are androgen-sensitive, while any detectable PSA level reflects the presence of androgen-insensitive prostate cancer cells. This was supported by a study which showed that patients who had biochemical relapse following 3 months of neoadjuvant androgen deprivation therapy and radical prostatectomy had greater PSA mRNA levels and more intense PSA immunostaining despite castrate levels of testosterone, than patients who did not relapse, yet they had similar levels of androgen receptor gene expression and protein staining [33]. The majority of the literature showed that PSA nadir is consistent in predicting disease prognosis. A higher PSA nadir level has been shown to be associated with biochemical or disease progression [4, 15, 19, 25, 31, 32, 34–37], prostate cancer-specific mortality [6, 7, 16, 22, 25, 38–40] and all-cause mortality [6, 15, 16, 24, 26, 29, 30, 41–44]. However, there is no absolute threshold level for PSA nadir being recognized by any regulatory agency, and cut-off values at 0.2 ng/mL, 1.0 ng/mL and 4.0 ng/mL have been proposed in various studies. In particular, the drop of PSA to < 4.0 ng/mL has commonly been recognized as PSA normalization, and similar to PSA nadir, PSA normalization was associated with better progression-free survival, cancer-specific survival and overall survival [35, 39, 43, 44]. However, PSA nadir may be affected by the pre-treatment PSA level, rendering difficulty in clinical application, and the PSA nadir may only be known after there is a PSA rise in subsequent follow-up.

4.3. Time to PSA nadir

Time to PSA nadir was defined as the duration needed for the PSA level to reach its nadir after the initiation of treatment. Upon hormonal therapy, one may expect the PSA level to drop to its nadir within a shorter period of time in case of hormone-sensitive prostate cancer, but the ability to have sustained continuous suppression over a longer period of time may be as important. The majority of the studies showed that a longer time to PSA nadir was associated with better outcomes including biochemical or disease progression, cancer-specific survival and overall survival [15, 16, 26, 29, 34, 36]. The other studies either showed the contrary or did not detect any associations between them [6, 22, 23, 31]. Due to the potential immortal time bias, the relationship between time to PSA nadir and survival has to be interpreted with caution [45]. For example, one must have survived 12 months in order to have a time to PSA nadir of 12 months. Hence, this immortal time bias favours a positive correlation between time to PSA nadir and survival outcomes. In order to minimize this potential bias, one study attempted to investigate the prognostic significance of time to PSA nadir using survival beyond time to PSA nadir as an alternative outcome measurement. It has been shown that a longer time to PSA nadir was associated with better survival beyond time to PSA nadir [45]. A longer time to PSA nadir was also shown to be associated with a lower PSA velocity after progression, but whether PSA velocity after progression can be a surrogate for survival is doubtful [46].

4.4. PSA doubling time

PSA doubling time can generally be interpreted as the time needed for the PSA level to double itself. It assumes an exponential increase in serum PSA and first-order kinetics and can be calculated by natural logarithm of 2 divided by the slope of the relationship between the logarithm of PSA and time of PSA measurement [47]. However, several other calculation models have been proposed, and there is no standardization in the calculation of PSA doubling time. A shorter PSA doubling time has been shown to predict metastasis after prior radical prostatectomy [27, 28, 47], disease progression [32, 48], prostate cancer-specific mortality [6, 7, 22, 23, 25, 40, 49–51] and all-cause mortality [6, 9, 24, 27, 38, 52–54]. The utility of PSA doubling time has been widespread, yet the inconsistencies in the methodologies in calculating PSA doubling time [55] and the complicated logarithm calculations involved limited its use in clinical practice. Small deviations from the different methods of calculations may also lead to wide variations in the calculated PSA doubling time [55]. In 2008, the Prostate Cancer Clinical Trials Working Group (PCWG2) discourages the use of PSA doubling time as the primary endpoint in clinical trials because its significance is uncertain [56]. A subsequent systematic review also concluded that the evidence on PSA doubling time is limited and there is no justification for the use of PSA doubling time to guide decision-making in subsequent treatment [57].

4.5. PSA progression

PSA progression is commonly used as an endpoint in clinical trials, and it was generally thought to represent disease progression and hence reflect the survival outcomes. However, in particular for metastatic disease, multiple definitions of PSA progression have been proposed; they rendered difficulties comparing the results between different studies and limited the generalization of the utility of PSA progression. In 1999, Prostate-specific Antigen Working Group (PCWG1) made consensus recommendations for different outcome measures in clinical trials in prostate cancer [58]. PCWG1 defined PSA progression as a >50% increase from nadir and an increase of at least 5 ng/mL, or back to baseline, whichever was lowest. In 2008, PCWG2 proposed another definition for PSA progression, recognizing that early changes in PSA should not be used for clinical decision-making [56]. For those with PSA decline from baseline, PSA progression was defined as an increase in PSA by ≥25% and ≥2 ng/mL above the nadir, which should be confirmed by a second value 3 or more weeks later; for those with no PSA decline, PSA progression was defined as an increase in PSA ≥25% and ≥2 ng/mL after 12 weeks. Hussain et al. [44] reviewed the data from two large-scale clinical trials, namely the Southwest Oncology Group (SWOG) 9346 trial on intermittent ADT and the SWOG 9916 trial on docetaxel. It was shown that both PCWG1 and PCWG2 definitions of PSA progression predicted a 2.4-fold increase in risk of death and a more than 4-fold increase in the risk of death if PSA progression occurred in the first 7 months. This important study demonstrated that PSA progression is a significant predictor of survival in patients who have newly diagnosed metastatic hormone-sensitive prostate cancer as well as in those with castration resistant prostate cancer treated with chemotherapy. The authors suggested that the PCWG2 definition might be more appealing as patients are identified with progression relatively earlier on. Pooling data from 9 cancer and leukaemia Group B trials [11], both PCWG1 and PCWG2 definitions of PSA progression were shown to be significant predictors of overall survival with hazard ratios of 1.44 (95% CI 1.28–1.62, $P < 0.001$) and 1.43 (95% CI 1.27–1.61, $P < 0.001$), respectively. The above evidence formed the basis of using PSA progression as the primary endpoint in various clinical trials.

4.6. PSA response

PSA response was determined by the degree of decline from its pre-treatment level. The PCWG1 [58] defined PSA response as a decline of >50% from baseline, measured twice 3–4 weeks apart. Several studies have shown that a PSA decline of >50% was associated with better cancer-specific survival [39, 59] and overall survival [17, 18, 60–62]. However, post hoc analyses in both SWOG 9916 [63] and TAX 327 [43] trials on the use of docetaxel showed that a PSA decline of >30% might be a better surrogate marker for survival than a PSA decline of >50% based on the proportion of treatment effect and the proportion of variation. A subsequent combined analysis on the SWOG 9346 and SWOG 9916 trials [44] showed that a PSA decline of >30% was associated with better overall survival. However, PCWG2 [56] advised against reporting PSA response rates in clinical trials. Concerns were raised about the strength of association between PSA decline and survival, and no criterion, be it >50% or >30% decline in PSA, has been shown prospectively to be a surrogate of clinical benefit [64]. Instead, PCWG2 recommended the use of waterfall plot to provide a broader and more sensitive display of data. On the other hand, following the discovery of AR-V7 splice variant [65], it was proposed that the lack of PSA response after initial hormonal manipulation might represent primary resistance to hormonal therapy. This is particularly important, as other non-hormonal treatment such as chemotherapy should be considered early on, based on the prediction of poor response to further hormonal manipulation.

5. Conclusions

PSA and PSA kinetics may provide additional information about the biological behaviour of prostate cancer and may aid the treatment decision in an individualized approach. One should be aware of the pros and cons of the different PSA-related parameters and should be cautious when interpreting the results from different studies. PSA and its kinetics should play an important role in the management of advanced prostate cancer, and generalization can only be achieved if definitions of the different parameters can be utilized in a more standardized manner. Among the different parameters discussed, PSA progression appeared to be the most consistent and reliable surrogate marker of survival and can serve as the primary endpoint in future clinical trials.

Author details

Jeremy Teoh[1,2*] and Ming-Kwong Yiu[1,2]

*Address all correspondence to: jeremyteoh@surgery.cuhk.edu.hk

1 Division of Urology, Department of Surgery, Prince of Wales Hospital, The Chinese University of Hong Kong, Hong Kong, China

2 Division of Urology, Department of Surgery, Queen Mary Hospital, The University of Hong Kong, Hong Kong, China

References

[1] Ablin RJ, Pfeiffer L, Gonder MJ, Soanes WA. Precipitating antibody in the sera of patients treated cryosurgically for carcinoma of the prostate. Exp Med Surg 1969; 27:406–10.

[2] Nadji M, Tabei SZ, Castro A, Chu TM, Murphy GP, Wang MC, et al. Prostatic-specific antigen: an immunohistologic marker for prostatic neoplasms. Cancer 1981; 48:1229–32.

[3] Stamey TA, Yang N, Hay AR, McNeal JE, Freiha FS, Redwine E. Prostate-specific antigen as a serum marker for adenocarcinoma of the prostate. N Engl J Med 1987; 317:909–16.

[4] Soga N, Arima K, Sugimura Y. Undetectable level of prostate specific antigen (PSA) nadir predicts PSA biochemical failure in local prostate cancer with delayed-combined androgen blockade. Jpn J Clin Oncol 2008; 38:617–22.

[5] Ross RW, Xie W, Regan MM, Pomerantz M, Nakabayashi M, Daskivich TJ, et al. Efficacy of androgen deprivation therapy (ADT) in patients with advanced prostate cancer: association between Gleason score, prostate-specific antigen level, and prior ADT exposure with duration of ADT effect. Cancer 2008; 112:1247–53.

[6] Chung CS, Chen MH, Cullen J, McLeod D, Carroll P, D'Amico AV. Time to prostate-specific antigen nadir after androgen suppression therapy for postoperative or postradiation PSA failure and risk of prostate cancer-specific mortality. Urology 2008; 71:136–40.

[7] Stewart AJ, Scher HI, Chen MH, McLeod DG, Carroll PR, Moul JW, et al. Prostate-specific antigen nadir and cancer–specific mortality following hormonal therapy for prostate-specific antigen failure. J Clin Oncol 2005; 23:6556–60.

[8] Kuriyama M, Wang MC, Lee CI, Papsidero LD, Killian CS, Inaji H, et al. Use of human prostate-specific antigen in monitoring prostate cancer. Cancer Res 1981; 41:3874–6.

[9] Armstrong AJ, Garrett-Mayer ES, Yang YC, de Wit R, Tannock IF, Eisenberger M. A contemporary prognostic nomogram for men with hormone-refractory metastatic prostate cancer: a TAX327 study analysis. Clin Cancer Res 2007; 13:6396–403.

[10] Berthold DR, Pond GR, Soban F, de Wit R, Eisenberger M, Tannock IF. Docetaxel plus prednisone or mitoxantrone plus prednisone for advanced prostate cancer: updated survival in the TAX 327 study. J Clin Oncol 2008; 26:242–5.

[11] Halabi S, Vogelzang NJ, Ou SS, Owzar K, Archer L, Small EJ. Progression-free survival as a predictor of overall survival in men with castrate-resistant prostate cancer. J Clin Oncol 2009; 27:2766–71.

[12] Smith MR, Cook R, Lee KA, Nelson JB. Disease and host characteristics as predictors of time to first bone metastasis and death in men with progressive castration-resistant nonmetastatic prostate cancer. Cancer 2011; 117:2077–85.

[13] Crook JM, O'Callaghan CJ, Duncan G, Dearnaley DP, Higano CS, Horwitz EM, et al. Intermittent androgen suppression for rising PSA level after radiotherapy. N Engl J Med 2012; 367:895–903.

[14] Saad F, Segal S, Eastham J. Prostate-specific antigen kinetics and outcomes in patients with bone metastases from castration-resistant prostate cancer treated with or without zoledronic acid. Eur Urol 2014; 65:146–53.

[15] Huang SP, Bao BY, Wu MT, Choueiri TK, Goggins WB, Huang CY, et al. Impact of prostate-specific antigen (PSA) nadir and time to PSA nadir on disease progression in prostate cancer treated with androgen-deprivation therapy. Prostate 2011; 71:1189–97.

[16] Huang SP, Bao BY, Wu MT, Choueiri TK, Goggins WB, Liu CC, et al. Significant associations of prostate-specific antigen nadir and time to prostate-specific antigen nadir with survival in prostate cancer patients treated with androgen-deprivation therapy. Aging Male 2012; 15:34–41.

[17] Kelly WK, Scher HI, Mazumdar M, Vlamis V, Schwartz M, Fossa SD. Prostate-specific antigen as a measure of disease outcome in metastatic hormone-refractory prostate cancer. J Clin Oncol 1993; 11:607–15.

[18] Dowling AJ, Czaykowski PM, Krahn MD, Moore MJ, Tannock IF. Prostate specific antigen response to mitoxantrone and prednisone in patients with refractory prostate cancer: prognostic factors and generalizability of a multicenter trial to clinical practice. J Urol 2000; 163:1481–5.

[19] Kwak C, Jeong SJ, Park MS, Lee E, Lee SE. Prognostic significance of the nadir prostate specific antigen level after hormone therapy for prostate cancer. J Urol 2002; 168:995–1000.

[20] Petrylak DP, Tangen CM, Hussain MH, Lara PN, Jr., Jones JA, Taplin ME, et al. Docetaxel and estramustine compared with mitoxantrone and prednisone for advanced refractory prostate cancer. N Engl J Med 2004; 351:1513–20.

[21] Berruti A, Mosca A, Tucci M, Terrone C, Torta M, Tarabuzzi R, et al. Independent prognostic role of circulating chromogranin A in prostate cancer patients with hormone-refractory disease. Endocr Relat Cancer 2005; 12:109–17.

[22] Rodrigues NA, Chen MH, Catalona WJ, Roehl KA, Richie JP, D'Amico AV. Predictors of mortality after androgen-deprivation therapy in patients with rapidly rising prostate-specific antigen levels after local therapy for prostate cancer. Cancer 2006; 107:514–20.

[23] D'Amico AV, McLeod DG, Carroll PR, Cullen J, Chen MH. Time to an undetectable prostate-specific antigen (PSA) after androgen suppression therapy for postoperative or postradiation PSA recurrence and prostate cancer-specific mortality. Cancer 2007; 109:1290–5.

[24] Daskivich TJ, Regan MM, Oh WK. Distinct prognostic role of prostate-specific antigen doubling time and velocity at emergence of androgen independence in patients treated with chemotherapy. Urology 2007; 70:527–31.

[25] Scholz M, Lam R, Strum S, Jennrich R, Johnson H, Trilling T. Prostate-cancer-specific survival and clinical progression-free survival in men with prostate cancer treated intermittently with testosterone-inactivating pharmaceuticals. Urology 2007; 70:506–10.

[26] Choueiri TK, Xie W, D'Amico AV, Ross RW, Hu JC, Pomerantz M, et al. Time to prostate-specific antigen nadir independently predicts overall survival in patients who have metastatic hormone-sensitive prostate cancer treated with androgen-deprivation therapy. Cancer 2009; 115:981–7.

[27] Antonarakis ES, Chen Y, Elsamanoudi SI, Brassell SA, Da Rocha MV, Eisenberger MA, et al. Long-term overall survival and metastasis-free survival for men with prostate-specific antigen-recurrent prostate cancer after prostatectomy: analysis of the Center for Prostate Disease Research National Database. BJU Int 2011; 108:378–85.

[28] Antonarakis ES, Feng Z, Trock BJ, Humphreys EB, Carducci MA, Partin AW, et al. The natural history of metastatic progression in men with prostate-specific antigen recurrence after radical prostatectomy: long-term follow-up. BJU Int 2012; 109:32–9.

[29] Sasaki T, Onishi T, Hoshina A. Nadir PSA level and time to PSA nadir following primary androgen deprivation therapy are the early survival predictors for prostate cancer patients with bone metastasis. Prostate Cancer Prostatic Dis 2011; 14:248–52.

[30] Miyamoto S, Ito K, Miyakubo M, Suzuki R, Yamamoto T, Suzuki K, et al. Impact of pretreatment factors, biopsy Gleason grade volume indices and post-treatment nadir

PSA on overall survival in patients with metastatic prostate cancer treated with step-up hormonal therapy. Prostate Cancer Prostatic Dis 2012; 15:75–86.

[31] Benaim EA, Pace CM, Lam PM, Roehrborn CG. Nadir prostate-specific antigen as a predictor of progression to androgen-independent prostate cancer. Urology 2002; 59:73–8.

[32] Keizman D, Huang P, Antonarakis ES, Sinibaldi V, Carducci MA, Denmeade S, et al. The change of PSA doubling time and its association with disease progression in patients with biochemically relapsed prostate cancer treated with intermittent androgen deprivation. Prostate 2011; 71:1608–15.

[33] Ryan CJ, Smith A, Lal P, Satagopan J, Reuter V, Scardino P, et al. Persistent prostate-specific antigen expression after neoadjuvant androgen depletion: an early predictor of relapse or incomplete androgen suppression. Urology 2006; 68:834–9.

[34] Hori S, Jabbar T, Kachroo N, Vasconcelos JC, Robson CN, Gnanapragasam VJ. Outcomes and predictive factors for biochemical relapse following primary androgen deprivation therapy in men with bone scan negative prostate cancer. J Cancer Res Clin Oncol 2011; 137:235–41.

[35] Oosterlinck W, Mattelaer J, Casselman J, Van Velthoven R, Derde MP, Kaufman L. PSA evolution: a prognostic factor during treatment of advanced prostatic carcinoma with total androgen blockade. Data from a Belgian multicentric study of 546 patients. Acta Urol Belg 1997; 65:63–71.

[36] Morote J, Trilla E, Esquena S, Abascal JM, Reventos J. Nadir prostate-specific antigen best predicts the progression to androgen-independent prostate cancer. Int J Cancer 2004; 108:877–81.

[37] Park SC, Rim JS, Choi HY, Kim CS, Hong SJ, Kim WJ, et al. Failing to achieve a nadir prostate-specific antigen after combined androgen blockade: predictive factors. Int J Urol 2009; 16:670–5.

[38] D'Amico AV, Chen MH, de Castro M, Loffredo M, Lamb DS, Steigler A, et al. Surrogate endpoints for prostate cancer-specific mortality after radiotherapy and androgen suppression therapy in men with localised or locally advanced prostate cancer: an analysis of two randomised trials. Lancet Oncol 2012; 13:189–95.

[39] Suzuki H, Okihara K, Miyake H, Fujisawa M, Miyoshi S, Matsumoto T, et al. Alternative nonsteroidal antiandrogen therapy for advanced prostate cancer that relapsed after initial maximum androgen blockade. J Urol 2008; 180:921–7.

[40] Park YH, Hwang IS, Jeong CW, Kim HH, Lee SE, Kwak C. Prostate specific antigen half-time and prostate specific antigen doubling time as predictors of response to androgen deprivation therapy for metastatic prostate cancer. J Urol 2009; 181:2520–4; discussion 5.

[41] Teoh JY, Tsu JH, Yuen SK, Chan SY, Chiu PK, Wong KW, et al. Survival outcomes of Chinese metastatic prostate cancer patients following primary androgen deprivation

therapy in relation to prostate-specific antigen nadir level. Asia Pac J Clin Oncol 2014. (Epub ahead of print).

[42] Hussain M, Tangen CM, Higano C, Schelhammer PF, Faulkner J, Crawford ED, et al. Absolute prostate-specific antigen value after androgen deprivation is a strong independent predictor of survival in new metastatic prostate cancer: data from Southwest Oncology Group Trial 9346 (INT-0162). J Clin Oncol 2006; 24:3984–90.

[43] Armstrong AJ, Garrett-Mayer E, Ou Yang YC, Carducci MA, Tannock I, de Wit R, et al. Prostate-specific antigen and pain surrogacy analysis in metastatic hormone-refractory prostate cancer. J Clin Oncol 2007; 25:3965–70.

[44] Hussain M, Goldman B, Tangen C, Higano CS, Petrylak DP, Wilding G, et al. Prostate-specific antigen progression predicts overall survival in patients with metastatic prostate cancer: data from Southwest Oncology Group Trials 9346 (Intergroup Study 0162) and 9916. J Clin Oncol 2009; 27:2450–6.

[45] Teoh JY, Tsu JH, Yuen SK, Chan SY, Chiu PK, Lee WM, et al. Prognostic significance of time to prostate-specific antigen (PSA) nadir and its relationship to survival beyond time to PSA nadir for prostate cancer patients with bone metastases after primary androgen deprivation therapy. Ann Surg Oncol 2015; 22:1385–91.

[46] Teoh JY, Tsu JH, Yuen SK, Chiu PK, Chan SY, Wong KW, et al. Association of time to prostate-specific antigen nadir and logarithm of prostate-specific antigen velocity after progression in metastatic prostate cancer with prior primary androgen deprivation therapy. Asian J Androl 2015. (Epub ahead of print).

[47] Pound CR, Partin AW, Eisenberger MA, Chan DW, Pearson JD, Walsh PC. Natural history of progression after PSA elevation following radical prostatectomy. JAMA 1999; 281:1591–7.

[48] Keizman D, Huang P, Carducci MA, Eisenberger MA. Contemporary experience with ketoconazole in patients with metastatic castration-resistant prostate cancer: clinical factors associated with PSA response and disease progression. Prostate 2012; 72:461–7.

[49] D'Amico AV, Halabi S, Tempany C, Titelbaum D, Philips GK, Loffredo M, et al. Tumor volume changes on 1.5 tesla endorectal MRI during neoadjuvant androgen suppression therapy for higher-risk prostate cancer and recurrence in men treated using radiation therapy results of the phase II CALGB 9682 study. Int J Radiat Oncol Biol Phys 2008; 71:9–15.

[50] Freedland SJ, Humphreys EB, Mangold LA, Eisenberger M, Dorey FJ, Walsh PC, et al. Risk of prostate cancer-specific mortality following biochemical recurrence after radical prostatectomy. JAMA 2005; 294:433–9.

[51] Svatek RS, Shulman M, Choudhary PK, Benaim E. Critical analysis of prostate-specific antigen doubling time calculation methodology. Cancer 2006; 106:1047–53.

http://dx.doi.org/10.5772/64180

[52] Semeniuk RC, Venner PM, North S. Prostate-specific antigen doubling time is associated with survival in men with hormone-refractory prostate cancer. Urology 2006; 68:565–9.

[53] Oudard S, Banu E, Scotte F, Banu A, Medioni J, Beuzeboc P, et al. Prostate-specific antigen doubling time before onset of chemotherapy as a predictor of survival for hormone-refractory prostate cancer patients. Ann Oncol 2007; 18:1828–33.

[54] Oudard S, Banu E, Medioni J, Scotte F, Banu A, Levy E, et al. What is the real impact of bone pain on survival in patients with metastatic hormone-refractory prostate cancer treated with docetaxel? BJU Int 2009; 103:1641–6.

[55] Daskivich TJ, Regan MM, Oh WK. Prostate specific antigen doubling time calculation: not as easy as 1, 2, 4. J Urol 2006; 176:1927–37.

[56] Scher HI, Halabi S, Tannock I, Morris M, Sternberg CN, Carducci MA, et al. Design and end points of clinical trials for patients with progressive prostate cancer and castrate levels of testosterone: recommendations of the Prostate Cancer Clinical Trials Working Group. J Clin Oncol 2008; 26:1148–59.

[57] Vickers AJ, Savage C, O'Brien MF, Lilja H. Systematic review of pretreatment prostate-specific antigen velocity and doubling time as predictors for prostate cancer. J Clin Oncol 2009; 27:398–403.

[58] Bubley GJ, Carducci M, Dahut W, Dawson N, Daliani D, Eisenberger M, et al. Eligibility and response guidelines for phase II clinical trials in androgen-independent prostate cancer: recommendations from the Prostate-Specific Antigen Working Group. J Clin Oncol 1999; 17:3461–7.

[59] Okihara K, Ukimura O, Kanemitsu N, Mizutani Y, Kawauchi A, Miki T, et al. Clinical efficacy of alternative antiandrogen therapy in Japanese men with relapsed prostate cancer after first-line hormonal therapy. Int J Urol 2007; 14:128–32.

[60] Smith DC, Dunn RL, Strawderman MS, Pienta KJ. Change in serum prostate-specific antigen as a marker of response to cytotoxic therapy for hormone-refractory prostate cancer. J Clin Oncol 1998; 16:1835–43.

[61] Small EJ, McMillan A, Meyer M, Chen L, Slichenmyer WJ, Lenehan PF, et al. Serum prostate-specific antigen decline as a marker of clinical outcome in hormone-refractory prostate cancer patients: association with progression-free survival, pain end points, and survival. J Clin Oncol 2001; 19:1304–11.

[62] Berthold DR, Pond GR, Roessner M, de Wit R, Eisenberger M, Tannock AI, et al. Treatment of hormone-refractory prostate cancer with docetaxel or mitoxantrone: relationships between prostate-specific antigen, pain, and quality of life response and survival in the TAX-327 study. Clin Cancer Res 2008; 14:2763–7.

[63] Petrylak DP, Ankerst DP, Jiang CS, Tangen CM, Hussain MH, Lara PN, Jr., et al. Evaluation of prostate-specific antigen declines for surrogacy in patients treated on SWOG 99-16. J Natl Cancer Inst 2006; 98:516–21.

[64] Scher HI, Morris MJ, Basch E, Heller G. End points and outcomes in castration-resistant prostate cancer: from clinical trials to clinical practice. J Clin Oncol 2011; 29:3695–704.

[65] Antonarakis ES, Lu C, Wang H, Luber B, Nakazawa M, Roeser JC, et al. AR-V7 and resistance to enzalutamide and abiraterone in prostate cancer. N Engl J Med 2014; 371:1028–38.

Chapter 4

Transperineal Targeted Biopsy with Real-Time Fusion Image of Multiparametric Magnetic Resonance Image and Transrectal Ultrasound Image for the Diagnosis of Prostate Cancer

Sunao Shoji

Additional information is available at the end of the chapter

http://dx.doi.org/10.5772/64603

Abstract

Objectives: To report clinical results of early experience of manually controlled targeted biopsy with real-time multiparametric magnetic resonance image (mpMRI)-transrectal ultrasound (TRUS) fusion images for the diagnosis of prostate cancer.

Methods: One hundred sixty-eight patients who were suspected of prostate cancer from mpMRI scans were recruited prospectively. We performed targeted biopsies for each cancer-suspicious lesion and 12 systematic biopsies using the BioJet® system. Pathological findings of targeted and systematic biopsies were analyzed.

Results: Median age of the 168 patients was 67 years (range: 52–89). Median preoperative prostate specific antigen (PSA) value was 6.9 ng/ml (range: 3.54–20). Median preoperative prostate volume was 37 ml (range: 22–68). The number of the cancer-detected cases was 99 (59%). The median biopsy time, included the MRI-TRUS fusion time and needle-punctured time without the anesthesia, was 8 minutes (range: 5–65). Cancer-detected rates of the systematic and targeted biopsy cores were 5.9 and 38%, respectively ($p < 0.0001$). In 25 patients who underwent radical prostatectomy, the geographic locations and pathological grades of clinically significant cancers and index lesions corresponded to the pathological results of the targeted biopsies.

Conclusion: The cancer cores detected by targeted biopsies with manually controlled targeted biopsy with real-time mpMRI-TRUS fusion image had significantly higher grades and larger length compared with those detected by the systematic biopsies. The further study of the comparisons with pathological findings of whole-gland specimens will give a larger role to the present biopsy method.

Keywords: prostate cancer, targeted biopsy, magnetic resonance image, transrectal ultrasound, fusion image

1. Introduction

Multiparametric magnetic resonance imaging (mpMRI) improves the imaging of prostate cancer lesion [1, 2], and several methods use MRI to guide the biopsy needle to target the cancer lesion. MRI-TRUS fusion image-guided biopsy achieved accurate prostate biopsy based on MRI, combining the superior sensitivity of MRI for targeting suspicious lesions with the practicality and familiarity of TRUS. MRI-TRUS fusion methods are used as visual registration [1, 3, 4] and fusion biopsy devices [5–9]. In visual registration, the TRUS operator identified the geographic location of the lesions in the prostate on the MRI, and then identify and biopsy viewing real-time TRUS [10]. In previous reports, the visual registration biopsy method improved accuracy over systematic biopsy [11–14]. However, the disadvantages of visual registration lie in human error when the targeted lesion was less than 10 mm in diameter [15]. Therefore, the visual registration is regarded as the prostate biopsy method for experts [10–14]. With the MRI-TRUS fusion devices, the stored MRI and real-time TRUS are superimposed using computer software to enable targeted biopsy of cancer-suspicious lesions [16]. MRI-TRUS fusion biopsy device "BioJet®" was approved by FDA after the evaluation of the accuracy with phantoms. We report the BioJet® experience of the manually controlled targeted biopsy using real-time fusion image from mpMRI and TRUS.

2. Methods

2.1. Population

From November 2013 to October 2015, after receiving the approval of institutional review board, the patients with PSA level greater than 4.0 ng/ml and less than 20 ng/ml were performed mpMRI prospectively. No patients had any previous history of prostate biopsy.

2.2. Multiparametric MRI

The MRI examination was carried out using a 1.5-Tesla magnet (Signa HDx®; GE Healthcare, Amersham Place, UK) with an 8-channel cardiac coil. T1-weighted fat-saturated axial fast spin-echo images (TR, 450 ms; TE, 8.8 ms; slice thickness, 3 mm; resolution, 0.9 × 1.3 mm) were obtained before injection. An intravenous bolus of 0.2 ml/kg of meglumine gadopentetate (Magnevist Syringe®; Bayer HealthCare Pharmaceuticals, Berlin, Germany) was then injected. All MRI examinations were performed using the same protocol, and included non-enhanced T2-weighted images (T2WI) (TR, 5000 ms; TE, 125 ms; slice thickness, 3 mm; resolution, 0.6 × 0.9 mm) acquired in the axial and sagittal planes, diffusion weighted image (DWI) and apparent diffusion coefficient (ADC) maps (b-value = 1500 s/mm^2), and dynamic-contrast-enhanced (DCE) MRI (resolution, 0.9 × 1.3 mm) using a fat-saturated T1-weighted fast-field echo sequence in the axial plane.

2.3. Image analysis

All mpMRI images, including T2WI, dynamic, DWI, and ADC map, were reviewed by two experienced radiologists with no prior clinical information. Suspicious areas, the so-called "regions of interest (ROI)", were provided a likelihood score that clinically significant cancer would be present for each ROI from 2 to 5 on the prostate imaging reporting and data system (PI-RAS) classification [17] based on Likert scale according to the European Society of Urogenital Radiology Prostate MR Guidelines 2012 [18]: 1, most probably benign; 2, probably benign; 3, intermediate; 4, probably malignant; and 5, highly suspicious of malignancy [17] The location of each area was determined based on dividing the prostate into 27 regions, as described by Dickson et al. [16]. MRIs were imported into the biopsy fusion system. Segmentation into a two-dimensional (2D) mpMRI was performed on the workstation to create a 3D model of the MRI, and then fused to the real-time TRUS.

2.4. Biopsy protocol

A cleaning enema and antibiotics were given before the biopsy. TRUS with power Doppler was performed using a Prosound $\alpha7$ (Hitachi Aloka Medical, Tokyo, Japan) equipped with a UST-678 transrectum composite probe, in the lithotomy position under spinal anesthesia. On the workstation, the operator fused the real-time TRUS image and 3D MRI model that included the prostate contour and ROI. After the elastic image fusion, an ultrasound probe was fixed to the arm that senses the 3D movement of the probe and exports the information to the workstation (**Figure 1a**). Using this device, the 2D image created from the 3D MRI model moves together with the real-time TRUS image on the workstation. The operator performed the biopsy using MRI-TRUS fusion image navigation (**Figure 1b**). During the procedure, the real-time ultrasound image is continuously available. The biopsy started with targeted biopsies to the center of cancer-suspicious lesions, and then 12 systematic biopsies were performed with transperineal technique in all patients. The biopsy used a standard brachytherapy grid with 5-mm spacing, with x-axis coordinates A through G and y-axis coordinates from 1 through 7, using D as the middle line urethral plane. An 18-gauge automatic biopsy gun with a specimen size of 22 mm (BARD® MAGNUM®, BARD MEDICAL, Covington, USA) was used to take biopsy cores. Using the interactive needle guide system, the biopsy template coordinates were shown on the monitor when the operator marked the target point of the ROI on the workstation (**Figure 2a, b**). The operator inserted the needle at the template coordinates and could get the prostate specimens by viewing the sagittal image of the prostate (**Figure 2c**). Immediately after each biopsy, the spatial punctured needle orbits were recorded in 2D TRUS image of axial and sagittal plane, and in the 3D model of MRI.

2.5. Pathological analysis

All biopsies were examined by expert pathologists. A significant cancer was defined as follows: at least one core with a Gleason score of 3 + 4 or 6 with a maximum cancer core length larger than 4 mm [19]. The pathological biopsy results were compared between systematic and targeted biopsies. The biopsy-proven index lesion of each patient was defined primarily as the lesion with the highest Gleason score, and secondarily as the lesion with the greatest cancer-involved core in terms of length or percentage. Geographic location of prostate cancer in the prostate [16] was compared with pathologic step-sectioned prostatectomy specimens in the patients who were performed with radical prostatectomy.

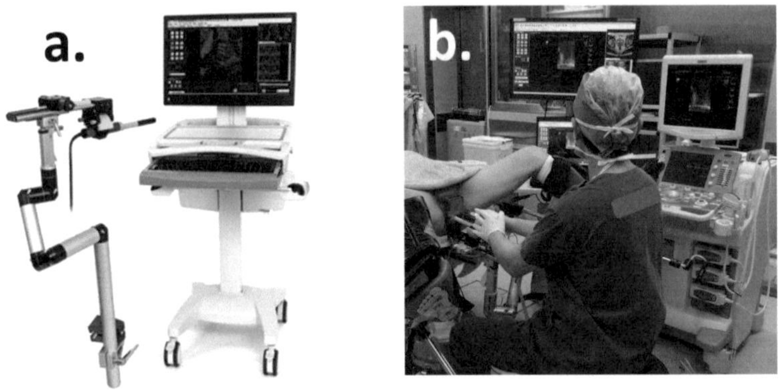

Figure 1. (a) BioJet system (D&K Technologies GmbH, Barum, Germany); (b) the set-up of prostate biopsy with BioJet system.

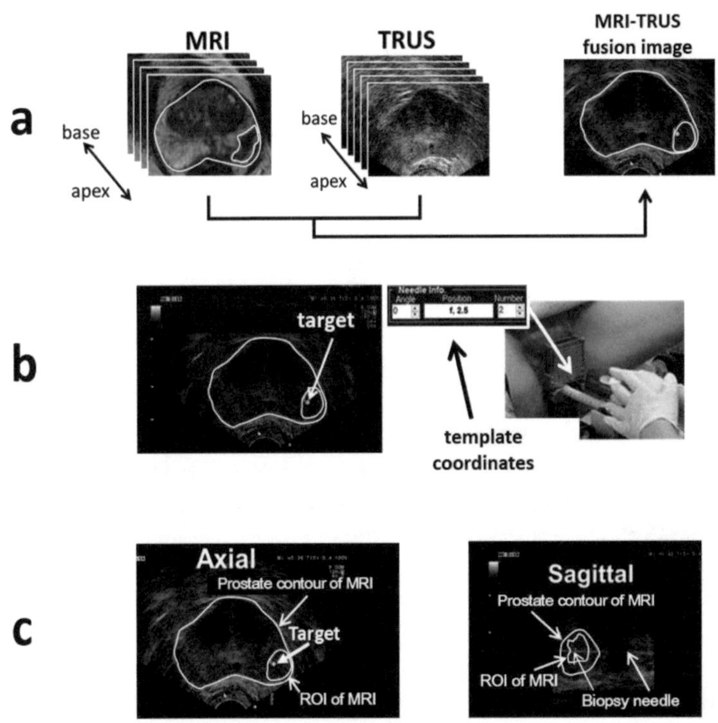

Figure 2. Process of prostate biopsy with BioJet system. (a) Fusion image from MRI and TRUS image. (b) Interactive needle guide system. (c) Real-time fusion images of axial and sagittal image.

http://dx.doi.org/10.5772/64603

2.6. Statistical analysis

All statistical analyses were performed using IBM SPSS® Statistics version 19 (IBM, Armonk, NY, USA). Among systematic and targeted biopsies, cancer-detected rate of biopsy, positive core length, positive core percentage, primary and secondary Gleason grade, and Gleason score were analyzed using the Mann-Whitney U-test. Changes in patient functional data were analyzed using paired *t*-tests. *P*-values of <0.05 were considered to indicate statistically significant differences.

3. Results

One-hundred sixty eight patients were suspected of prostate cancer with 2 to 5 of PI-RAD classification. The median age of the 168 patients was 67 years (range: 52–89). The median preoperative PSA value was 6.9 ng/ml (range: 3.54–20). The median preoperative prostate volume was 37 ml (range: 22–68). In the resected prostate specimen of 25 patients, the geographic locations and pathological grades of clinically significant cancers and index lesions corresponded to the results of the targeted biopsies.

The results of the prostate biopsies are shown in **Table 1**. The number of the cancer-detected cases was 99 (59%). The median biopsy time included the MRI-TRUS fusion time and needle-punctured time without the anesthesia, which was 8 minutes (range: 5–65). For the systematic and targeted biopsy cores, the total number of cores were 2016 and 372, respectively; the cancer-detected rates, the median positive core lengths, the median positive core percents, the median primary Gleason grades, the median secondary Gleason grades, and the median Gleason scores in systematic and targeted biopsy cores were significantly different.

	Target biopsy	Systematic biopsy	*P*-value
No. of biopsy cores	372	2016	n.d.
Rates of cancer detection	38%	5.9%	$p < 0.0001$
Rates of significant cancer detection	35%	1.4%	$p < 0.0001$
Median positive core lengths	8 mm (range: 1–22)	2 mm (range: 1–8)	$p < 0.0001$
Median positive core percents	60% (range: 5–100)	12% (range: 5–40)	$p < 0.0001$
Median primary Gleason grades	3 (3–5)	3 (3–4)	$p < 0.0001$
Median secondary Gleason grades	3 (3–5)	3 (3–4)	$p = 0.0020$
Median Gleason scores	6.5 (6–9)	6 (6–7)	$p = 0.0012$

Table 1. Biopsy results.

In targeted lesions of transition zone (TZ) ($n = 146$) and peripheral zone (PZ) ($n = 226$), the rate of cancer detection was 28% (n = 40) and 45% (n = 101), respectively. The rates of cancer detection and the corresponding scores on the PI-RAD in TZ and PZ are shown in **Table 2**.

	No. of target	PI-RADS classification	Rates of cancer detection		Rates of significant cancer detection
TZ + PZ	372	2 (*n* = 70)	38% (*n* = 141)	4.3% (*n* = 3)	0% (*n* = 0)
		3 (*n* = 126)		13% (*n* = 16)	10% (*n* = 13)
		4 (*n* = 110)		61% (*n* = 67)	58% (*n* = 64)
		5 (*n* = 71)		77% (*n* = 55)	77% (*n* = 55)
TZ	146	2 (*n* = 28)	28% (*n* = 40)	7.1% (*n* = 2)	0% (*n* = 0)
		3 (*n* = 40)		15% (*n* = 6)	10% (*n* = 4)
		4 (*n* = 48)		24% (*n* = 12)	21% (*n* = 10)
		5 (*n* = 35)		56% (*n* = 20)	56% (*n* = 20)
PZ	226	2 (*n* = 42)	45% (*n* = 101)	2.4% (*n* = 1)	0% (*n* = 0)
		3 (*n* = 86)		12% (*n* = 10)	11% (*n* = 9)
		4 (*n* = 62)		88% (*n* = 55)	87% (*n* = 54)
		5 (*n* = 36)		97% (*n* = 35)	97% (*n* = 35)

TZ, transition zone; PZ, peripheral zone; PI-RADS, prostate imaging and reporting data system.

Table 2. The rates of cancer detection and the corresponding scores on the PI-RAD in transition zone and peripheral zone.

4. Discussion

Our results showed that cancer detection rates using targeted biopsies were significantly better than using systematic biopsies ($p < 0.0001$). Positive core length ($p < 0.0001$), positive core percent ($p < 0.0001$), primary ($p < 0.0001$) and secondary ($p = 0.0020$) Gleason grade, and Gleason score ($p = 0.0012$) were also significantly different between targeted and systematic biopsies. In addition, all biopsy-proven significant cancers were detected in ROIs, and the index lesions corresponded to the largest-sized ROIs. Based on these results, the targeted biopsy method was superior to systematic biopsy, and clinically significant cancers with a spatial relationship were detected accurately in the present study. Although the resected prostate specimens only comprised 25 cases, accuracy of the locations and pathological grades was reliable in our study.

In the present study, we used the T2WI for segmentation of the ROI, but the decision concerning the selection of ROI was made using multiparametric MRI factors, such as T2WI, DCE, DWI, and ADC maps because T2WI is sensitive but not specific for prostate cancer detection [1]. In mpMRI, the image values of its component techniques are different. T2WI provides the best depiction of the prostate's zonal anatomy and capsule in mpMRI and thus is used for prostate cancer detection and localization [18]. DCE is the most common imaging method for evaluating vascularity in the tumor [20]. DWI involves the quantification of free water motion [21] and allows ADC maps to be calculated, enabling qualitative and quantitative assessment of prostate cancer aggressiveness. Lower ADC corresponds to greater restriction in free water motion, likely on the basis of increased cellularity compared with normal prostate tissue, and cancer shows a lower ADC value than normal prostate tissue [21]. Furthermore, ADC values correlate with Gleason scores [22–24]. However, some normal prostatic tissues, especially in the TZ, such as benign prostatic hyperplasia, chronic inflammation, and atrophic tissue, have similar findings of prostate cancer [16]. Indeed, the detection of prostate cancer in TZ was found difficulty in a previous study [23]. In our results, the cancer detection rate of the patients with a PI-RAD classification of 4 or 5 in TZ (39%) was inferior to that in PZ (92%).

The present device allows manually controlled targeted biopsy using real-time MRI-TRUS fusion images by the sensor arm of 3D movement. In addition, the fusion function has elastic fusion functions. The axial and sagittal view of US and MRI was useful to fuse the images of MRI and TRUS easily during the procedure. In addition, the present biopsy was performed with transperineal technique. Using the transperineal technique with the device, the biopsies were performed accurately to the ROIs. However, our study has limitations. First, our study did not compare biopsy results with pathological findings from whole-gland specimens. Therefore, although locations and pathological grades of clinically significant cancers and index lesions corresponded to the targeted biopsy results, it is difficult to exclude the possibility that a clinically important cancer has been missed without pathological analysis of whole-gland specimens.

In conclusion, cancers detected by targeted biopsies using manual controlled targeted biopsy with real-time fusion image of mpMRI and TRUS had a significantly higher grade and larger length compared with systematic biopsies. In present study, the cancer detection rate in TZ was significantly lower than in PZ. However, further study would contribute to set the cutoff point of PI-RADS scores in TZ and PZ to detect the prostate cancer at high frequency. The further study of the comparisons with pathological findings of whole-gland specimens will give a larger role to the present biopsy method.

Author details

Sunao Shoji

Address all correspondence to: sunashoj@mail.goo.ne.jp

Department of Urology, Tokai University Hachioji Hospital, Hachioji, Tokyo, Japan

References

[1] Moore CM, Kasivisvanathan V, Eggener S, et al. Standards of reporting for MRI-targeted biopsy studies (START) of the prostate: recommendations from an International Working Group. European Urology. 2013;64(4):544–552.

[2] Sciarra A, Barentsz J, Bjartell A, et al. Advances in magnetic resonance imaging: how they are changing the management of prostate cancer. European Urology. 2011;59(6): 962–977.

[3] Hambrock T, Somford DM, Hoeks C, et al. Magnetic resonance imaging guided prostate biopsy in men with repeat negative biopsies and increased prostate specific antigen. The Journal of Urology. 2010;183(2):520–527.

[4] Kasivisvanathan V, Dufour R, Moore CM, et al. Transperineal magnetic resonance image targeted prostate biopsy versus transperineal template prostate biopsy in the detection of clinically significant prostate cancer. The Journal of Urology. 2013;189(3): 860–866.

[5] Natarajan S, Marks LS, Margolis DJ, et al. Clinical application of a 3D ultrasound-guided prostate biopsy system. Urologic Oncology. 2011;29(3):334–342.

[6] Fiard G, Hohn N, Descotes JL, Rambeaud JJ, Troccaz J, Long JA. Targeted MRI-guided prostate biopsies for the detection of prostate cancer: initial clinical experience with real-time 3-dimensional transrectal ultrasound guidance and magnetic resonance/ transrectal ultrasound image fusion. Urology. 2013;81(6):1372–1378.

[7] Mozer P, Roupret M, Le Cossec C, et al. First round of targeted biopsies with magnetic resonance imaging/ultrasound-fusion images compared to conventional ultrasound-guided trans-rectal biopsies for the diagnosis of localised prostate cancer. BJU International. 2014; 115(1): 50–57.

[8] Wysock JS, Rosenkrantz AB, Huang WC, et al. A prospective, blinded comparison of magnetic resonance (MR) imaging-ultrasound fusion and visual estimation in the performance of MR-targeted prostate biopsy: the PROFUS Trial. European Urology. 2014; 66(2):343:351.

[9] Marks L, Young S, Natarajan S. MRI-ultrasound fusion for guidance of targeted prostate biopsy. Current Opinion in Urology. 2013;23(1):43–50.

[10] Moore CM, Robertson NL, Arsanious N, et al. Image-guided prostate biopsy using magnetic resonance imaging-derived targets: a systematic review. European Urology. 2013;63(1):125–140.

[11] Haffner J, Lemaitre L, Puech P, et al. Role of magnetic resonance imaging before initial biopsy: comparison of magnetic resonance imaging-targeted and systematic biopsy for significant prostate cancer detection. BJU International. 2011;108(8 Pt 2):E171–E178.

[12] Park BK, Park JW, Park SY, et al. Prospective evaluation of 3-T MRI performed before initial transrectal ultrasound-guided prostate biopsy in patients with high prostate-specific antigen and no previous biopsy. AJR American Journal of Roentgenology. 2011;197(5):W876–W881.

[13] Sciarra A, Panebianco V, Ciccariello M, et al. Value of magnetic resonance spectroscopy imaging and dynamic contrast-enhanced imaging for detecting prostate cancer foci in

men with prior negative biopsy. Clinical Cancer Research: An Official Journal of the American Association for Cancer Research. 2010;16(6):1875–1883.

[14] Labanaris AP, Engelhard K, Zugor V, Nutzel R, Kuhn R. Prostate cancer detection using an extended prostate biopsy schema in combination with additional targeted cores from suspicious images in conventional and functional endorectal magnetic resonance imaging of the prostate. Prostate Cancer and Prostatic Diseases. 2010;13(1):65–70.

[15] Sonn GA, Margolis DJ, Marks LS. Target detection: magnetic resonance imaging-ultrasound fusion-guided prostate biopsy. Urologic Oncology. 2014;32(6):903–911.

[16] Dickinson L, Ahmed HU, Allen C, et al. Magnetic resonance imaging for the detection, localisation, and characterisation of prostate cancer: recommendations from a European consensus meeting. European Urology. 2011;59(4):477–494.

[17] Rothke M, Blondin D, Schlemmer HP, Franiel T. PI-RADS classification: structured reporting for MRI of the prostate. RoFo: Fortschritte auf dem Gebiete der Rontgenstrahlen und der Nuklearmedizin. 2013;185(3):253–261.

[18] Barentsz JO, Richenberg J, Clements R, et al. ESUR prostate MR guidelines 2012. European Radiology. 2012;22(4):746–757.

[19] Harnden P, Naylor B, Shelley MD, Clements H, Coles B, Mason MD. The clinical management of patients with a small volume of prostatic cancer on biopsy: what are the risks of progression? A systematic review and meta-analysis. Cancer. 2008;112(5): 971–981.

[20] Collins DJ, Padhani AR. Dynamic magnetic resonance imaging of tumor perfusion. Approaches and biomedical challenges. IEEE Engineering in Medicine and Biology Magazine: The Quarterly Magazine of the Engineering in Medicine & Biology Society. 2004;23(5):65–83.

[21] Gibbs P, Liney GP, Pickles MD, Zelhof B, Rodrigues G, Turnbull LW. Correlation of ADC and T2 measurements with cell density in prostate cancer at 3.0 Tesla. Investigative Radiology. 2009;44(9):572–576.

[22] Turkbey B, Shah VP, Pang Y, et al. Is apparent diffusion coefficient associated with clinical risk scores for prostate cancers that are visible on 3-T MR images? Radiology. 2011;258(2):488–495.

[23] Oto A, Kayhan A, Jiang Y, et al. Prostate cancer: differentiation of central gland cancer from benign prostatic hyperplasia by using diffusion-weighted and dynamic contrast-enhanced MR imaging. Radiology. 2010;257(3):715–723.

[24] Zelhof B, Pickles M, Liney G, et al. Correlation of diffusion-weighted magnetic resonance data with cellularity in prostate cancer. BJU International. 2009;103(7):883–888.

Chapter 5

Oligometastatic Disease in Prostate Cancer: Advances in Diagnosis and Treatment

Weranja Ranasinghe and Raj Persad

Additional information is available at the end of the chapter

http://dx.doi.org/10.5772/63370

Abstract

Prostate cancer (PC) is the second most common cancer in men and the fifth leading cause of death in men worldwide in 2012 [1]. Oligometastatic disease is defined as the presence of five or fewer metastatic or recurrent lesions that could be treated by local therapy to achieve long-term survival or cure [2]. Androgen deprivation therapy is currently the accepted treatment of metastatic PC. However, the identification of oligometastatic disease in PC with the improvements in diagnostic imaging has lead to early treatment of these isolated metastases showing some benefit [3]. In this chapter, we aim to discuss the newer modalities used in the identification of oligometastatic disease in PC and the advances in treatment.

Keywords: Oligometastases, prostate cancer, diagnosis, treatment

1. Introduction

Although oligometastases forms a recent vogue in prostate cancer, the concept of 'oligometastases' was originally described by Hellman and Weichselbaum in 1995 [4]. They theorised that metastases occurred as a 'metastatic progression' from localised disease to widespread systemic disease [5]. As such, in some patients with limited metastases, they described an 'oligometastatic state' which occurs as a transitional state between localised and systemic disease [5]. Therefore, rather than classifying all metastatic prostate cancer in to a universal cohort with poor outcomes, this defined a group of patients who could be identified and treated with potentially favourable results.

1.1. Definitions

The nomenclature in 'oligometastases' is often used inter changeably and can be sometimes confusing. The term 'oligometastasis' usually refers to metastases (from tumours early in the chain of progression) limited in number and location because the facility for metastatic growth has not been fully developed and the site for growth is restricted, while 'oligometastatic disease' is defined as solitary or few detectable metastatic lesions (<5 metastases) that are usually confined to a single organ [5]. Although sometimes oligometastases can refer to synchronous or metachronous disease, it should be stressed that the key feature determining the behaviour of oligometastases is its metastatic potential. As such, 'true oligometastases' are defined as oligometastases with limited metastatic potential, while 'induced oligometastases' occur following successful systemic treatment have more extensive malignant capacities and were spared from eradication by pharmacological means, local immunological conditions or from the development of resistant clones [6].

In prostate cancer, induced oligometastases can be further divided into those with a rising PSA following primary therapy who has oligometastases on imaging or those with castrate-resistant prostate cancer (CRPC) with a rising PSA level and image-detected oligometastases [7].

2. The evidence for treatment of oligometastases

Treatment of liver metastases in colorectal cancer, lung metastases from a variety of cancers and adrenal metastases in lung cancer have demonstrated in improved survival and in some cases even cure; forming the basis of treating oligometastases in cancers [6]. Currently, androgen deprivation therapy is the optimal treatment for widespread metastatic prostate cancer. Studies have demonstrated that those men on androgen deprivation therapy for ≤3 metastases had much superior outcomes compared to those with larger number of metastases [8, 9]. A further study demonstrated that men with prostate cancer who developed ≤5 metastatic sites had better survival than those with >5 lesions [10]. With the recent shift, the landscape of prostate cancer diagnostics and treatments has changed significantly offering the opportunity to accurately identify and treats the oligometastases. Treatment of oligometastases in prostate cancer can offer better local cancer control and reduce the systematic metastatic potential and its complications by reducing seeding of established metastases control of the overall disease burden and perhaps even cure [7]. In addition, the treatment of oligometastatic disease in prostate cancer delays the need for androgen deprivation and its associated systemic side effects.

3. Biology of oligometastases

As described in Paget's 'seed and soil' hypothesis, metastases occur due to an interaction between the tumour cell and the targeted organ, which supports the secondary growth of the primary tumour cells [6, 11]. This is a complex and selective process which promotes tumour growth by tumour diversity due to the genetic instability of the tumour cells due to the telomere erosion, mutations in tumour-suppressor and DNA-repair genes, and intrinsic tumour metabolism (aerobic glycolysis) that is toxic to surrounding normal cell and suppression of the host immunity [6]. A number of genes contribute to this metastatic process such as metastasis 'initiation' genes; metastasis 'progression' genes and metastasis 'virulence' genes by altering cell adhesion, intravasation, survival in the circulation, extravasation, seeding in a distant site, invasion, and development of the appropriate microenvironment in host organs and provides a selective advantage of the primary tumour cells to be preserved and amplified during tumour progression [6]. As such, these primary tumour cells that have limited capability in one or more of the necessary biological requirements for metastasis form the basis of oligometastases [6].

4. Advances in imaging modalities: identification of oligometastases in prostate cancer

4.1. The conventional modalities: computed tomography (CT) and skeletal scintigraphy (^{99M}Tc-MDP bone scan)

CT of the abdomen and pelvis forms the main modality of staging patients with intermediate or high-risk disease generating valuable information of local advancement, lymph node and bony involvement of prostate cancer [12] (**Figure 1**). Studies have demonstrated its specificity and positive predictive value up to 100%, but its sensitivity remains poor [13]. As such, CT is gradually being superseded by MRI and the combination PET/CT in recurrent prostate cancer and oligometastatic disease.

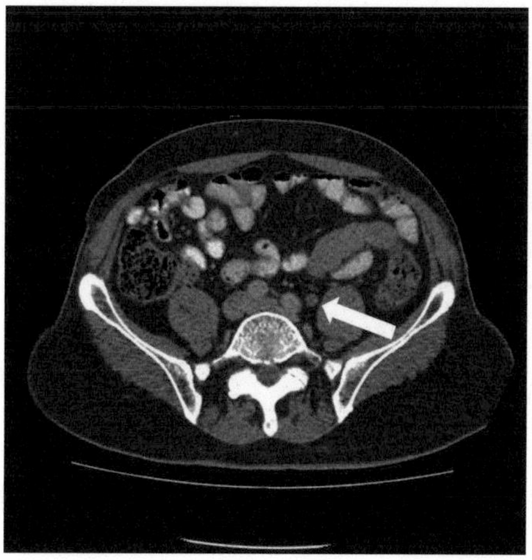

Figure 1. The CT scan of the abdomen and pelvis demonstrates a pelvic lymph node denoted by the white arrow.

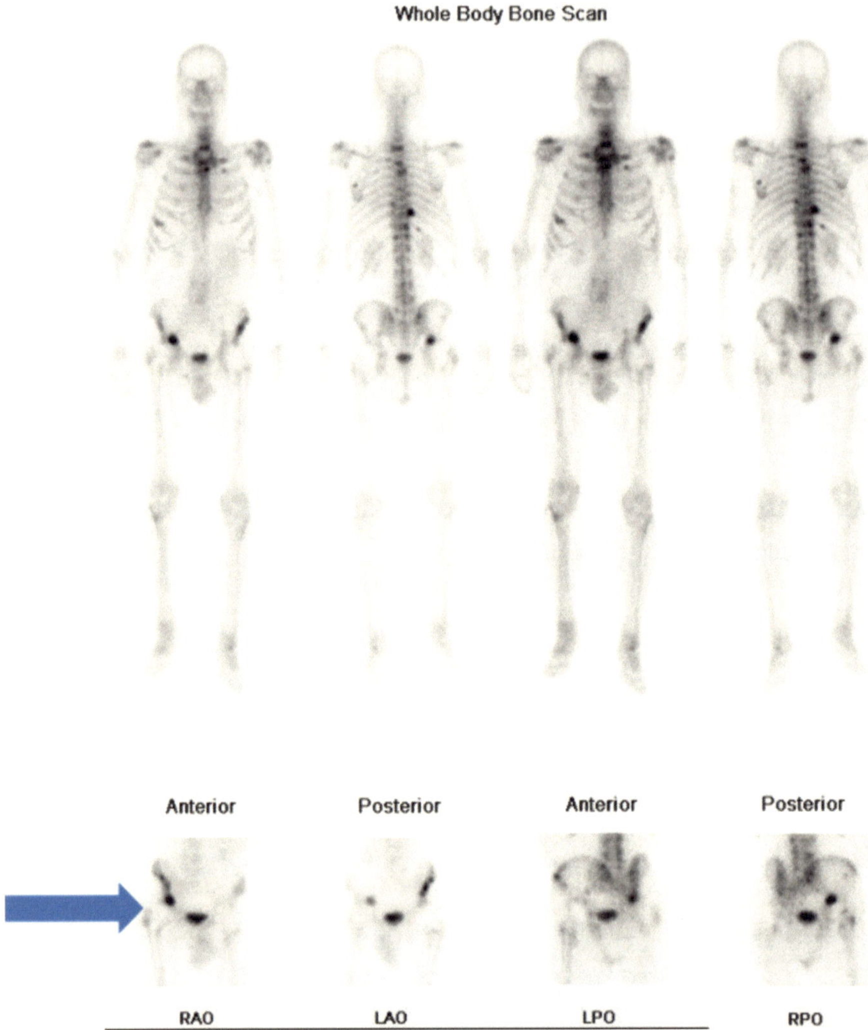

Figure 2. The isotope bone scan demonstrates uptake at the right acetabulum (blue arrow) with several areas of focal uptake in the axial skeleton, in the ribs and in the left scapula.

^{99m}Tc-methylene diphosphonate (MDP) bone scan is the main imaging modality used to assess the burden of skeletal disease in patients with PC in intermediate or high-risk PC or those with symptoms of bony metastases [12] (**Figure 2**). However, bone scintigraphy can be non-specific and can show increase bone uptake in degenerative joint disease, benign fractures and inflammation in addition to metastases [14]. However, further functional and anatomical details can be obtained by integrating the SPECT/CT along with skeletal scintigraphy. While the negative predictive value of the bone scan is estimated between 87 and 100% in the literature, its diagnostic yield is highly dependent on the PSA level and clinical stage [12]. As such bone scans have a poor yield in the early detection of prostate cancer recurrences post-definitive treatment.

4.2. The newer imaging modalities

4.2.1. Multi-parametric magnetic resonance imaging (MP-MRI)

MP-MRI forms an integral role in diagnosis of prostate cancer and localisation for prostatic biopsy. In addition, it is a very useful tool in determining extra prostatic extension, lymph nodes or bony metastases in prostate cancer.

A number of studies have demonstrated promising results in detecting local recurrences post-radical prostatectomy using MP-MRI. In patients with biochemical recurrence post-radical prostatectomy, MP-MRI can help determine loco-regional relapse and small amounts of healthy residual glandular tissue, scar/fibrosis and granulation tissue, and it may even enable assessment of the aggressiveness of nodule recurrence by means of ADC values and help identify tumour deposits and target treatment [15]. One study demonstrated sensitivities and specificities of 84–88 and 89–100%, respectively in detection of recurrences post-radical prostatectomy using MP-MRI [16].

One of the limitations of MRI is the poor detection of pelvic lymph nodes at PSA levels <0.5 ng/mL, threshold usually used for salvage therapy. One of the main reasons for this being that 70% of lymph-node metastases in prostate cancer is <8 mm [17]. In 2008, a meta-analysis of 24 studies demonstrated that both CT and MRI scans were both poor at detecting pelvic lymph-node metastases and there were no differences between the modalities [18]. In fact, they concluded that reliance on either CT or MRI will misrepresent the patient's true status regarding nodal metastases, and thus misdirect the therapeutic strategies offered to the patient [18]. However, there have been significant advances in better anatomical imaging since the introduction of MP–MRI scans and technology such as lymphotropic nanoparticle–enhanced MRI can improve the lymph–node detection as well as for biopsy targeting and guidance of salvage treatment [19].

The increasing use of whole body MP-MRI may be the future of staging patients with oligo-metastatic prostate cancer, as this can also be used to detect bony metastases with good accuracy [20]. However, this technology is currently mainly limited due to cost and needs further validation.

4.2.2. Positron emission tomography (PET) scan

Positron emission tomography (PET) scan is a functional scan which commonly uses 18F-labeled sodium fluoride (18F-NaF) and 18F-labeled 2-fluoro-2-deoxy-Dglucose (18F-FDG) as a radiotracer to detect a metabolic process associated with PC and is fused with a CT to determine the anatomic location of this process. Despite the role of 18F–FDG PET/CT in detecting occult metastatic disease in men with biochemical recurrence, and the high detection rates of osseous metastases with 18F–NaF PET/CT compared to standard imaging [21], they are still not recommended as first-line imaging modalities due to poor sensitivities in at low PSA levels and in high-grade tumours [12, 22–24].

A recent meta-analysis by Evangelista et al. concluded that Choline PET and PET/CT represent high sensitivity and specificity techniques for the detection of loco-regional and distant metastases in prostate cancer patients with recurrence of disease demonstrating a pooled sensitivity of 85.6% and a pooled specificity of 92.6% for all sites of disease (prostatic fossa, lymph nodes and bone) [25]. They further demonstrated a pooled sensitivity of 100% (95% CI 90.5–100%) and pooled specificity of 81.8% (95% CI 48.2–97.7%) for lymph-node metastases [25]. In accordance, majority of the studies investigating recurrent oligometastatic prostate cancer utilised Choline PET as the imaging modality of choice [26].

4.2.3. Prostate specific membrane antigen PET/CT (PSMA PET/CT)

68Ga-PSMA-ligand PET/CT utilises the prostate specific membrane antigen which is significantly upregulated in prostate cancer. Although the data for PSMA PET/CT scan in recurrence of prostate cancer is limited, the early results have been promising. 68Ga-PSMA–PET improves detection of lymph nodes, bone or visceral metastases compared with standard imaging (**Figures 3** and **4**). One study demonstrated a specificity of 98.9% and sensitivity 65% for detection of pelvic lymph-node disease in prostate cancer with PSMA PET, much better than standard imaging modalities [27]. Furthermore, PSMA–PET–MRI or PSMA–PET–CT enables a complete staging procedure to be performed by a single examination compared with the standard staging combination of CT and bone scan.

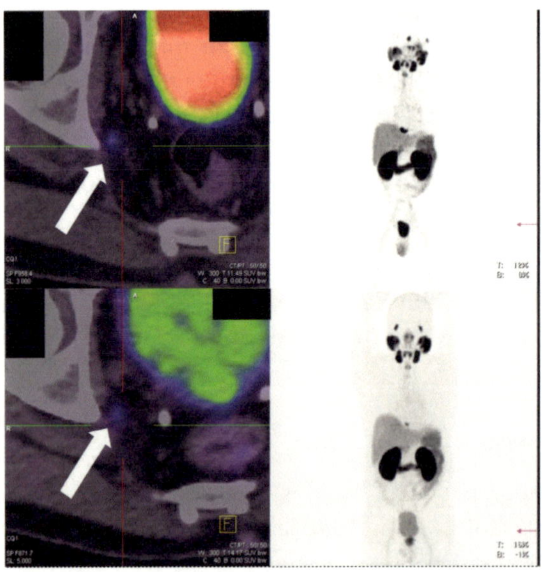

Figure 3. The PSMA PET scan demonstrates uptake of the tracer in an internal iliac node denoted by the white arrow.

One study using data from 319 patients showed a sensitivity, specificity, negative predictive value and positive predictive value of PSMA PET/CT of 76.6, 100, 91.4 and 100%, respectively, in the detection of recurrent prostate cancer [28]. The PSMA detection of recurrent prostate cancer improved with higher PSA levels and the use of androgen deprivation therapy [28]. A further study of 248 patients replicated the accuracy of PSMA-PET with an overall detection rate of 89.5% with a mean PSA value of 1.99 ng/ml [29]. As such, PSMA PET/CT is increasingly being used in studies focussed on oligometastatic disease and may form the cornerstone in detection and management of oligometastatic disease.

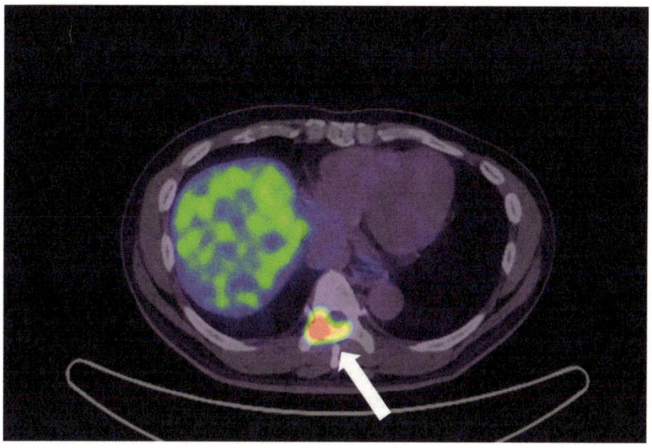

Figure 4. The PSMA PET scan demonstrates uptake of the tracer in a spine at the T9 level denoted by the white arrow.

5. Advances in treatment: treatment of oligometastatic prostate cancer

The conventional treatment of metastatic prostate cancer of androgen deprivation therapy is associated with a number of systemic side effects most importantly cardiovascular disease, and a large majority of patients will develop resistance to androgen deprivation. As such, metastases directed treatment of oligometastatic disease provides opportunity to select and treat this group of patients, delay the need for androgen deprivation or perhaps even cure.

5.1. Synchronous oligometastatic prostate cancer

5.1.1. Radical prostatectomy

Based on the responses seen by cytoreductive therapy in other cancers such as ovarian, breast and renal cell carcinoma, a few recent studies have investigated the role of radical prostatectomy in metastatic prostate cancer. Using the SEER database of 8185 men with stage IV M1 prostate cancer, Culp et al. demonstrated that a reduction in cancer specific mortality in men undergoing radical prostatectomy or brachytherapy [30]. They demonstrated a 44.8% improvement in 5-year overall survival and 27.1% improvement disease-specific survival in this cohort undergoing radical prostatectomy compared with those who did not have surgery or radiotherapy [30]. However, there were a few significant limitations in this study including the use of systemic therapy. A further study by Engel et al. replicated these findings using the Munich Cancer registry data demonstrating an improved survival in those who underwent a radical prostatectomy in the presence of lymph-node metastases [31]. While these results appear to be promising, in the absence of prospective randomised controlled study data, radical prostatectomy for oligometastatic disease should be currently considered experimental.

5.2. Recurrent disease: oligometastases after primary curative therapy

5.2.1. Salvage lymph-node dissection

Salvage lymph-node dissection in the setting of oligometastatic prostate cancer is limited to a number of cohort studies, with the largest being 59 patients [32]. Recently, a systematic review combined the results of these smaller series and reported on the results of 151 patients undergoing salvage pelvic, retroperitoneal or pelvic and retroperitoneal lymph-node dissection for oligometastatic disease [26]. Majority of the studies performed an open salvage lymph-node dissection with a median two positive nodes removed with 49 patients receiving post-operative prophylactic nodal irradiation and adjuvant ADT in 54% [26].

In the reported largest series with the longest follow-up of 59 patients undergoing salvage lymph-node dissection for oligometastatic prostate cancer, Suardi et al. reported a 8-year biochemical recurrence free survival rate of 23% and an overall 8-year clinical recurrence free survival of 38% and cancer specific mortality free survival rate of 81% [32]. They found that the PSA level at salvage LND, biochemical recurrence and the presence of retroperitoneal lymph-node metastases all influenced clinical recurrence post-operative clinical recurrence [32]. Jilg et al., in their study of 47 patients undergoing salvage LND, reported a clinical progression-free survival of 25.6% and cancer specific survival of 77.7% at 5 years [33]. Notably, the initial disease recurrence post-salvage lymph-node dissection occurred again in lymph nodes in 47–59% in these studies [26].

A large proportion of patients (55%) undergoing salvage lymph-node dissection developed complications with the majority being Clavien grade ≤ 2 [26]. The most common complications were lymphorrhoea (13%), fever (17%), ileus (10%), and a lymphocele requiring drainage (8%). Grade 3a complications were observed in 11% of the patients. Only one case of grade 3b complication (lymphocele requiring surgical drainage) was reported [26].

The current role of salvage lymph-node dissection in oligometastatic disease remains experimental and more robust long-term data are needed prior to being utilised as an established treatment modality in this setting.

5.2.2. Stereotactic radiotherapy (SBRT)

SBRT is external beam radiotherapy which is used to deliver a high dose of radiation very precisely to an extra cranial target within the body, as a single dose or a small number of fractions, thus reducing the amount of normal tissue irradiated and potentially offering complete ablation of all tissue in the treated area [34]. Therefore, it is a less invasive alternative to surgery in treating lymph-node recurrence and bony metastases in prostate cancer.

Similar to salvage lymph-node dissection, the evidence is based on small cohort studies. In one of the larger studies of 50 men with recurrence, post-definitive therapy for Schick et al.

demonstrated that a short duration androgen deprivation with and high-dose irradiation to the metastatic lesions median follow-up of 31 months (range 9–89) the 3-year biochemical relapse-free survival, clinical failure-free survival, and overall survival rates were 54.5, 58.6 and 92%, respectively [35]. In a contrasting large cohort of 50 patients receiving SBRT with a median follow up of 2 years, Decaestecker et al. reported a 35% progression free survival at 2 years [36]. The differences in progression-free survival rates are attributed to the use of adjuvant ADT and prophylactic nodal irradiation used in the study by Schick, offering better progression-free survival [31]. A further interesting observation between the studies was the pattern of first progression where, 75% presented with oligometastases in the series of Decaestecker et al. compared with only 10% in the series of Schick et al. The recurring patents then went on to receive second or third course of SBRT in the former study [36]. A short PSA doubling time before SBRT predicted worse PFS in the study by Decaestecker et al. [36]. A recent retrospective series of 19 men who had biochemical recurrence post-local therapy for prostate cancer with oligometastases (≤3 metachronous metastases) demonstrated a 21 months' median distant progression-free survival with 3- and 5-year DPFS of 31 and 15%, respectively [37]. Also importantly, this study demonstrated a delay of androgen deprivation by 28 months [37].

A further study by Tabata et al. demonstrated overall survival rates of up to 90.5% in patients receiving radiotherapy for oligometastatic disease of the bones with long-term pain control in oligometastatic disease and no spinal cord compression or pathological fractures occurring at the radiated sites [38]. CyberKnife-based stereotactic ablative radiotherapy is newer modality being utilised in oligometastatic disease with early studies also demonstrating good local control and relatively good PSA response [39].

The toxicity rates of SBRT six studies were reviewed in their analysis by Ost et al. [26]. Sixteen per cent of patients had late complications with the majority being grade 2 toxicity, mainly gastrointestinal in 8.5%, with one case of grade 3 toxicity (macroscopic haematuria) [26].

6. Conclusion

The concept of oligometastases in prostate cancer offers a newer approach to patients with the presence of five or fewer metastatic or recurrent lesions that could be treated by local therapy to achieve long-term survival or cure. Furthermore, it offers the advantage of delaying the need for androgen deprivation therapy and its associated side effects. Treatment of oligometastatic prostate cancer relies on early diagnosis in order to offer the best outcomes for these patients. Therefore, improvements in prostate cancer diagnostics such as choline PET, whole-body multi-parametric MRI, PSMA PET can provide early identification of this group of patients, while surgical and targeted radio-ablative techniques can deliver advanced therapeutics to the targeted regions. While the future management strategies appear promising for oligometastatic prostate cancer, it currently remains experimental.

Acknowledgements

We would like to thank Dr Chew-Lin Yip for the images used in this manuscript.

Author details

Weranja Ranasinghe[1*] and Raj Persad[2]

*Address all correspondence to: weranja@gmail.com

1 Boxhill Hospital, Melbourne, Australia

2 University Hospitals Bristol NHS Foundation Trust, Bristol, UK

References

[1] Ferlay J, Soerjomataram I, Dikshit R, Eser S, Mathers C, Rebelo M, et al. Cancer incidence and mortality worldwide: sources, methods and major patterns in GLOBOCAN 2012. Int J Cancer. 2015;136(5):E359–E386.

[2] Niibe Y, Chang JY. Novel insights of oligometastases and oligo-recurrence and review of the literature. Pulm Med. 2012;2012:261096.

[3] Yao HH, Hong M, Corcoran NM, Siva S, Foroudi F. Advances in local and ablative treatment of oligometastasis in prostate cancer. Asia Pac J Clin Oncol. 2014;10(4):308–321.

[4] Hellman S, Weichselbaum RR. Oligometastases. J Clin Oncol. 1995;13(1):8–10.

[5] Reyes DK, Pienta KJ. The biology and treatment of oligometastatic cancer. Oncotarget. 2015;6(11):8491–8524.

[6] Weichselbaum RR, Hellman S. Oligometastases revisited. Nat Rev Clin Oncol. 2011;8(6):378–382.

[7] Reeves F, Murphy D, Evans C, Bowden P, Costello A. Targeted local therapy in oligometastatic prostate cancer: a promising potential opportunity after failed primary treatment. BJU Int. 2015;116(2):170–172.

[8] Ost P, Decaestecker K, Lambert B, Fonteyne V, Delrue L, Lumen N, et al. Prognostic factors influencing prostate cancer-specific survival in non-castrate patients with metastatic prostate cancer. Prostate. 2014;74(3):297–305.

[9] Schweizer MT, Zhou XC, Wang H, Yang T, Shaukat F, Partin AW, et al. Metastasis-free survival is associated with overall survival in men with PSA-recurrent prostate cancer

treated with deferred androgen deprivation therapy. Ann Oncol. 2013;24(11):2881–2886.

[10] Singh D, Yi WS, Brasacchio RA, Muhs AG, Smudzin T, Williams JP, et al. Is there a favorable subset of patients with prostate cancer who develop oligometastases? Int J Radiat Oncol, Biol, Phys. 2004;58(1):3–10.

[11] Paget S. The distribution of secondary growths in cancer of the breast. 1889. Cancer Metastasis Rev. 1989;8(2):98–101.

[12] Heidenreich A, Bastian PJ, Bellmunt J, Bolla M, Joniau S, van der Kwast T, et al. EAU guidelines on prostate cancer. part 1: screening, diagnosis, and local treatment with curative intent-update 2013. Eur Urol. 2014;65(1):124–137.

[13] Abuzallouf S, Dayes I, Lukka H. Baseline staging of newly diagnosed prostate cancer: a summary of the literature. J Urol. 2004;171(6 Pt 1):2122–2127.

[14] Tombal B, Lecouvet F. Modern detection of prostate cancer's bone metastasis: is the bone scan era over? Adv Urol. 2012;2012:893193.

[15] Picchio M, Mapelli P, Panebianco V, Castellucci P, Incerti E, Briganti A, et al. Imaging biomarkers in prostate cancer: role of PET/CT and MRI. Eur J Nucl Med Mol Imaging. 2015;42(4):644–655.

[16] Casciani E, Polettini E, Carmenini E, Floriani I, Masselli G, Bertini L, et al. Endorectal and dynamic contrast-enhanced MRI for detection of local recurrence after radical prostatectomy. AJR Am J Roentgenol. 2008;190(5):1187–1192.

[17] Wang L, Hricak H, Kattan MW, Schwartz LH, Eberhardt SC, Chen HN, et al. Combined endorectal and phased-array MRI in the prediction of pelvic lymph node metastasis in prostate cancer. AJR Am J Roentgenol. 2006;186(3):743–748.

[18] Hovels AM, Heesakkers RA, Adang EM, Jager GJ, Strum S, Hoogeveen YL, et al. The diagnostic accuracy of CT and MRI in the staging of pelvic lymph nodes in patients with prostate cancer: a meta-analysis. Clin Radiol. 2008;63(4):387–395.

[19] Fortuin AS, Smeenk RJ, Meijer HJ, Witjes AJ, Barentsz JO. Lymphotropic nanoparticle-enhanced MRI in prostate cancer: value and therapeutic potential. Curr Urol Rep. 2014;15(3):389.

[20] Eiber M, Holzapfel K, Ganter C, Epple K, Metz S, Geinitz H, et al. Whole-body MRI including diffusion-weighted imaging (DWI) for patients with recurring prostate cancer: technical feasibility and assessment of lesion conspicuity in DWI. J Magn Reson Imaging. 2011;33(5):1160–1170.

[21] Even-Sapir E, Metser U, Mishani E, Lievshitz G, Lerman H, Leibovitch I. The detection of bone metastases in patients with high-risk prostate cancer: 99mTc-MDP Planar bone scintigraphy, single- and multi-field-of-view SPECT, 18F-fluoride PET, and 18F-fluoride PET/CT. J Nucl Med. 2006;47(2):287–297.

[22] Igerc I, Kohlfurst S, Gallowitsch HJ, Matschnig S, Kresnik E, Gomez-Segovia I, et al. The value of 18F-choline PET/CT in patients with elevated PSA-level and negative prostate needle biopsy for localisation of prostate cancer. Eur J Nucl Med Mol Imaging. 2008;35(5):976–983.

[23] Hacker A, Jeschke S, Leeb K, Prammer K, Ziegerhofer J, Sega W, et al. Detection of pelvic lymph node metastases in patients with clinically localized prostate cancer: comparison of [18F]fluorocholine positron emission tomography-computerized tomography and laparoscopic radioisotope guided sentinel lymph node dissection. J Urol. 2006;176(5):2014–2018; discussion 8–9.

[24] Husarik DB, Miralbell R, Dubs M, John H, Giger OT, Gelet A, et al. Evaluation of [(18)F]-choline PET/CT for staging and restaging of prostate cancer. Eur J Nucl Med Mol Imaging. 2008;35(2):253–263.

[25] Evangelista L, Zattoni F, Guttilla A, Saladini G, Zattoni F, Colletti PM, et al. Choline PET or PET/CT and biochemical relapse of prostate cancer: a systematic review and meta-analysis. Clin Nucl Med. 2013;38(5):305–314.

[26] Ost P, Bossi A, Decaestecker K, De Meerleer G, Giannarini G, Karnes RJ, et al. Metastasis-directed therapy of regional and distant recurrences after curative treatment of prostate cancer: a systematic review of the literature. Eur Urol. 2015;67(5):852–863.

[27] Maurer T, Gschwend JE, Rauscher I, Souvatzoglou M, Haller B, Weirich G, et al. Diagnostic efficacy of gallium-PSMA positron emission tomography compared to conventional imaging in lymph node staging of 130 consecutive patients with intermediate to high risk prostate cancer. J Urol. 2015.

[28] Afshar-Oromieh A, Avtzi E, Giesel FL, Holland-Letz T, Linhart HG, Eder M, et al. The diagnostic value of PET/CT imaging with the (68)Ga-labelled PSMA ligand HBED-CC in the diagnosis of recurrent prostate cancer. Eur J Nucl Med Mol Imaging. 2015;42(2): 197–209.

[29] Eiber M, Maurer T, Souvatzoglou M, Beer AJ, Ruffani A, Haller B, et al. Evaluation of hybrid (6)(8)ga-psma ligand pet/ct in 248 patients with biochemical recurrence after radical prostatectomy. J Nucl Med. 2015;56(5):668–674.

[30] Culp SH, Schellhammer PF, Williams MB. Might men diagnosed with metastatic prostate cancer benefit from definitive treatment of the primary tumor? A SEER-based study. Eur Urol. 2014;65(6):1058–1066.

[31] Engel J, Bastian PJ, Baur H, Beer V, Chaussy C, Gschwend JE, et al. Survival benefit of radical prostatectomy in lymph node-positive patients with prostate cancer. EurUrol. 2010;57(5):754–761.

[32] Suardi N, Gandaglia G, Gallina A, Di Trapani E, Scattoni V, Vizziello D, et al. Long-term outcomes of salvage lymph node dissection for clinically recurrent prostate

cancer: results of a single-institution series with a minimum follow-up of 5 years. Eur Uro. 2015;67(2):299–309.

[33] Jilg CA, Rischke HC, Reske SN, Henne K, Grosu AL, Weber W, et al. Salvage lymph node dissection with adjuvant radiotherapy for nodal recurrence of prostate cancer. J Urol. 2012;188(6):2190–2197.

[34] Tree AC, Khoo VS, Eeles RA, Ahmed M, Dearnaley DP, Hawkins MA, et al. Stereotactic body radiotherapy for oligometastases. Lancet Oncol. 2013;14(1):e28–37.

[35] Schick U, Jorcano S, Nouet P, Rouzaud M, Vees H, Zilli T, et al. Androgen deprivation and high-dose radiotherapy for oligometastatic prostate cancer patients with less than five regional and/or distant metastases. Acta Oncol. 2013;52(8):1622–1628.

[36] Decaestecker K, De Meerleer G, Lambert B, Delrue L, Fonteyne V, Claeys T, et al. Repeated stereotactic body radiotherapy for oligometastatic prostate cancer recurrence. Radiat Oncol. 2014;9:135.

[37] Ost P, Jereczek-Fossa BA, As NV, Zilli T, Muacevic A, Olivier K, et al. Progression-free survival following stereotactic body radiotherapy for oligometastatic prostate cancer treatment-naive recurrence: a multi-institutional analysis. Eur Urol. 2016;69(1):9–12.

[38] Tabata K, Niibe Y, Satoh T, Tsumura H, Ikeda M, Minamida S, et al. Radiotherapy for oligometastases and oligo-recurrence of bone in prostate cancer. Pulm Med. 2012;2012:541656.

[39] Napieralska A, Miszczyk L, Stapor-Fudzinska M. CyberKnife stereotactic ablative radiotherapy as an option of treatment for patients with prostate cancer having oligometastatic lymph nodes: single-center study outcome evaluation. Technol Cancer Res Treat. 2015.

Chapter 6

Targeted Therapy for Metastatic Prostate Cancer with Radionuclides

Hojjat Ahmadzadehfar

Additional information is available at the end of the chapter

http://dx.doi.org/10.5772/64016

Abstract

Progression to androgen-independent status is the main cause of death in patients with metastatic prostate cancer. Prostate-specific membrane antigen (PSMA) is anchored in the cell membrane of prostate epithelial cells. PSMA is highly expressed on prostate epithelial cells and strongly upregulated in prostate cancer. Therefore, it is an appropriate target for diagnosis and therapy of prostate cancer and its metastases. There is growing knowledge about promising response and low toxicity profile of radioligand therapy of metastatic castration-resistant prostate cancer using Lutetium-177-labeled PSMA ligands. For patients with only bone metastases, there are different radionuclides which have been used for decades. In this chapter, different methods of targeted radionuclide therapy of metastatic prostate cancer are described.

Keywords: PSMA, prostate cancer, radioligand therapy, metastatic disease, PSA, bone metastasis, radionuclide therapy

1. Introduction

Almost all patients with metastatic prostate cancer (PC) will initially respond to well-established and innovative anti-androgen treatments including the two recently approved hormone therapy agents, enzalutamide and abiraterone [1, 2], which significantly improve overall survival. However, progression to androgen-independent status is the main cause of death in these patients [3]. Most deaths related to PC are due to metastatic disease, which results from any combination of blood, lymphatic, or local spread. Targeted radionuclide therapy is an attractive and quickly developing therapy option for many different cancers, such as lymphoma, melanoma, and neuroendocrine tumors [4–7]. Radionuclide therapies should be targeted, because this procedure always involves the administration of unsealed sources of radioactivity.

Most therapeutic tracers utilize β-particle emissions due to the ability of these particles to penetrate tissues. The deposition of energy in tissue by β-emitters results in cellular damage. Among the β-emitters, there are several choices regarding the energy of the β-emission. Lower energy β-particles can travel a few cell diameters, or at most in the submillimeter range. Higher energy β-particles, such as those emitted by Yttrium-90 (^{90}Y) or Lutetium-177 (^{177}Lu), have excellent tissue penetration with a range beyond the source of several millimeters [8, 9]. The only routinely used α-emitter for the treatment of metastatic disease is Radium-223 (^{223}Ra), which has been approved for the treatment of bone metastases in patients with prostate cancer and symptomatic disease with no known visceral metastases [10]. The physical half-life of therapeutic radionuclide is an important consideration and an underlying principle for therapy planning [11].

2. PSMA as a target

Prostate-specific membrane antigen (PSMA), also known as folate hydrolase I or glutamate carboxypeptidase II, is a type II transmembrane protein anchored in the cell membrane of prostate epithelial cells [12]. Several biological characteristics make PSMA an outstanding target for drug development. PSMA is highly expressed on prostate epithelial cells and strongly upregulated in PC. PSMA expression levels are directly correlated to androgen independence, metastasis, and PC progression [13]; thus, PSMA is an attractive target for the diagnosis and therapy of metastasized PC. Its target specificity is maintained after radiolabeling with ^{68}Ga [12, 14].

A commonly used radionuclide is ^{68}Ga-PSMA-11, which has been successfully used for the imaging of PC with high sensitivity and specificity, even in patients with very low prostate-specific antigen (PSA) levels (<2 ng/ml) [15]. Direct comparison studies support the superiority of ^{68}Ga-PSMA-11 in lymph node assessment over CT 3D volumetric-based lymph node assessments [16] and in overall disease assessment compared to ^{18}F-methylcholine, especially in patients with low PSA levels [17]. These positive results will lead to or have already led to a paradigm shift in the use of imaging in primary staging of PC. In a recent study by Hijazi et al., the diagnostic accuracy of ^{68}Ga-PSMA-11 in the preoperative assessment of nodal metastases was very high for macrometastases and even micrometastases in lymph nodes. Correlating imaging and tissue specimens of 213 removed nodes provided 94% sensitivity, 99% specificity, 89% positive predictive value, and 99.5% negative predictive value [18].

3. PSMA radioimmunotherapy

After rather unsuccessful therapy with the ^{90}Y-CYT-356 monoclonal antibody (mAb) recognizing the intracellular domain of PSMA [19], Phase I and II clinical trials utilizing the PSMA mAb J591, radiolabeled with ^{177}Lu or ^{90}Y, have shown promising results [20–23].

J591 is an anti-PSMA mAb that binds with 1 nM affinity to the extracellular domain of PSMA [24, 25]. Milowsky et al. [26] treated 29 patients in the ^{90}Y-J591 Phase I trial; patients received therapeutic doses of 185, 370, 555, 647.5, and 740 MBq/m^2 ^{90}Y-J591. Dose-limiting toxicity was seen at 740 MBq/m^2, with two patients experiencing thrombocytopenia with nonlife-threatening bleeding episodes requiring platelet transfusions. The 647.5 MBq/m^2 dose was determined to be the maximum tolerated dose (MDT).

Bander et al. [21] treated 35 patients with progressing androgen-independent PC with ^{177}Lu-J591, and 16 of these patients received up to three doses. Myelosuppression was dose-limiting at 2775 MBq/m^2, and the 2590 MBq/m^2 dose was determined to be the single-dose MTD. Repeat dosing at 1665–2220 MBq/m^2 was associated with dose-limiting myelosuppression [21]. The authors reported good targeting of all known sites of bone and soft tissue metastases in all patients. They found no clear relationship between a history of prior chemotherapy treatment and the degree of toxicity. Biological activity was seen with four patients experiencing ≥50% declines in PSA levels lasting from 3 to 8 months. An additional 16 patients (46%) experienced PSA stabilization for a median of 60 days [21]. Tagawa et al. presented the results of a Phase II study of radionuclide therapy with the ^{177}Lu-PSMA mAb J591 [20], which was based on two published Phase I studies investigating this agent [21, 26]. In this study [20], 47 hormone-refractory patients (55.3% also had received chemotherapy) were treated with ^{177}Lu-J591. They compared two different doses (2405 vs. 2590 MBq/m^2). About 11% of patients experienced a ≥50% decline in PSA, 36.2% experienced a ≥30% decline in PSA, and 59.6% experienced any PSA decline following a single therapy. All experienced reversible hematological toxicity, with Grade 4 thrombocytopenia occurring in 46.8% without significant hemorrhage. Grade 4 neutropenia happened in a total of 25.5% of patients, with one episode of febrile neutropenia. The 2590 MBq/m^2 dose resulted in not only 30% more of PSA decline (46.9 vs. 13.3%, $P = 0.048$) and longer survival (21.8 vs. 11.9 months, $P = 0.03$), but also more Grade 4 hematological toxicity and platelet transfusions. mAb are large molecules, and therefore show poor permeability in solid tumors and slow clearance from the circulation. This combination leads to suboptimal targeting and an increased absorbed dose in the bone marrow, narrowing the therapeutic window [27]. Thus, radionuclide treatment with ^{90}Y-J591 and ^{177}Lu-J591 is limited by myelosuppression and nonhematological toxicity, with a maximum tolerated activity per cycle of 650 and 2450 MBq/m^2, respectively.

4. PSMA radioligand therapy with a small-molecule inhibitor

The synthesis and design of a series of small-molecule inhibitors of PSMA have been described by Maresca et al. [28]. On the basis of the work of this group, Hillier et al. [29] performed a preclinical evaluation of two radiopharmaceuticals, ^{123}I-MIP-1072 and ^{123}I-MIP-1095, which were designed to target PSMA in PC cells and tissue. In a recent published study from the Heidelberg group, Zechmann et al. showed the utility of ^{131}I-MIP-1095 PSMA [27]. Therapy with ^{131}I-MIP-1095 PSMA was performed in 25 patients. The patients received a single therapeutic dose of ^{131}I-MIP-1095 (mean activity 4.8 GBq, range 2.0–7.2 GBq). Erythrocyte counts fell below the normal range at the nadir in 21 patients, with 17 patients having lower values prior to therapy. In 14 patients, white blood cell counts fell below the normal range after therapy (one with Grade 3 toxicity). However, five of these 14 patients had levels below normal, prior to therapy (four Grade 1, one Grade 2); 11 patients had a reduction in platelet count below normal after therapy (two Grade 3), and one had a value below normal (Grade 2), prior to therapy. The changes in hematological parameters were not related to the activity administered. The onset of the myelosuppression occurred within 6 weeks after treatment with a quite variable time to recovery, in some cases requiring up to 3–6 months for recovery. White blood cells typically recovered within several weeks, whereas platelets required several months to recover [12, 27]. In contrast to mAb, the low-molecular-weight compounds, with higher permeability into solid tumors, offered a significant advantage in achieving higher uptake per gram of tumor tissue and a higher percentage of specific binding. Moreover, small molecules displayed more rapid tissue distribution and faster blood clearance compared with intact immunoglobulins. These properties often lead to a higher target to nontarget tissue ratio, which is important for successful application of therapeutic absorbed doses [27].

^{131}I has a long half-life of 8.02 days and has a β-particle range in soft tissue of just 0.8 mm. Due to its γ-emitting properties and long half-life, ^{131}I is less attractive from a radiation safety point of view. ^{90}Y has a half-life of 64 h, but only undergoes high-energy β-emission, resulting in a long mean β-particle range of 3.6 mm and a maximum range of 10 mm in soft tissue. Due to its long β-particle range, collateral damage to surrounding tissues is quite high [30].

Recently, a novel theranostic drug, ^{177}Lu-PSMA 617, which is a DOTA-derivative of the Glu–urea–Lys motif, has been developed for the treatment of patients with metastatic PC [29, 31]. ^{177}Lu has a half-life of 6.7 days and undergoes low-energy β-particle emission with a mean range of 1 mm and a maximum range of 2–4 mm in soft tissue. So, the practical issues surrounding radiation safety with ^{131}I and the limited collateral damage to surrounding tissues compared to ^{90}Y make ^{177}Lu-labeled radionuclide treatment the most attractive option from a physics point of view. Ahmadzadehfar et al. [32] reported on the first 10 consecutive patients who were treated with ^{177}Lu-PSMA-617 in their department (University Hospital Bonn and Muenster, Germany). They showed that 8 weeks after the therapy in these 10 patients, seven patients showed a PSA decline, of whom six experienced a more than 30% and five a more than 50% decline. Three patients showed progressive disease according to the PSA increase. No patients experienced any side effects immediately after injection of ^{177}Lu-PSMA 617 [32]. Relevant hematotoxicity (Grade 3 or 4) occurred 7 weeks after the administration in just one patient. These encouraging results showed again the efficacy of radionuclide therapy in patients who have no other approved therapeutic option. A later study by the group from Bonn showed the efficacy and safety of ^{177}Lu-PSMA 617 therapy in patients who had undergone two cycles of therapy [8]. In this study, 46 cycles of ^{177}Lu-PSMA 617 were performed in 24 consecutive hormone and/or chemorefractory patients. Twenty-two patients received two cycles of therapy. Twenty-two patients had a history of or were on therapy with enzalutamide and/or abiraterone. Twelve patients had received ^{223}Ra (1–6 cycles; median 5 cycles). All patients had multiple bone metastases, and the majority of them also had lymph node metastases. The mean and median PSA levels prior to therapy were 628.3 and 522 ng/ml, respectively (range: 17.1–2360 ng/ml). It was found that 8 weeks after the first cycle of ^{177}Lu-PSMA therapy, 19/24 patients (79.1%) experienced a PSA decline, out of whom 13 experienced a decline of more than 30% and 10 more than 50% (41.6%). Five patients showed progressive disease according to an increase in PSA. Two months after the second cycle in 22 patients who underwent two cycles of ^{177}Lu-PSMA therapy, 15/22 patients (68.2%) experienced a PSA decline in comparison to the baseline PSA value, of whom 15 experienced a decline of more than 30%, and 13 (60%) of more than 50%. Seven patients showed progressive disease according to an increase in PSA or disease progression. Again, in this study, the patients received radioligand therapy as the last therapeutic option [8]. Interestingly, although a majority of prostate cancer patients at such an advanced stage of disease with massive bone marrow infiltration suffer from anemia, relevant hematotoxicity (Grade 3) occurred during the observation period (within 2 months after the last cycle) in just two patients. Apart from some Grade 1 or 2 hematotoxicity, the majority of patients did not show any hematotoxicity during the observation period. Some patients who needed blood transfusions prior to the first cycle needed fewer transfusions after radioligand therapy with ^{177}Lu-PSMA 617 because of the regression of bone marrow involvement [33]. The Nordrhein–Westfalen study group recently published the results of single-dose administration of ^{177}Lu-PSMA 617 in 74 patients. They showed a PSA decline in 47 patients (64%); of these, 23 (31%) had a PSA decline >50%; 35 (47%) had stable disease with a PSA decline from <50% to an increase of <25%; and 17 (23%) showed progressive disease with a PSA increase >25%. Response and tolerability of a single dose of 177Lu-PSMA-617 in patients with metastatic castration-resistant prostate cancer: a multicenter retrospective analysis.

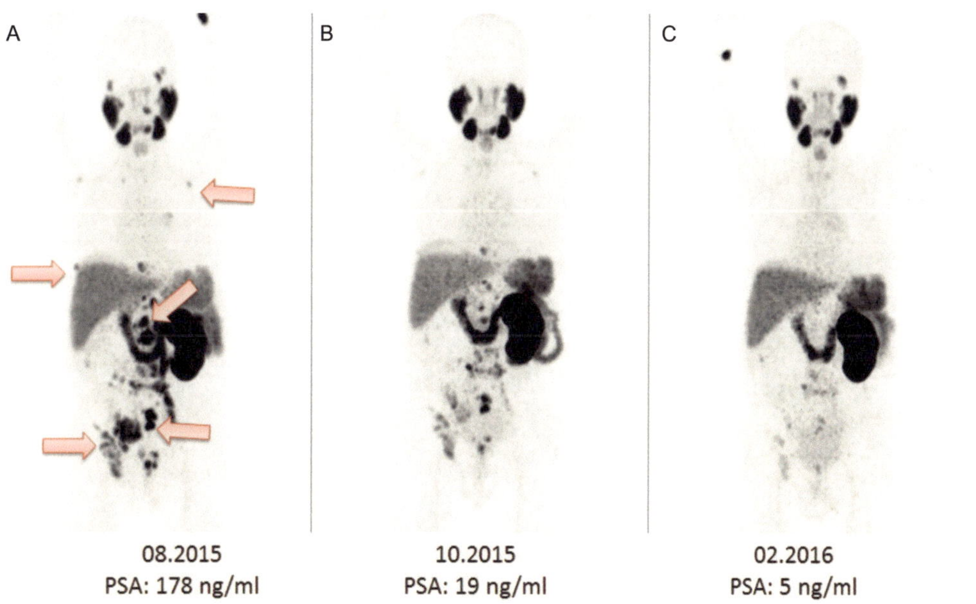

Figure 1. (**A**) 68Ga-PSMA PET scan of a 66-year-old hormone- and chemorefractory patient with multiple bone and lymph node metastases (*pink arrows*), with a history of chemotherapy, abiraterone, and ^{223}Ra therapies. (**B**) The follow-up PET scan prior to the second cycle shows a partial response with regression of the metastases and PSA decline. (**C**) The PET scan, 2 months after the third cycle of Lu-PSMA therapy, which shows a very good response with further decline of PSA.

Rahbar K, Schmidt M, Heinzel A, Eppard E, Bode A, Yordanova A, Claesener M, Ahmadzadehfar H. J Nucl Med. 2016 Apr 7. pii: jnumed.116.173757. [Epub ahead of print]

Further research into the efficacy of this therapy is needed. Rahbar et al. showed for the first time the overall survival benefit of RLT in comparison to a historical collective. They showed that the estimated median survival was 29.4 weeks, significantly longer than the survival in the historical control group at 19.7 weeks [hazard ratio: 0.44 (95% confidence interval: 0.20–0.95); $P = 0.031$] [34] (**Figure 1**).

5. Treatment of bone metastases with radionuclides

Bone metastases, a major cause of morbidity and mortality in patients with castration-resistant prostate cancer, are associated with pain, pathological fractures, spinal cord compression, and decreased survival [35]. The major mechanism of pain from small metastases appears to be the stimulation of nerve endings in the endosteum by a variety of chemical mediators. Larger bone metastases produce stretching of the periosteum, which leads to pain [36]. The incidence of bone metastases in patients with prostate cancer, according to autopsy studies, is 65–85% [37].

Bone pain palliation with radionuclides has a very long history of using different β-emitters such as phosphorus-32 (^{32}P) [38], strontium-89 (^{89}Sr) [38], rhenium-186-hydroxyethylidene diphosphonate (^{186}Re-HEDP) [39], ^{188}Re-HEDP, samarium-153-EDTMP (^{153}Sm-EDTMP) [39], and recently, lutetium-177-EDTMP (^{177}Lu-EDTMP) [40] and ^{177}Lu-BPAMD [41]. The only approved α-emitter is radium-223 (^{223}Ra) [42].

Calcium analogues	Attached to phosphate
Strontium-89	Phosphorus-32
Radium-223	Samarium-153-EDTMP
	Rhenium-186-HEDP
	Rhenium-188-HEDP
	Lutetium-177-EDTMP
	Lutetium-177-BPAMD

Table 1. Different radionuclides for bone palliation.

Bone-seeking radionuclides are classified into two groups: calcium analogues and radionuclides attached to phosphate (**Table 1**). Different radionuclides have different physical characteristics, which are shown in **Table 2**.

	Emission type	t½ (days)	Maximum energy (MeV)	Max tissue penetration range (mm)
Phosphorus-32	β	14.3	1.7	8.5
Strontium-89	β	50.5	1.46	7
Samarium-153	β and γ	1.9	0.81	4
Rhenium-186	β and γ	3.7	1.07	5
Rhenium-188	β and γ	0.7	2.1	10
Lutetium-177	β and γ	6.7	0.498	1.8
Radium-223	αand γ	11.4	27.78	0.1

All, but Radium-223, are β-emitters.

Table 2. Summary of the main physical properties of different radionuclides in clinical use for pain palliation.

5.1. ^{32}Phosphorus

^{32}P decays by 1.7 MeV (E_{max}) β-emission and has a physical half-life of 14.3 days, with a maximum tissue penetration of 8.5 mm (**Table 2**) [43]. During treatment with ^{32}P, pain relief was reported by 50–87% of patients treated with 200–800 MBq of ^{32}P administered daily in 20–80 MBq fractions after androgen priming. Pain reduction occurred within 5–14 days, with a mean response duration of 2–4 months [38, 44, 45] (**Table 3**). The main disadvantage of ^{32}P therapy is dose-limiting myelosuppression with reversible pancytopenia maximal at 5–6 weeks after administration [46].

Radiopharmaceutical	activity	Typical response time	Typical response duration	Retreatment interval
Phosphorus-32	444 MBq (fractionated)	14 days	10 weeks	<3 months
Strontium-89 chloride	150–200 MBq	14–28 days	12–26 weeks	<3 months
Samarium-153-EDTMP	37 MBq/kg	2–7 days	8 weeks	<2 months
Rhenium-186-HEDP	1.3 GBq	2–7 days	8–10 weeks	<2 months
Rhenium-188-HEDP	1.3–4.4 GBq	2–7 days	8 weeks	2 months

Refs. [93–95].

Table 3. Bone-seeking radionuclides.

5.2. ^{89}Strontium

$^{89}SrCl^2$ is an element that behaves like calcium and localizes in bone, primarily in areas of osteoblastic activity. It decays by 1.4 MeV (E_{max}) β-emission, with a long physical half-life of 50.5 days. The maximum penetration range in tissue is about 7 mm. Excretion is predominantly renal, dictated by the skeletal tumor burden and glomerular filtration rate [47, 48].

The biological half-life in normal bone is around 14 days, compared with more than 50 days in osteoblastic metastases. The first studies using ^{89}Sr demonstrated efficacy for pain reduction as high as 80%. Complete response rates vary widely among studies and have been reported in 8–77% of cases. The overall response rate varied from 33 to 82% [49–54]. It was the first radiopharmaceutical to be approved for systemic radionuclide therapy in the palliation of painful bone metastases. The standard recommended dose of ^{89}Sr is 150–200 MBq (**Table 3**). It was shown to be as effective as both local field and hemibody external-beam radiotherapy in relieving existing bone pain, but delayed the development of new pain at preexisting, clinically silent sites [45, 55].

Toxicity is limited with the common development of thrombocytopenia, with the nadir between the 4th and 6th weeks. Recovery is typically slow over the next 6 weeks, dictated by skeletal tumor extent and bone marrow reserve [45].

The largest study was published by Robinson et al. In this study, 622 patients were included (466 with prostate cancer). About 15% of patients showed complete pain relief, and a partial response was documented in 81% [56–58]. Tu et al. [59] reported improved survival using six weekly administrations of $^{89}SrCl^2$ combined with doxorubicin after induction chemotherapy, compared with six weekly administrations of doxorubicin alone; however, the follow-up Phase II trial of the same study group did not confirm the positive effect of this combination therapy on overall survival [60].

A nonrandomized study using 12 weekly administrations of estramustine phosphate, vinblastine, and $^{89}SrCl^2$ recorded effective, durable symptom palliation, more than a 50% reduction in PSA in 48% of treated patients, and reduced demand for subsequent palliative radiotherapy [61]. Several patient characteristics could predict a favorable response to ^{89}Sr. A normal serum hemoglobin level prior to treatment is associated with a higher pain response rate [62]. Other predictors of a poor pain response were low performance status, higher serum PSA, more extensive osseous metastases, and a poor PSA response [63–66].

5.3. ^{186}Rhenium-HEDP

^{186}Re is a medium-energy β-emitter with a physical half-life of 89 h. ^{186}Re-1,1-hydroxyethylidene diphosphonate (^{186}Re-HEDP) is a surface bone-seeking radiopharmaceutical used for internal radiotherapy. The maximum tolerated activity is 2960 MBq, but for routine use the recommended activity is 1285 MBq. Peak skeletal uptake occurs 3 h after intravenous administration [67, 68]. An early study by Maxon et al. [69] using 1285 MBq of ^{186}Re-HEDP documented overall pain relief in 80% of patients, with a mean duration of 7 weeks in hormone refractory PC patients (**Table 3**) [70]. Eighty to ninety percent of patients reported improved symptoms after a single ^{186}Re-HEDP administration. The response was typically rapid, occurring within 24–48 h of activity administration. Placebo-controlled, randomized studies have confirmed the efficacy of ^{186}Re-HEDP [70, 71]. ^{186}Re-HEDP undergoes rapid urinary excretion and rapid blood clearance (plasma half-life of 41 h) [70]. For the standard applied activity of 1285 MBq, ^{186}Re-HEDP provided a median radiation-absorbed dose of 26 Gy to bone metastases and 1.73 Gy to the red bone marrow [70]. The tumor to marrow dose ratios had a high therapeutic index, with a mean value of 34:1 [69]. Toxicity was limited to temporary myelosuppression, with platelet and neutrophil nadirs at 4 weeks after therapy. Recovery occurred within 8 weeks and was usually complete [72].

5.4. ^{188}Rhenium-HEDP

^{188}Re has a short physical half-life of 16.8 h and a maximum β-particle energy of 2.1 MeV with a 15% γ-component of 155 keV. The maximum β-range in tissue is approximately 10 mm [73]. Blood clearance is rapid after injection, with 41% renal clearance within 8 h of administration. Absorbed doses for bone metastases are in the range of 3.83 ± 2 mGy/MBq, in comparison with 0.61 ± 0.2 mGy/MBq for bone marrow and 0.07 ± 0.02 mGy/MBq for the whole body. The mean effective whole-body half-life is 11.6 ± 2.1 h compared with 15.9 ± 3.5 h in bone metastases [45]. ^{188} Re is of special interest in clinical applications because of its excellent availability and cost-effectiveness, as it is the product of a ^{188}W (^{188}W/^{188}Re) generator [74].

The short physical half-life and high dose rate are predicted to lead to a rapid symptom response. Fractionated therapy has been shown to prolong response duration and progression-free survival (PFS). Palmedo et al. [73] randomly assigned 64 patients to two different groups for radionuclide therapy with ^{188}Re-HEDP; patients in group A received a single injection, while patients in group B received two injections with an 8-week interval. In both groups, toxicity was low, with moderate thrombopenia and leukopenia. Repeated ^{188}Re-HEDP therapies (group B) were more effective for pain palliation compared to group A, with a response rate and time of response of 92% and 5.66 months, respectively (P = 0.006 and P = 0.001). In group B, 11/28 patients (39%) had a PSA decline of more than 50% for at least 8 weeks, compared with 2/30 patients (7%) in group A. The median times to progression in group A and group B were 2.3 months (0–12.2 months) and 7.0 months (0–24.1 months), respectively (P = 0.0013), and the median overall survival times were 7.0 months (range, 1.3–36.7 months) and 12.7 months (range, 4.1–32.2 months), respectively (P = 0.043) [74].

Liepe et al. [75] reported moderate transient bone marrow toxicity with a decrease in the number of platelets from a baseline value of 286 ± 75 × 10^9/l to a maximum of 218 ± 83 × 10^9/l with the nadir at 3 weeks. This study group found no evidence of either local or systemic intolerance to treatment with ^{188}Re-HEDP, while a flare reaction with an increase in pain within 14 days after therapy was noted in 16% of patients [75].

Biersack et al. [76] also showed the positive effect of repeated therapy on overall survival. They retrospectively analyzed 60 hormone-refractory patients classified into three different groups according to the number of therapies. Group A comprised patients who had received only one therapy (19 patients), group B included patients who had received two therapies (19 patients), and group C included patients who had received three or more therapies (22 patients). All patients had bone pain and presented with more than five lesions documented by a bone scan. Mean survival after the initial therapy improved from 4.5 months in group A to 9.98 months in group B and 15.7 months in group C [76].

5.5. ^{153}Samarium-EDTMP

^{153}Sm-EDTMP has a lower β-emission energy [0.81 MeV (20%), 0.71 MeV (49%), and 0.64 MeV (30%)], a 28% abundance of γ-emission at 103 keV (28%) and a physical half-life of 46.3 h. ^{153}Sm forms a stable complex with ethylenediamine tetramethylene phosphonate (EDTMP).

Clearance is bi-exponential after administration, comprising rapid bone uptake (half-life of 5.5 min) and plasma renal clearance (half-life of 65 min) [77].

A dose escalation study with 10–36 MBq/kg of ^{153}Sm-EDTMP reported a pain relief rate of 65%, with a duration range from 4 to 35 weeks [78]. A further dose escalation study in 52 patients using administered activities from 37 to 111 MBq/kg had a response rate of 74% with a median duration of 10 weeks [79]. Larger studies with more than 100 patients showed a median therapeutic efficacy of 80%. In a randomized, double-blind, placebo trial ($n = 152$), pain relief was found in 65% of patients after ^{153}Sm-EDTMP treatment compared to 45% in the placebo group [80]. A significant decrease in pain between ^{153}Sm-EDTMP and placebo was reported after 1 week, and the analgesic intake was significantly reduced after 3 and 4 weeks. Two large studies using ^{153}Sm-EDTMP with more than 550 patients reported response rates of 73 and 86% [81, 82].

5.6. Comparing the pain response between different radionuclides

Dickie et al. compared ^{89}Sr with ^{153}Sm in 57 prostate cancer patients. They found no difference in the pain response rate and toxicity [83]. van der Poel et al. compared ^{186}Re with ^{89}Sr and reported no differences in the response rate or toxicity [54]. A nonrandomized comparison of ^{188}Re-HEDP and ^{153}Sm-EDTMP in patients with painful metastases from prostate and breast cancer by Liepe et al. [84] showed a comparable response and toxicity with both agents. Liepe et al. also performed a comparative study of ^{188}Re-HEDP, ^{186}Re-HEDP, ^{153}Sm-EDTMP, and $^{89}SrCl^2$ in the treatment of painful bone metastases. They reported that all radiopharmaceuticals were effective in pain palliation, without the induction of severe side effects or significant differences in therapeutic efficacy or toxicity [39].

5.7. ^{223}Radium dichloride

^{223}Ra, an α-emitter, has a half-life of 11.4 days, with a total emitted energy of about 28 MeV. It is the only FDA-approved radiopharmaceutical for the treatment of bone metastases of PC with positive impact on overall survival according to a prospective randomized study [10]. It is a bone stromal-targeted radiopharmaceutical that undergoes α-emission. The α-particle is considerably more destructive to tumor cells than the β-particle. ^{223}Ra has a very high linear energy transfer, and only one to five hits per cell can be fatal. Double-strand breaks are induced even in quiescent cells and at low oxygen levels [85].

The penetration range of α-particles (<100 μm) in tissue is much smaller than that of previously described β-emitters in this chapter; so, despite the high energy, because of the short penetration range, bone marrow damage is minimal [86]. Nonhematological toxicities are more commonly observed, and are mild to moderate in intensity. The most common side effects are diarrhea, fatigue, nausea, vomiting, and bone pain, some of which are dose-related [87–89]. These side effects are easily manageable with symptomatic and supportive treatments [90].

Parker et al. [89] performed a randomized, double-blind, dose-finding, Phase II study that included 122 PC patients who were randomized to be treated with three injections of ^{223}Ra at 6-week intervals, at doses of 25 kBq/kg ($n = 41$), 50 kBq/kg ($n = 39$), or 80 kBq/kg ($n = 42$). They compared the proportion of patients in each group with confirmed PSA decline of ≥50%. No patient in the 25 kBq/kg dose group showed a significant PSA decline ≥50%. In the 50 kBq/kg dose group, only two patients (6%) showed a significant PSA decline, whereas in five patients (13%) in the 80 kBq/kg dose group, a significant PSA decline was reported ($P = 0.0297$). A ≥50% decrease in the bone alkaline phosphatase level was reported in 6 patients (16%), 24 patients (67%), and 25 patients (66%), in the 25, 50, and 80 kBq/kg dose groups, respectively ($P < 0.0001$). The most common treatment-related adverse events (≥10%) occurring up to week 24 across all dose groups were diarrhea (21%), nausea (16%), and anemia (14%). No difference in the incidence of hematological events was seen among the dose groups. They concluded that ^{223}Ra had a dose-dependent effect on serum markers of PC activity, suggesting that controlling bone disease with ^{223}Ra may affect cancer-related outcomes [89].

The ALSYMPCA trial (ALpharadin in SYMptomatic Prostate CAncer) is the first randomized Phase III study demonstrating improved survival with a bone-seeking radioisotope [42]. The number of PC patients recruited was 921. All patients were required to have progressed with symptomatic bone metastases, with at least two or more metastases on bone scintigraphy with no known visceral metastases. Randomization was 2:1 in a double-blind fashion to receive six cycles of intravenous ^{223}Ra every 4 weeks with best standard of care or six infusions of placebo with best standard of care. This study demonstrated a significant prolongation of survival (14.9 vs. 11.3 months, respectively; $P < 0.001$). Apart from this, the frequency of skeletal-related events was reduced in the ^{223}Ra group, and the median time to a skeletal-related event increased (15.6 vs. 9.8 months; $P < 0.001$). ^{223}Ra was well-tolerated with low rates of grade 3/4 neutropenia (1.8 vs. 0.8%) and thrombocytopenia (4 vs. 2%) [42].

Etchebehere et al. retrospectively reviewed 110 patients with metastatic PC treated with ^{223}Ra. The end points of this study were overall survival, bone event-free survival, progression-free survival (PFS), and bone marrow failure. They evaluated the following parameters prior to the first therapy cycle: hemoglobin (Hb), PSA, alkaline phosphatase (ALP), ECOG status, pain score, prior chemotherapy, and external beam radiation therapy (EBRT). Furthermore during/after ^{223}Ra, the PSA doubling time (PSADT), the total number of radium cycles (RaTot), and the use of chemotherapy, EBRT, enzalutamide, and abiraterone were evaluated. A significant reduction of alkaline phosphatase and pain score occurred throughout the ^{223}Ra cycles. The risk of progression was associated with declining ECOG status and decrease in PSADT. RaTot, initial ECOG(Eastern Cooperative Oncology Group) status, ALP, initial pain score, and the use of abiraterone were associated with OS ($P \leq 0.008$), PFS ($P \leq 0.003$), and BeFS ($P \leq 0.020$). RaTot, initial ECOG status, ALP, and initial pain score were significantly associated with bone marrow failure ($P \leq 0.001$), as well as Hb ($P < 0.001$) and EBRT ($P = 0.009$). In the multivariable analysis, only RaTot and abiraterone remained significantly associated with OS ($P < 0.001$ and $P = 0.033$, respectively), PFS ($P < 0.001$ and $P = 0.041$, respectively), and BeFS ($P < 0.001$ and $P = 0.019$, respectively). Additionally, RaTot ($P = 0.027$) and EBRT ($P = 0.013$) remained significantly associated with bone marrow failure. They concluded that the concomitant use of abiraterone and ^{223}Ra seems to have a beneficial effect, while EBRT may increase the risk of bone marrow failure [91].

Recently, Pacilio et al. [90] performed a dosimetry study and showed that the lesion uptake of ^{223}Ra was significantly correlated with that of ^{99m}Tc-MDP. The D_{RBE} (RBE, relative biological effectiveness; D_{RBE}, RBE-weighted absorbed dose) to lesions per unit administered activity was much higher than that of other bone-seeking radiopharmaceuticals, but considering a standard administration of 21 MBq (six injections of 50 kBq/kg to a 70-kg patient), the mean cumulative value of D_{RBE} was about 19 Gy, and was therefore in a similar range as other radiopharmaceuticals.

Nilsson et al. [92] reported the quality-of-life results of the ALSYMPCA study. It was found that improved survival with ^{223}Ra was accompanied by significant quality-of-life benefits, including a higher percentage of patients with meaningful quality-of-life improvements and a slower decline in quality-of-life over time.

6. Conclusion

A pain response is seen in approximately one-half of patients treated with radionuclides for painful osseous metastases of prostate cancer. The ALSYMPCA study showed an OS benefit with ^{223}Ra treatment. However, it should be mentioned that this study was supported by the company, Bayer. The other radiopharmaceuticals which are mentioned in this chapter were not tested in prospective multicenter trials with a large number of patients. This means that β-emitters could also have an OS benefit, which was shown in only a few studies. A combination of hormone therapy with bone-targeted therapy may be more effective than a single therapy approach. Different combinations of therapies are being studied at the moment. PSMA-targeted therapy has so far shown very promising results. According to the published studies, ^{177}Lu-PSMA therapy after ^{223}Ra is feasible and safe.

Author details

Hojjat Ahmadzadehfar

Address all correspondence to: Hojjat.ahmadzadehfar@ukb.uni-bonn.de; nuclearmedicine@gmail.com

Department of Nuclear Medicine, University Hospital Bonn, Bonn, Germany

References

[1] Scher HI, Fizazi K, Saad F, Taplin ME, Sternberg CN, Miller K, de Wit R, Mulders P, Chi KN, Shore ND, Armstrong AJ, Flaig TW, Flechon A, Mainwaring P, Fleming M, Hainsworth JD, Hirmand M, Selby B, Seely L, de Bono JS. Increased survival with

enzalutamide in prostate cancer after chemotherapy. *The New England Journal of Medicine* 2012; 367: 1187–97.

[2] Ryan CJ, Smith MR, Fizazi K, Saad F, Mulders PF, Sternberg CN, Miller K, Logothetis CJ, Shore ND, Small EJ, Carles J, Flaig TW, Taplin ME, Higano CS, de Souza P, de Bono JS, Griffin TW, De Porre P, Yu MK, Park YC, Li J, Kheoh T, Naini V, Molina A, Rathkopf DE. Abiraterone acetate plus prednisone versus placebo plus prednisone in chemotherapy-naive men with metastatic castration-resistant prostate cancer (COU-AA-302): final overall survival analysis of a randomised, double-blind, placebo-controlled phase 3 study. *The Lancet Oncology* 2015; 16: 152–60.

[3] Wei Q, Li M, Fu X, Tang R, Na Y, Jiang M, Li Y. Global analysis of differentially expressed genes in androgen-independent prostate cancer. *Prostate Cancer and Prostatic Diseases* 2007; 10: 167–74.

[4] Kraeber-Bodere F, Bodet-Milin C, Rousseau C, Eugene T, Pallardy A, Frampas E, Carlier T, Ferrer L, Gaschet J, Davodeau F, Gestin JF, Faivre-Chauvet A, Barbet J, Cherel M. Radioimmunoconjugates for the treatment of cancer. *Seminars in Oncology* 2014; 41: 613–22.

[5] Mier W, Kratochwil C, Hassel JC, Giesel FL, Beijer B, Babich JW, Friebe M, Eisenhut M, Enk A, Haberkorn U. Radiopharmaceutical therapy of patients with metastasized melanoma with the melanin-binding benzamide 131I-BA52. *Journal of Nuclear Medicine: Official Publication, Society of Nuclear Medicine* 2014; 55: 9–14.

[6] van der Zwan WA, Bodei L, Mueller-Brand J, de Herder WW, Kvols LK, Kwekkeboom DJ. GEPNETs update: radionuclide therapy in neuroendocrine tumors. *European Journal of Endocrinology/European Federation of Endocrine Societies* 2015; 172: R1–8.

[7] Bodei L, Kidd M, Paganelli G, Grana CM, Drozdov I, Cremonesi M, Lepensky C, Kwekkeboom DJ, Baum RP, Krenning EP, Modlin IM. Long-term tolerability of PRRT in 807 patients with neuroendocrine tumours: the value and limitations of clinical factors. *European Journal of Nuclear Medicine and Molecular Imaging* 2015; 42: 5–19.

[8] Ahmadzadehfar H, Eppard E, Kurpig S, Fimmers R, Yordanova A, Schlenkhoff CD, Gartner F, Rogenhofer S, Essler M. Therapeutic response and side effects of repeated radioligand therapy with 177Lu-PSMA-DKFZ-617 of castrate-resistant metastatic prostate cancer. Oncotarget. 2016 Mar 15;7(11):12477-88. doi: 10.18632/oncotarget.7245.

[9] Ahmadzadehfar H, Biersack HJ, Ezziddin S. Radioembolization of liver tumors with yttrium-90 microspheres. *Seminars in Nuclear Medicine* 2010; 40: 105–21.

[10] Parker C, Sartor O. Radium-223 in prostate cancer. *The New England Journal of Medicine* 2013; 369: 1659–60.

[11] Ahmadzadehfar H, Sabet A, Biersack H, Risse J. Therapy of hepatocellular carcinoma with iodine-131-lipidiol. In: Lau J, ed. *Hepatocellular Carcinoma - Clinical Research* 2012.

[12] Haberkorn U, Eder M, Kopka K, Babich JW, Eisenhut M. New strategies in prostate cancer: prostate-specific membrane antigen (PSMA) ligands for diagnosis and therapy.

Clinical Cancer Research: An Official Journal of the American Association for Cancer Research 2016; 22: 9–15.

[13] Santoni M, Scarpelli M, Mazzucchelli R, Lopez-Beltran A, Cheng L, Cascinu S, Montironi R. Targeting prostate-specific membrane antigen for personalized therapies in prostate cancer: morphologic and molecular backgrounds and future promises. *Journal of Biological Regulators and Homeostatic Agents* 2014; 28: 555–63.

[14] Banerjee SR, Pullambhatla M, Byun Y, Nimmagadda S, Green G, Fox JJ, Horti A, Mease RC, Pomper MG. 68Ga-labeled inhibitors of prostate-specific membrane antigen (PSMA) for imaging prostate cancer. *Journal of Medicinal Chemistry* 2010; 53: 5333–41.

[15] Eiber M, Maurer T, Souvatzoglou M, et al. Evaluation of hybrid ^{68}Ga-PSMA ligand PET/CT in 248 patients with biochemical recurrence after radical prostatectomy. *Journal of Nuclear Medicine* 2015; 56: 668–74.

[16] Giesel FL, Fiedler H, Stefanova M, et al. PSMA PET/CT with Glu-urea-Lys-(Ahx)-[^{68}Ga(HBED-CC)] versus 3D CT volumetric lymph node assessment in recurrent prostate cancer. *European Journal of Nuclear Medicine and Molecular Imaging* 2015; 42: 1794–800.

[17] Morigi JJ, Stricker PD, van Leeuwen PJ, et al. Prospective comparison of 18f-fluoromethylcholine versus 68Ga-PSMA PET/CT in prostate cancer patients who have rising PSA after curative treatment and are being considered for targeted therapy. *Journal of Nuclear Medicine* 2015; 56: 1185–90.

[18] Hijazi S, Meller B, Leitsmann C, et al. Pelvic lymph node dissection for nodal oligometastatic prostate cancer detected by 68Ga-PSMA-positron emission tomography/computerized tomography. *Prostate* 2015; 75: 1934–40.

[19] Deb N, Goris M, Trisler K, Fowler S, Saal J, Ning S, Becker M, Marquez C, Knox S. Treatment of hormone-refractory prostate cancer with 90Y-CYT-356 monoclonal antibody. *Clinical Cancer Research : An Official Journal of the American Association for Cancer Research* 1996; 2: 1289–97.

[20] Tagawa ST, Milowsky MI, Morris M, Vallabhajosula S, Christos P, Akhtar NH, Osborne J, Goldsmith SJ, Larson S, Taskar NP, Scher HI, Bander NH, Nanus DM. Phase II study of Lutetium-177-labeled anti-prostate-specific membrane antigen monoclonal antibody J591 for metastatic castration-resistant prostate cancer. *Clinical Cancer Research: An Official Journal of the American Association for Cancer Research* 2013; 19: 5182–91.

[21] Bander NH, Milowsky MI, Nanus DM, Kostakoglu L, Vallabhajosula S, Goldsmith SJ. Phase I trial of 177lutetium-labeled J591, a monoclonal antibody to prostate-specific membrane antigen, in patients with androgen-independent prostate cancer. *Journal of Clinical Oncology: Official Journal of the American Society of Clinical Oncology* 2005; 23: 4591–601.

[22] Vallabhajosula S, Goldsmith SJ, Hamacher KA, Kostakoglu L, Konishi S, Milowski MI, Nanus DM, Bander NH. Prediction of myelotoxicity based on bone marrow radiation-

absorbed dose: radioimmunotherapy studies using 90Y- and 177Lu-labeled J591 antibodies specific for prostate-specific membrane antigen. *Journal of Nuclear Medicine: Official Publication, Society of Nuclear Medicine* 2005; 46: 850-8.

[23] Vallabhajosula S, Goldsmith SJ, Kostakoglu L, Milowsky MI, Nanus DM, Bander NH. Radioimmunotherapy of prostate cancer using 90Y- and 177Lu-labeled J591 monoclonal antibodies: effect of multiple treatments on myelotoxicity. *Clinical Cancer Research: An Official Journal of the American Association for Cancer Research* 2005; 11: 7195s–200s.

[24] Liu H, Moy P, Kim S, Xia Y, Rajasekaran A, Navarro V, Knudsen B, Bander NH. Monoclonal antibodies to the extracellular domain of prostate-specific membrane antigen also react with tumor vascular endothelium. *Cancer Research* 1997; 57: 3629–34.

[25] Smith-Jones PM, Vallabahajosula S, Goldsmith SJ, Navarro V, Hunter CJ, Bastidas D, Bander NH. In vitro characterization of radiolabeled monoclonal antibodies specific for the extracellular domain of prostate-specific membrane antigen. *Cancer Research* 2000; 60: 5237–43.

[26] Milowsky MI, Nanus DM, Kostakoglu L, Vallabhajosula S, Goldsmith SJ, Bander NH. Phase I trial of yttrium-90-labeled anti-prostate-specific membrane antigen monoclonal antibody J591 for androgen-independent prostate cancer. *Journal of Clinical Oncology: Official Journal of the American Society of Clinical Oncology* 2004; 22: 2522–31.

[27] Zechmann CM, Afshar-Oromieh A, Armor T, Stubbs JB, Mier W, Hadaschik B, Joyal J, Kopka K, Debus J, Babich JW, Haberkorn U. Radiation dosimetry and first therapy results with a (124)I/(131)I-labeled small molecule (MIP-1095) targeting PSMA for prostate cancer therapy. *European Journal of Nuclear Medicine and Molecular Imaging* 2014; 41: 1280–92.

[28] Maresca KP, Hillier SM, Femia FJ, Keith D, Barone C, Joyal JL, Zimmerman CN, Kozikowski AP, Barrett JA, Eckelman WC, Babich JW. A series of halogenated heterodimeric inhibitors of prostate specific membrane antigen (PSMA) as radiolabeled probes for targeting prostate cancer. *Journal of Medicinal Chemistry* 2009; 52: 347–57.

[29] Hillier SM, Maresca KP, Femia FJ, Marquis JC, Foss CA, Nguyen N, Zimmerman CN, Barrett JA, Eckelman WC, Pomper MG, Joyal JL, Babich JW. Preclinical evaluation of novel glutamate-urea-lysine analogues that target prostate-specific membrane antigen as molecular imaging pharmaceuticals for prostate cancer. *Cancer Research* 2009; 69: 6932–40.

[30] Yeong CH, Cheng MH, Ng KH. Therapeutic radionuclides in nuclear medicine: current and future prospects. *Journal of Zhejiang University Science B* 2014; 15: 845–63.

[31] Kratochwil C, Giesel FL, Eder M, Afshar-Oromieh A, Benesova M, Mier W, Kopka K, Haberkorn U. [Lu]Lutetium-labeled PSMA ligand-induced remission in a patient with metastatic prostate cancer. *European Journal of Nuclear Medicine and Molecular Imaging* 2015; 42: 987–8.

[32] Ahmadzadehfar H, Rahbar K, Kurpig S, Bogemann M, Claesener M, Eppard E, Gartner F, Rogenhofer S, Schafers M, Essler M. Early side effects and first results of radioligand therapy with (177)Lu-DKFZ-617 PSMA of castrate-resistant metastatic prostate cancer: a two-centre study. *EJNMMI Research* 2015; 5: 114.

[33] Schlenkhoff CD, Gaertner F, Essler M, Schmidt M, Ahmadzadehfar H. Positive influence of 177Lu PSMA-617 therapy on bone marrow depression caused by metastatic prostate cancer. Clin Nucl Med. 2016 Jun;41(6):478-80. doi: 10.1097/RLU.0000000000001195.

[34] Rahbar K, Bode A, Weckesser M, Avramovic N, Claesener M, Stegger L, Bögemann M. Radioligand therapy with 177Lu-PSMA-617 as a novel therapeutic option in patients with metastatic castration resistant prostate cancer. Clin Nucl Med. 2016 Apr 15. [Epub ahead of print].

[35] Mundy GR. Metastasis to bone: causes, consequences and therapeutic opportunities. *Nature Reviews Cancer* 2002; 2: 584–93.

[36] Crawford ED, Kozlowski JM, Debruyne FM, Fair WR, Logothetis CJ, Balmer C, Robinson RG, Porter AT, Kirk D. The use of strontium 89 for palliation of pain from bone metastases associated with hormone-refractory prostate cancer. *Urology* 1994; 44: 481–5.

[37] Koslowski J, Ellis W, Grayhack J. Advanced prostatic carcinoma early versus late endocrine therapy. *Urologic Clinics of North America* 1991; 18: 15–24.

[38] Nair N. Relative efficacy of 32P and 89Sr in palliation in skeletal metastases. *Journal of Nuclear Medicine: Official Publication, Society of Nuclear Medicine* 1999; 40: 256–61.

[39] Liepe K, Kotzerke J. A comparative study of 188Re-HEDP, 186Re-HEDP, 153Sm-EDTMP and 89Sr in the treatment of painful skeletal metastases. *Nuclear Medicine Communications* 2007; 28: 623–30.

[40] Yuan J, Liu C, Liu X, Wang Y, Kuai D, Zhang G, Zaknun JJ. Efficacy and safety of 177Lu-EDTMP in bone metastatic pain palliation in breast cancer and hormone refractory prostate cancer: a phase II study. *Clinical Nuclear Medicine* 2013; 38: 88–92.

[41] Meckel M, Nauth A, Timpe J, Zhernosekov K, Puranik AD, Baum RP, Rosch F. Development of a [177Lu]BPAMD labeling kit and an automated synthesis module for routine bone targeted endoradiotherapy. *Cancer Biotherapy & Radiopharmaceuticals* 2015; 30: 94–9.

[42] Parker C, Nilsson S, Heinrich D, Helle SI, O'Sullivan JM, Fossa SD, Chodacki A, Wiechno P, Logue J, Seke M, Widmark A, Johannessen DC, Hoskin P, Bottomley D, James ND, Solberg A, Syndikus I, Kliment J, Wedel S, Boehmer S, Dall'Oglio M, Franzen L, Coleman R, Vogelzang NJ, O'Bryan-Tear CG, Staudacher K, Garcia-Vargas J, Shan M, Bruland OS, Sartor O. Alpha emitter radium-223 and survival in metastatic prostate cancer. *The New England Journal of Medicine* 2013; 369: 213–23.

[43] Silberstein EB. The treatment of painful osseous metastases with phosphorus-32-labeled phosphates. *Seminars in Oncology* 1993; 20: 10–21.

[44] Burnet NG, Williams G, Howard N. Phosphorus-32 for intractable bony pain from carcinoma of the prostate. *Clinical Oncology (The Royal College of Radiologists)* 1990; 2: 220–3.

[45] Lewington VJ. Bone-seeking radionuclides for therapy. *Journal of Nuclear Medicine : Official Publication, Society of Nuclear Medicine* 2005; 46 Suppl 1: 38S–47S.

[46] Silberstein EB, Elgazzar AH, Kapilivsky A. Phosphorus-32 radiopharmaceuticals for the treatment of painful osseous metastases. *Seminars in Nuclear Medicine* 1992; 22: 17–27.

[47] Blake GM, Zivanovic MA, Blaquiere RM, Fine DR, McEwan AJ, Ackery DM. Strontium-89 therapy: measurement of absorbed dose to skeletal metastases. *Journal of Nuclear Medicine: Official Publication, Society of Nuclear Medicine* 1988; 29: 549–57.

[48] Blake GM, Zivanovic MA, McEwan AJ, Ackery DM. Sr-89 therapy: strontium kinetics in disseminated carcinoma of the prostate. *European Journal of Nuclear Medicine* 1986; 12: 447–54.

[49] Lewington VJ, McEwan AJ, Ackery DM, Bayly RJ, Keeling DH, Macleod PM, Porter AT, Zivanovic MA. A prospective, randomised double-blind crossover study to examine the efficacy of strontium-89 in pain palliation in patients with advanced prostate cancer metastatic to bone. *European Journal of Cancer* 1991; 27: 954–8.

[50] Laing AH, Ackery DM, Bayly RJ, Buchanan RB, Lewington VJ, McEwan AJ, Macleod PM, Zivanovic MA. Strontium-89 chloride for pain palliation in prostatic skeletal malignancy. *British Journal of Radiology* 1991; 64: 816–22.

[51] Mertens WC, Stitt L, Porter AT. Strontium 89 therapy and relief of pain in patients with prostatic carcinoma metastatic to bone: a dose response relationship? *American Journal of Clinical Oncology* 1993; 16: 238–42.

[52] Mertens WC, Porter AT, Reid RH, Powe JE. Strontium-89 and low-dose infusion cisplatin for patients with hormone refractory prostate carcinoma metastatic to bone: a preliminary report. *Journal of Nuclear Medicine: Official Publication, Society of Nuclear Medicine* 1992; 33: 1437–43.

[53] Buchali K, Correns HJ, Schuerer M, Schnorr D, Lips H, Sydow K. Results of a double blind study of 89-strontium therapy of skeletal metastases of prostatic carcinoma. *European Journal of Nuclear Medicine* 1988; 14: 349–51.

[54] van der Poel HG, Antonini N, Hoefnagel CA, Horenblas S, Valdes Olmos RA. Serum hemoglobin levels predict response to strontium-89 and rhenium-186-HEDP radionuclide treatment for painful osseous metastases in prostate cancer. *Urologia Internationalis* 2006; 77: 50–6.

[55] Quilty PM, Kirk D, Bolger JJ, Dearnaley DP, Lewington VJ, Mason MD, Reed NS, Russell JM, Yardley J. A comparison of the palliative effects of strontium-89 and external beam radiotherapy in metastatic prostate cancer. *Radiotherapy and Oncology: Journal of the European Society for Therapeutic Radiology and Oncology* 1994; 31: 33–40.

[56] Robinson RG, Blake GM, Preston DF, McEwan AJ, Spicer JA, Martin NL, Wegst AV, Ackery DM. Strontium-89: treatment results and kinetics in patients with painful metastatic prostate and breast cancer in bone. *Radiographics: A Review Publication of the Radiological Society of North America, Inc* 1989; 9: 271–81.

[57] Robinson RG, Preston DF, Schiefelbein M, Baxter KG. Strontium 89 therapy for the palliation of pain due to osseous metastases. *JAMA* 1995; 274: 420–4.

[58] Liepe K, Kotzerke J. Internal radiotherapy of painful bone metastases. *Methods* 2011; 55: 258–70.

[59] Tu SM, Millikan RE, Mengistu B, Delpassand ES, Amato RJ, Pagliaro LC, Daliani D, Papandreou CN, Smith TL, Kim J, Podoloff DA, Logothetis CJ. Bone-targeted therapy for advanced androgen-independent carcinoma of the prostate: a randomised phase II trial. *Lancet* 2001; 357: 336–41.

[60] Bilen MA, Johnson MM, Mathew P, Pagliaro LC, Araujo JC, Aparicio A, Corn PG, Tannir NM, Wong FC, Fisch MJ, Logothetis CJ, Tu SM. Randomized phase 2 study of bone-targeted therapy containing strontium-89 in advanced castrate-sensitive prostate cancer. *Cancer* 2015; 121: 69–76.

[61] Akerley W, Butera J, Wehbe T, Noto R, Stein B, Safran H, Cummings F, Sambandam S, Maynard J, Di Rienzo G, Leone L. A multiinstitutional, concurrent chemoradiation trial of strontium-89, estramustine, and vinblastine for hormone refractory prostate carcinoma involving bone. *Cancer* 2002; 94: 1654–60.

[62] Windsor PM. Predictors of response to strontium-89 (Metastron) in skeletal metastases from prostate cancer: report of a single centre's 10-year experience. *Clinical Oncology (Royal College of Radiologists)* 2001; 13: 219–27.

[63] Oosterhof GO, Roberts JT, de Reijke TM, Engelholm SA, Horenblas S, von der Maase H, Neymark N, Debois M, Collette L. Strontium(89) chloride versus palliative local field radiotherapy in patients with hormonal escaped prostate cancer: a phase III study of the European Organisation for Research and Treatment of Cancer, Genitourinary Group. *European Urology* 2003; 44: 519–26.

[64] Dafermou A, Colamussi P, Giganti M, Cittanti C, Bestagno M, Piffanelli A. A multi-centre observational study of radionuclide therapy in patients with painful bone metastases of prostate cancer. *European Journal of Nuclear Medicine* 2001; 28: 788–98.

[65] Porter AT, McEwan AJ, Powe JE, Reid R, McGowan DG, Lukka H, Sathyanarayana JR, Yakemchuk VN, Thomas GM, Erlich LE, et al. Results of a randomized phase-III trial to evaluate the efficacy of strontium-89 adjuvant to local field external beam irradiation

in the management of endocrine resistant metastatic prostate cancer. *International Journal of Radiation Oncology, Biology, Physics* 1993; 25: 805–13.

[66] Zyskowski A, Lamb D, Morum P, Hamilton D, Johnson C. Strontium-89 treatment for prostate cancer bone metastases: does a prostate-specific antigen response predict for improved survival? *Australasian Radiology* 2001; 45: 39–42.

[67] de Klerk JM, Zonnenberg BA, van het Schip AD, van Dijk A, Han SH, Quirijnen JM, Blijham GH, van Rijk PP. Dose escalation study of rhenium-186 hydroxyethylidene diphosphonate in patients with metastatic prostate cancer. *European Journal of Nuclear Medicine* 1994; 21: 1114–20.

[68] de Klerk JM, van het Schip AD, Zonnenberg BA, van Dijk A, Quirijnen JM, Blijham GH, van Rijk PP. Phase 1 study of rhenium-186-HEDP in patients with bone metastases originating from breast cancer. *Journal of Nuclear Medicine: Official Publication, Society of Nuclear Medicine* 1996; 37: 244–9.

[69] Maxon HR, Deutsch EA, Thomas SR, Libson K, Lukes SJ, Williams CC, Ali S. Re-186(Sn) HEDP for treatment of multiple metastatic foci in bone: human biodistribution and dosimetric studies. *Radiology* 1988; 166: 501–7.

[70] Maxon HR, 3rd, Schroder LE, Thomas SR, Hertzberg VS, Deutsch EA, Scher HI, Samaratunga RC, Libson KF, Williams CC, Moulton JS, et al. Re-186(Sn) HEDP for treatment of painful osseous metastases: initial clinical experience in 20 patients with hormone-resistant prostate cancer. *Radiology* 1990; 176: 155–9.

[71] Han SH, de Klerk JM, Tan S, van het Schip AD, Derksen BH, van Dijk A, Kruitwagen CL, Blijham GH, van Rijk PP, Zonnenberg BA. The PLACORHEN study: a double-blind, placebo-controlled, randomized radionuclide study with (186)Re-etidronate in hormone-resistant prostate cancer patients with painful bone metastases. Placebo Controlled Rhenium Study. *Journal of Nuclear Medicine: Official Publication, Society of Nuclear Medicine* 2002; 43: 1150–6.

[72] O'Sullivan JM, McCready VR, Flux G, Norman AR, Buffa FM, Chittenden S, Guy M, Pomeroy K, Cook G, Gadd J, Treleaven J, Al-Deen A, Horwich A, Huddart RA, Dearnaley DP. High activity Rhenium-186 HEDP with autologous peripheral blood stem cell rescue: a phase I study in progressive hormone refractory prostate cancer metastatic to bone. *British Journal of Cancer* 2002; 86: 1715–20.

[73] Palmedo H, Guhlke S, Bender H, Sartor J, Schoeneich G, Risse J, Grunwald F, Knapp FF, Jr., Biersack HJ. Dose escalation study with rhenium-188 hydroxyethylidene diphosphonate in prostate cancer patients with osseous metastases. *European Journal of Nuclear Medicine* 2000; 27: 123–30.

[74] Palmedo H, Manka-Waluch A, Albers P, Schmidt-Wolf IG, Reinhardt M, Ezziddin S, Joe A, Roedel R, Fimmers R, Knapp FF, Jr., Guhlke S, Biersack HJ. Repeated bone-targeted therapy for hormone-refractory prostate carcinoma: tandomized phase II trial with the new, high-energy radiopharmaceutical rhenium-188 hydroxyethylidenedi-

phosphonate. *Journal of Clinical Oncology: Official Journal of the American Society of Clinical Oncology* 2003; 21: 2869–75.

[75] Liepe K, Kropp J, Runge R, Kotzerke J. Therapeutic efficiency of rhenium-188-HEDP in human prostate cancer skeletal metastases. *British Journal of Cancer* 2003; 89: 625–9.

[76] Biersack HJ, Palmedo H, Andris A, Rogenhofer S, Knapp FF, Guhlke S, Ezziddin S, Bucerius J, von Mallek D. Palliation and survival after repeated (188)Re-HEDP therapy of hormone-refractory bone metastases of prostate cancer: a retrospective analysis. *Journal of Nuclear Medicine: Official Publication, Society of Nuclear Medicine* 2011; 52: 1721–6.

[77] Singh A, Holmes RA, Farhangi M, Volkert WA, Williams A, Stringham LM, Ketring AR. Human pharmacokinetics of samarium-153 EDTMP in metastatic cancer. *Journal of Nuclear Medicine: Official Publication, Society of Nuclear Medicine* 1989; 30: 1814–8.

[78] Turner JH, Claringbold PG. A phase II study of treatment of painful multifocal skeletal metastases with single and repeated dose samarium-153 ethylenediaminetetramethylene phosphonate. *European Journal of Cancer* 1991; 27: 1084–6.

[79] Collins C, Eary JF, Donaldson G, Vernon C, Bush NE, Petersdorf S, Livingston RB, Gordon EE, Chapman CR, Appelbaum FR. Samarium-153-EDTMP in bone metastases of hormone refractory prostate carcinoma: a phase I/II trial. *Journal of Nuclear Medicine: Official Publication, Society of Nuclear Medicine* 1993; 34: 1839–44.

[80] Sartor O, Reid RH, Hoskin PJ, Quick DP, Ell PJ, Coleman RE, Kotler JA, Freeman LM, Olivier P. Samarium-153-Lexidronam complex for treatment of painful bone metastases in hormone-refractory prostate cancer. *Urology* 2004; 63: 940–5.

[81] Tian JH, Zhang JM, Hou QT, Oyang QH, Wang JM, Luan ZS, Chuan L, He YJ. Multicentre trial on the efficacy and toxicity of single-dose samarium-153-ethylene diamine tetramethylene phosphonate as a palliative treatment for painful skeletal metastases in China. *European Journal of Nuclear Medicine* 1999; 26: 2–7.

[82] Enrique O, Zhongyun P, Parma EP, Pusuwan P, Riccabona G, Tian J-H, Obaldo J, Padhy AK. Efficacy and toxicity of Sm-153 EDTMP in the palliative treatment of painful bone metastases. *World Journal of Nuclear Medicine* 2002; 1: 21–7.

[83] Dickie GJ, Macfarlane D. Strontium and samarium therapy for bone metastases from prostate carcinoma. *Australasian Radiology* 1999; 43: 476–9.

[84] Liepe K, Runge R, Kotzerke J. The benefit of bone-seeking radiopharmaceuticals in the treatment of metastatic bone pain. *Journal of Cancer Research and Clinical Oncology* 2005; 131: 60–6.

[85] Anderson RM, Stevens DL, Sumption ND, Townsend KM, Goodhead DT, Hill MA. Effect of linear energy transfer (LET) on the complexity of alpha-particle-induced chromosome aberrations in human CD34+ cells. *Radiation Research* 2007; 167: 541–50.

[86] Hafeez S, Parker C. Radium-223 for the treatment of prostate cancer. *Expert Opinion on Investigational Drugs* 2013; 22: 379–87.

[87] Nilsson S, Larsen RH, Fossa SD, Balteskard L, Borch KW, Westlin JE, Salberg G, Bruland OS. First clinical experience with alpha-emitting radium-223 in the treatment of skeletal metastases. *Clinical Cancer Research: An Official Journal of the American Association for Cancer Research* 2005; 11: 4451–9.

[88] Nilsson S, Franzen L, Parker C, Tyrrell C, Blom R, Tennvall J, Lennernas B, Petersson U, Johannessen DC, Sokal M, Pigott K, Yachnin J, Garkavij M, Strang P, Harmenberg J, Bolstad B, Bruland OS. Bone-targeted radium-223 in symptomatic, hormone-refractory prostate cancer: a randomised, multicentre, placebo-controlled phase II study. *The Lancet Oncology* 2007; 8: 587–94.

[89] Parker CC, Pascoe S, Chodacki A, O'Sullivan JM, Germa JR, O'Bryan-Tear CG, Haider T, Hoskin P. A randomized, double-blind, dose-finding, multicenter, phase 2 study of radium chloride (Ra 223) in patients with bone metastases and castration-resistant prostate cancer. *European Urology* 2013; 63: 189–97.

[90] Pacilio M, Ventroni G, De Vincentis G, Cassano B, Pellegrini R, Di Castro E, Frantellizzi V, Follacchio GA, Garkavaya T, Lorenzon L, Ialongo P, Pani R, Mango L. Dosimetry of bone metastases in targeted radionuclide therapy with alpha-emitting (223)Ra-dichloride. *European Journal of Nuclear Medicine and Molecular Imaging* 2016; 43: 21–33.

[91] Etchebehere EC, Milton DR, Araujo JC, Swanston NM, Macapinlac HA, Rohren EM. Factors affecting (223)Ra therapy: clinical experience after 532 cycles from a single institution. *European Journal of Nuclear Medicine and Molecular Imaging* 2016; 43: 8–20.

[92] Nilsson S, Cislo P, Sartor O, Vogelzang NJ, Coleman RE, O'Sullivan JM, Reuning-Scherer J, Shan M, Zhan L, Parker C. Patient-reported quality of life analysis of radium-223 dichloride from the phase 3 ALSYMPCA study. Ann Oncol. 2016 May; 27(5):868-74. doi: 10.1093/annonc/mdw065.

[93] Falkmer U, et al. A systematic overview of radiation therapy effects in skeletal metastases. *Acta Oncology* 2003; 42(5-6): 620–33.

[94] Lewington. Bone-seeking radionuclides for therapy. *Journal of Nuclear Medicine* 2005; 46: 38S–47S.

[95] Bauman G et al. Radiopharmaceuticals for the palliation of painful bone metastasis-a systemic review. *Radiother Oncol* 2005;75(3):258-70.

Chapter 7

Samarium-153 Therapy and Radiation Dose for Prostate Cancer

Yasemin Parlak, Gul Gumuser and Elvan Sayit

Additional information is available at the end of the chapter

http://dx.doi.org/10.5772/64670

Abstract

Prostate cancer (PC) is one of the most frequent malignancies in Western countries. At initial diagnosis, bone metastases are present in 15–30% of cases. These metastases cause some complications including bone fracture, hypercalcemia, and bone pain, which significantly affect patients' quality of life. Radionuclide treatment was created as an alternative to external palliative radiotherapy in the treatment of bone pain arising from bone metastasis of PC. The basic principle of the radionuclide treatment of pain is that the uptake of radioactive material is kept in a high amount that is enough to constitute a proper clinical impact in the tumor, and it is kept at a low dose enough to avoid the occurrence of significant adverse effects in other organs (commonly in the bone marrow). Samarium-153 ethylenediaminetetramethylenephosphonic acid (153Sm-EDTMP) is a radiopharmaceutical compound that has an affinity for skeletal tissue and concentrates in areas of increased bone turnover, localizes in the skeleton, and is excreted via glomerular filtration. Medical staff preparing and administering radiopharmaceuticals in nuclear medicine, whether for diagnostic imaging or for therapeutic application, may receive significant radiation doses to their hands, particularly the fingers. Sm-153 treatment can be used as an effective and safe treatment alternative in the management of metastatic bone pain. Radiation protection of the public and the environment after Sm-153 EDTMP therapy is important.

Keywords: Sm-153 therapy, radiation dose, bone palliation, prostate cancer, radionuclide therapy

1. Introduction

Prostate cancer is one of the most common malignancies worldwide and the third most common cause of death from cancer in men. In advanced prostate cancer, spread of the disease to the skeleton occurs in the majority of patients, with skeletal metastases being predominantly osteoblastic in nature [1, 2]. Bone metastasis is a common sequela of solid malignant tumors such as prostate, breast, lung, and renal cancers, which can lead to various complications, including fractures, hypercalcemia, and bone pain, as well as reduced performance status and quality of life [3]. A multidisciplinary approach is often required not only to differentiate the specific cause of the pain but also for appropriate patient management. Several radiopharmaceuticals for treating painful bone metastases have been developed [3]. Radiation is of proven benefit for pain palliation, and there is growing interest in the therapeutic potential of bone-seeking radiopharmaceuticals [4]. Radionuclide therapy has been proposed as an alternative modality for the management of bone pain. These radiopharmaceuticals localize preferentially in active bone and, mainly, at metastatic lesions, allowing site-directed radiotherapy [1].

The basic principle of the radionuclide treatment of pain is that the uptake of radioactive material is kept in a high amount that is enough to constitute a proper clinical impact in the tumor, and it is kept at a low dose enough to avoid the occurrence of significant adverse effects in other organs (commonly in the bone marrow where more side effects were seen) [5]. One of the most important advantages of the pain treatment with radionuclide agents is the repeatability of the procedure [3]. The radioactive isotopes of P-32 and Sr-39 are the initial radiopharmaceuticals in radionuclide treatment of painful bone metastasis and most recently, Sm-153[4]. Sm-153 EDTMP is an effective treatment of painful bone metastases from different neoplasms. However, there are few studies describing clinical experience with this therapeutic modality. Medical staff preparing and administering radiopharmaceuticals in nuclear medicine, whether for diagnostic imaging or for therapeutic application, may receive significant radiation doses to their hands, particularly to the fingers. People occupationally exposed to radiation must have the relevant technical knowledge and competence, that is, must at least be aware of radiation protection rules and dose-optimized work practices.

The aim of this chapter was to evaluate the efficacy of Sm-153 EDTMP. The objective is to evaluate extremity doses and dose distributions across the hands of the medical staff working in Nuclear Medicine departments.

2. Main text

2.1. Prostate cancer

Prostate cancer is the most commonly diagnosed male malignancy. Prostate cancer is the most prevalent nonskin cancer among men in the United States and is the second leading cause of cancer deaths in men [6].

Prostate-specific membrane antigen (PSMA) is a cell surface protein with a significantly increased expression in prostate cancer cells when compared to other PSMA-expressing tissues such as the small intestine, renal tubular cells, or salivary glands. It therefore provides a promising target for prostate cancer–specific imaging and therapy. Recently, procedures have been developed to label PSMA with 68Ga, 99mTc, and radioiodine for positron emission tomography (PET) or single photon emission computed tomography (SPECT) imaging and therapy [7].

Choline-PET/CT is the most promising whole-body imaging modality in detecting distant metastases of prostate cancer, because of its ability to depict small pathological lymph nodes and bone metastases with a high sensitivity, specificity, and accuracy. This feature is of primary importance on management of patients with prostate cancer and for evaluating their prognosis, thanks to the possibility to assess in a single session both anatomic and metabolic information about the disease [8]. There are several papers about the role of Ch-PET in primary prostate cancer detection and its role in staging prostatic disease before treatment. However, since the Ch uptake can occur in some benignant conditions, such as prostatitis or prostatic hyperplasia, the role of this technique in this field is still not well clear.

The 11C-Ch is characterized by a short half-life (approximately 20.4 min), and for this reason, its use is allowed only in centers provided with a cyclotron. In consideration of the logistical limitations of the use of 11C-Ch, Ch was subsequently labeled with 18F, which, thanks to the increased half-life (109.8 min), allows storage and transport. However, 18F-Ch radiotracer is characterized by an increased urinary excretion compared to 11C-Ch [9].

Bone metastases are the most common and severe complication in patients diagnosed with primary tumors. Skeletal metastases are clinically significant because of associated symptoms, complications such as pathological fracture significance for staging, treatment, and prognosis. It develops in up to 70% of patients diagnosed with prostate cancer and breast cancer. Skeletal-related events can reduce the health-related quality of life secondary to debilitating pain, paralysis, loss of mobility, and hospitalization. Systemic palliative-targeted therapy with suitable radiopharmaceuticals has emerged as a particularly appealing and efficient treatment modality for patients with multiple skeletal metastases [9].

There are essentially three main types of particulate radiations that are of interest for palliative treatment of bone metastasis using radiopharmaceuticals: beta (β^-) particles, alpha (α) particles, and Auger electrons. Traditionally, tumor-targeted radiotherapy has used β^--emitting radionuclides. However, high-energy β^- particles, with a range of several millimeters in tissues, can irradiate cells nearby the targeted tumor. Conversely, α particles (typical penetration range of <100 μm) and Auger electrons (penetration range of several nanometers to micrometers) have shorter penetration ranges and higher linear energy transfer (LET) [9].

In recent years, several reports have been published describing the use of multiple radionuclides in the context of palliative treatment of bone metastases.

2.2. Radionuclide therapy

Pain is the most common symptom in the prostate cancer patients. The incidence and severity of pain in the last period of the life is increasing. Patients and their relatives may adversely be affected from the quality of life as a major fear source. However, pain related to prostate cancer can be treated effectively about 85–90% by applying correct approaches. The remaining 5–15% of patients with pain can be achieved by applying appropriate surgical techniques. The severity and frequency of pain in cancer patients depends on many factors such as age of the patients, the stage of the disease, and the site of bone metastases. For effective pain treatment, accompanying medical and psychosocial problems of the patients should be evaluated, and then, appropriate treatment should be done [10].

In recent years, there has been a much greater emphasis on "radionuclide therapies" that are designed to damage only the cancerous cells. At present, effective targeted radiopharmaceutical therapeutics have been developed. Radionuclide therapy uses ionizing radiation to minimize tumors and kill cancer cells. The basic principles in the treatment of radioactive elements in nuclear medicine, to benefit from the devastating effects generated in the cells. Therefore, many radionuclides have oncological applications of many proven efficacy and safety. Radionuclide therapy uses radioactive isotopes, administered either orally or intravenously, to deliver highly targeted therapy for a range of disorders, enabling the delivery of a high dose to the target, while minimizing normal tissue toxicity [11].

In targeted radionuclide therapy, the biological effect is obtained by energy absorbed from the radiation emitted by the radionuclide. Whereas the radionuclides used for diagnostic nuclear medicine procedures emit gamma rays, which can penetrate highly into the body, the radionuclides used for radionuclide therapy must emit radiation with a comparatively short range. Radionuclides emitted beta particles, alpha particle, and Auger electrons for radionuclide therapy use due to short range and high ionization capability. In some cases, mixed emitters are used to perform both imaging and therapy with the same radionuclide (e.g., Samarium-153) [11].

Various radiopharmaceuticals have been advanced for the treatment of painful bone metastases (**Table 1**). The physical characteristics of these radionuclides are different and have specific benefits. These radionuclides are administered intravenously or orally and localize the painful bone metastases with a high target-to-nontarget tissue ratio and a very low concentration in the normal bone, especially bone marrow. The therapeutic suitability of the radionuclides is important. So the penetration range of the radionuclides is concerned with the energy of the electrons. The applications of the radiopharmaceuticals are easily performed without the need for expensive high-technology equipment. Thus, these agents can be applicable not only in major medical centers but also in minor hospitals, and the workers have to be educated to comply with Nuclear Regulatory Commission requirements. These agents target not only osteoblastic lesions but also lesions containing osteolytic and osteoblastic components. Most of the patients who are treated observed reduce of pain, thus reducing their need for analgesics and improving the quality of life and mobility [3, 4].

The studies regarding metastatic bone pain have particularly focused on the metastases of hormone refractory prostate cancer, which was resistant to the treatment of opioid analgesic. While radiotherapy is more appropriate in the palliative treatment of localized, regional metastatic lesions, this management is less applicable in the treatment of diffuse metastatic lesions. The type of metastatic bone pain is different from other somatic pains, such as visceral, neuropathic, arthritic, and neuropathic pain. While the severity of pain is less intensive initially, it will progress a chronicle process including acute pain episodes with increasing severity subsequently. In this process, the pathophysiology of pain cannot be clearly explained, and various theories have been proposed [12].

Isotopes	T1/2 (days)	Max. energy (MeV)	Gamma-emission, keV (%)	Abundance (%)	Soft-tissue range (mm) (maximum/minimum)
P-32	14.3	1.7			8/3
Sr-89	50.5	1.4			2.4
Re-186	3.7	1.07	137	9	2.4
Re-188	16.9	2.1	155		3
Sm-153	1.9	0.81	103	29	0.6

Table 1. Physical properties of therapy isotopes for bone pain palliation.

A study reported that the maximal pain response to the treatment occurred at 4–6 weeks after the treatment [13]. In another study, Silberstein [14] declared that the complete or partial response to 153Sm treatment was obtained in 62–74% of patients, and this response was commonly seen 5–10 days after the treatment.

The study investigated the efficacy of 153Sm treatment; complete response rate was found 12.4% and the partial response rate was found 73.4%.

Gul et al. determine the reduction in the analgesic consumption and improvement in the performance and mobility score of the patients (10).

Alleviating of pain can occurred about within 2–7 days depending on the agent after the first injection. The repeating injections should be performed as soon as possible after the occurrence of pain recurrence, if bone marrow reserve is adequate. The clinical usage of radionuclides is not only limited to the opioid resistant pain. As the result of some trials, it was obviously clear that the expected long-term efficacy and tolerance could be achieved without requirement of opioid analgesics. The primary goal of the treatment is to provide better quality of life in daily activities by minimal drug usage [3].

2.2.1. *Therapy radionuclides for bone pain palliation*

In the past few years, several radiopharmaceuticals have been improved with bone-seeking properties that provide palliation of pain to multiple bone metastasis. The most of these are beta electrons, depositing highly their energy over up to millimeters in the surrounding tissues. A few of the therapeutic radionuclides emit small amounts of gamma-radiation, allowing for a scintigraphic imaging. The commonly used radiopharmaceutical for pain palliation is samarium-153 HEDP. Hematopoietic suppression is the major side effect of radionuclide therapies, with leukopenia and thrombocytopenia more likely to be clinically significant than anemia. The physical properties of radiopharmaceuticals are discussed in detail in the following sections.

2.2.2. *Phosphorus-32*

Phosphorus-32 is pure beta-emitting radionuclide with a physical half-life of 14.3 days. The average beta particle energy is 695 keV. The mean and maximum particle ranges in tissue of phosphorus are 3 and 8 mm, respectively. P-32 is used orthophosphate compound as palliative treatment purposes. Approximately 85% of the total phosphate pool is located in the skeleton bound as inorganic phosphate to the hydroxyapatite matrix. From five to ten percentage of administered activity is excreted via the kidneys within the first 24 h. Total bone doses in the range 0.4–1.7 cGy/MBq have been reported [4, 15].

2.2.3. *Strontium-89*

Strontium-89 is a pure beta-emitter with a beta particle energy of 1.46 MeV and a physical half-life of 50.5 days [15]. It localizes in bone primarily in areas of osteoblastic activity. It is an mean particle range in tissue of 2.4 mm. The fix dose is 148 MBq (4 mCi). The radiation dose of metastatic foci is about 1000–5000 cGy. Bone marrow radiation dose is approximately ten percent of metastatic foci. 89Sr can be effective at relieve pain from bone metastases, particularly for metastatic prostate or breast cancer [4].

2.2.4. *Rhenium-186*

Rhenium-186 is a beta- and gamma-emitting radionuclide. The maximum beta particle energy is 1.07 MeV. Re-186 has a 137 keV, 9% abundance gamma-photon with a physical half-life of 89.3 h. It is forms a stable diphosphonate chelate with hydroxyethylidene diphosphonate (HEDP). Rhenium-186 HEDP has rapid urinary excretion. It is excreted about 70% of dose within 6 h in the urine [4].

2.2.5. *Sn-117m*

Sn-117m is gamma-emitting radionuclide with 159 keV. Physical half-life of Sn-117m is 13.6 days. It is decays by short-range conversion electrons. Bone marrow toxicity of this radionuclide is low because of its short range. Therefore, Sn-117m can be used to treat bone tumors and rheumatoid arthritis [16].

2.2.6. *Samarium-153*

Samarium-153 is a reactor which produced high radionuclidic purity by neutron bombardment of enriched 152Sm oxide [3]. Samarium-153 is a beta-emitter with a short half-life (46.7 h), which also emits gamma-photons suitable for imaging at 103 keV. Samarium-153 principal radiation emission data are shown in **Table 2**. The isotope is chelated to ethylene diamine tetramethylene phosphonate (EDTMP), which targets the bone matrix as a polyphosphonate (**Figures 1** and **2**). The therapeutic doses administered to patients about 50% settle in the bone excretion are through the kidneys. The proportion of skeletal uptake is the highest for the bone-seeking radiopharmaceuticals. The effective range of 153Sm is 2–3 mm in bone [1]. 153Sm-EDTMP is indicated for the relief of pain in patients with osteoblastic metastatic bone lesions at a standard dose of 37 MBq/kg to a maximum of 5550 MBq [1, 2]. Clinical benefit is reported by 60–80% of patients within 2 weeks of administration, frequently within 48 h, with a response duration of 4–40 weeks [4].

Radiation	Energy (keV)	Abundance (%)
Beta	640	30
Beta	710	50
Beta	810	20
Gamma	103	29

*Maximum energies are listed for beta emissions, and the average beta particle energy is 233 keV

Table 2. Samarium-153 principal radiation emission data.

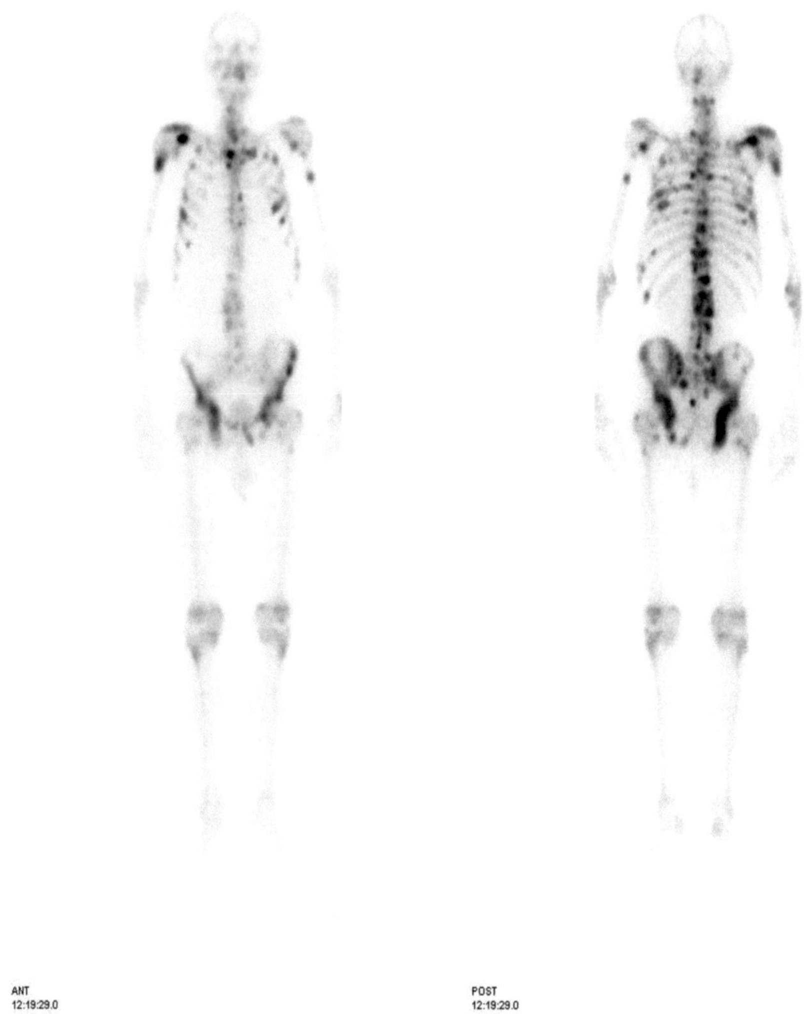

Figure 1. A bone scintigraphy that was obtained before the 153Sm-EDTMP treatment.

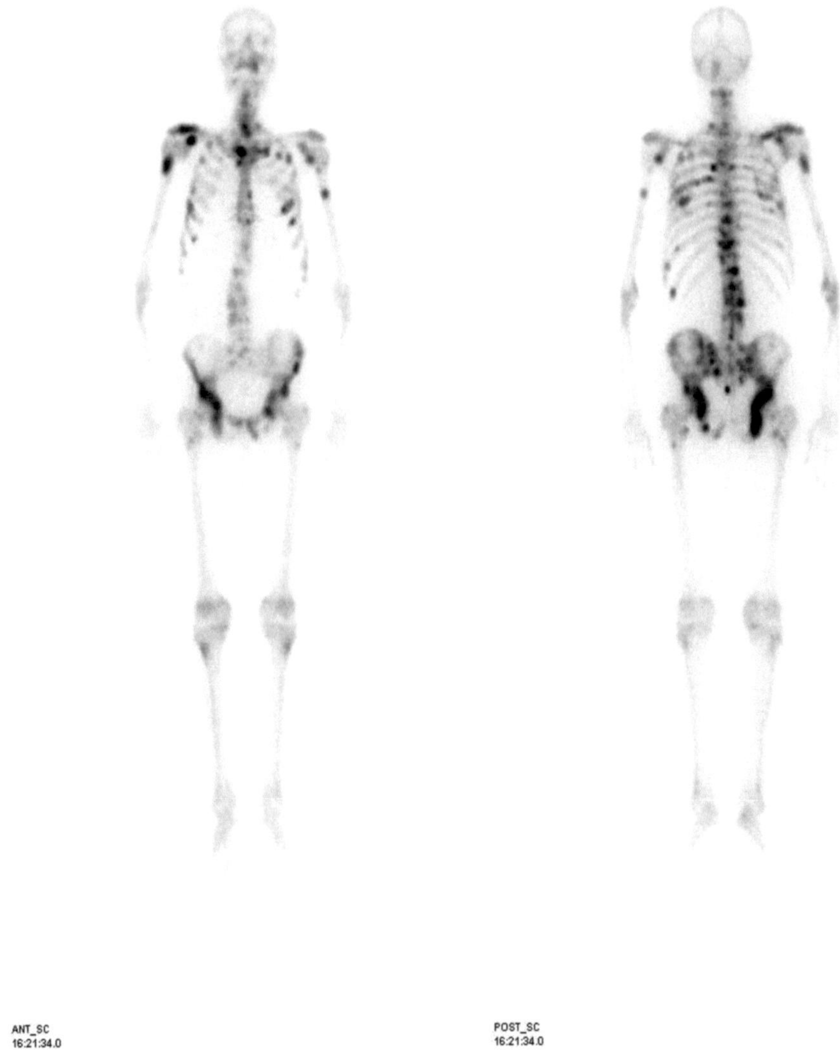

Figure 2. A bone scintigraphy that was obtained after the 153Sm-EDTMP treatment.

This treatment can be repeated several times to the patients. Repeat dosing with 153Sm is both safe and effective. The studied reports showed that the patients with symptomatic bone metastases receiving multiple doses of 153Sm have no significant differences in pain reduction or in myelosuppression after a second or third treatment [17].

Pregnancy, lactation, acute spinal cord compression, single metastatic lesion, renal failure, the long bone that holds more than 50% of the affected bone metastases, risk of fracture and in the presence of disseminated intravascular coagulation are the contraindications of pain palliation with 153Sm therapy.

2.2.7. Radiation dose

The diagnostic and therapeutic procedures have been continuously increasing in most of the nuclear medicine facilities. The risk of radiation exposure of staff is of importance due to increasing procedures. The radiation sources of nuclear medicine Departments are preparing and administering of the radiopharmaceuticals. The workers may receive significant radiation dose to their whole body, especially to the hands.

Therapeutic nuclear medicine requires special consideration due to the high doses of radiation. Therapeutic radionuclides have usually beta electrons. Owing to 153Sm-EDTMP's intermediate beta-energy and low tissue penetration, the bone marrow, for the most part, is spared throughout the skeleton. For protection, two radiation safety consideration needs to be paid attention. One of them, external radiation dose of 153Sm, the interaction of high-energy beta particles with high atomic number materials (e.g., lead) will lead to the production of high-energy X-rays (Bremsstrahlung). Parlak et al. reported that external radiation dose of 153Sm is high for the first 8 h (**Figure 3**). They suggest that hospitalizing the patients treated with Sm-153 therapy in an isolated room for 8 h would be helpful for radiation protection of the public. On the other hand, radiation safety consideration is the contamination by excretion of the 153Sm. The variability of isolation times indicates a strong dependency of effective half-life on biological excretion and shows no relationship with administered activity. Certainly, this variability reveals the need to determine these parameters for each patient [1].

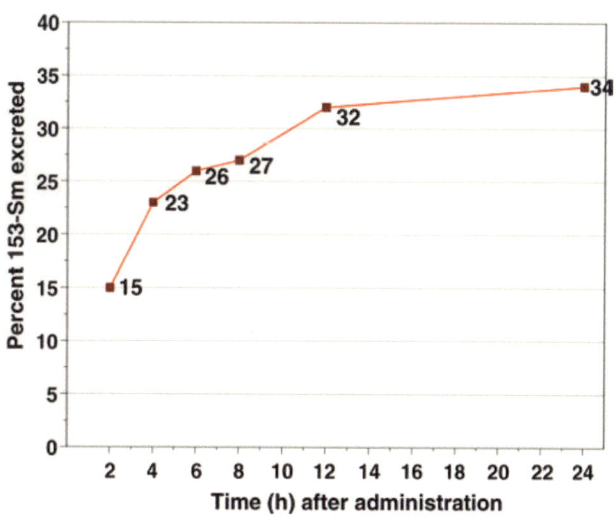

Figure 3. Excretion of 153Sm-EDTMP through the urinary tract in the first 24 h.

Developments in nuclear medicine show that applications involving beta-emitters will probably increase further. Data on the beta-radiation dose equivalents for the staff performing such treatments are limited. For this reason, additional measures should be provided for the training and continuing education of the staff in order to avoid any further increase in extremity doses.

Author details

Yasemin Parlak*, Gul Gumuser and Elvan Sayit

*Address all correspondence to: yasemin.gultekin@hotmail.com

Department of Nuclear Medicine, Medical School, Celal Bayar University, Manisa, Turkey

References

[1] Parlak Y, Gumuser G, Sayit E, Samarium-153 therapy for prostate cancer: the evaluation of urine activity, staff exposure and dose rate from patients. Radiat Prot Dosimetry 2015;163(4):468–472. doi: 10.1093/rpd/ncu237. Epub 2014 Jul 25

[2] Damber JE, Aus G. Prostate cancer. Lancet 2008;371:1710–1721

[3] Serafini AN. Therapy of metastatic bone pain. J Nucl Med 2001;42(6):895–906

[4] Lewington VJ. Cancer therapy using bone-seeking isotopes. Phys Med Biol 1996;41:2027–2042

[5] Sahin M, Basoglu T, Bernay I. Radyonuklid Palyatif Agri Tedavisi. On Dokuz Mayis Universitesi Tip Dergisi 1989;15:263–269

[6] Hanchette CL ,Schwartz GG. Geographic patterns of prostate cancer mortality. Evidence for a protective effect of ultraviolet radiation. Cancer. 1992;70(12):2861–2869.

[7] Afshar-Oromieh A, Zechmann CM, Malcher A, Eder M, Eisenhut M, Linhart HG, Holland-Letz T, Hadaschik BA, Giesel FL, Debus J, Haberkorn U. Comparison of PET imaging with a 68Ga-labelled PSMA ligand and 18F-choline-based PET/CT for the diagnosis of recurrent prostate cancer. Eur J Nucl Med Mol Imaging 2014;41:11–20

[8] Valeria Panebianco, Flavio Barchetti, Daniela Musio, Francesca De Felice, Camilla Proietti, Elena Lucia Indino, Valentina Megna, Orazio Schillaci, Carlo Catalano, and Vincenzo Tombolini. Advanced imaging for the early diagnosis of local recurrence prostate cancer after radical prostatectomy. BioMed Res Int, 2014;2014;12, Article ID 827265

[9] Guerra Liberal FDC, Tavares AAS, João Manuel RS. Tavares N. Palliative treatment of metastatic bone pain with radiopharmaceuticals: a perspective beyond Strontium-89 and Samarium-153. Appl Radiat Isot 2016;110:87–99

[10] Gul SS, Sonmez O, Deveci EK, Ilce HT, Ergonenc JS. Quantitative assessment of radionuclide pain palliation: case report. Türk Onkoloji Dergisi 2013;28(2):75–80

[11] Coronado M, Redondo A, Coya J, Espinosa E, Couto RM, Zamora P, Marin MD, Castelo B, Lillo ME, Frutos L, Barón MG, and Curto LM. Clinical role of Sm-153 EDTMP in the

http://dx.doi.org/10.5772/64670

treatment of painful bone metastatic disease. Clinical Nuclear Medicine 2006;31:605–610

[12] Clines GA, Guise TA. Molecular mechanisms and treatment of bone metastasis. Expert Rev Mol Med 2008;10:e7

[13] Deng H et al. Radiopharmaceutical (Sm-153-EDTMP) therapy of skeletal metastases: clinical application in 350 patients. J Radiol 2002 P:1637-1644, Volume:44

[14] Silberstein EB. Systemic radiopharmaceutical therapy of painful osteoblastic metastases. Semin Radiat Oncol. 2000;10(3):240–249

[15] Pandit-Taskar N, Batraki M, Divgi CR. Radiopharmaceutical therapy for palliation of bone pain from osseous metastases. J Nucl Med 2004;45:1358–1365

[16] Williams JE. New research developments increase therapeutic options for thyroid cancer and bone pain palliation. J Nucl Med 1997;38:19–20

[17] Tomblyn M. The role of bone-seeking radionuclides in the palliative treatment of patients with painful osteoblastic skeletal metastases. Cancer Control 2012;19(2):137–144

Chapter 8

Redefining Androgen Receptor Function: Clinical Implications in Understanding Prostate Cancer Progression and Therapeutic Resistance

Miltiadis Paliouras, Carlos Alvarado and Mark Trifiro

Additional information is available at the end of the chapter

http://dx.doi.org/10.5772/64392

Abstract

The current description of the function of the human androgen receptor (AR), as a transcription factor directing androgen responsive gene expression, is limited in scope and thus is unable to account for the varied cellular and physiological transformation observed in the development and progression of prostate cancer (CaP). The chapter will focus on four important aspects of AR and CaP investigations: (1) a description of AR somatic mutations and the perils of AR-directed therapeutics; (2) our characterization of AR protein interactors that have imbued new functional properties for AR linked to prostatic disease; (3) review of the advances made and shortcomings of AR mouse models in describing CaP onset and progression; and (4) speculate as to the mechanisms by which new mutations can originate and initiate disease onset.

Keywords: androgen receptor, prostate cancer, somatic mutations, interactome, mouse models, gain-of-function properties, therapeutic resistance, mutational landscape

1. Introduction

Advanced DNA sequencing technology and the information garnered from it has ushered a new era especially poignant to the genetics of cancer. In present and next-generation sequencing methodologies in conjunction with the establishment of consortiums (COSMIC: and TCGA: http://cancer.sanger.ac.uk/cosmic and TCGA: tcga-data.nci.nih.gov/tcga), whose major efforts are to characterize the cancer genome of a large number of cancers in a systematic fashion, modern cancer genetics has come to the forefront. These "mutational landscapes" have redefined cancer genetics and will dramatically direct cancer research for decades to come [1–10].

Modern cancer genetics has now unequivocally demonstrated extensive somatic DNA alterations many times more than previously envisioned [11–14]. Although dependent on specific tumor types, somatic mutations are in the order of tens of thousands; the present-day technology most likely underestimates the true number of mutations as mutations occurring in less than 10–15% of cells cannot be detected. Advances in single-cell DNA analysis now suggest that indeed many more mutations do exist at in smaller number of cells [15, 16]. More importantly, there is an advanced degree of intertumoral heterogeneity where the same tumor types in different patients share only a few DNA alterations [17, 18]. As well intratumoral heterogeneity is extensive, where in the same individual's tumor, there are many different DNA alterations in specific subpopulation of cells. Also, the DNA sequence defined for a specific tumor is a composite sequence, where an amalgamation of small "bits" of DNA sequence, whose origins are from many different cells, is aligned to generate the "tumor" DNA genome; where in reality, no individual tumor cell most likely has that defined sequence.

Cataloging sequence alterations are the mainstay on present-day consortiums, important in defining tumor heterogeneity and also to help understand what potential effects these alterations may have on neoplastic initiation and evolution. Many mutations evoke specific gain of function properties implying driver capabilities [19]. The true understanding of these mutations is an extremely daunting task; defining these new gain-of-function properties is presently done in the context of the somatically mutated protein in question without any of the mutations of other proteins present; to truly account for real gain of function properties would require the presence of all mutations. The possible permutations and combinations of tens-of-thousands mutations on many proteins and the outcome on cellular physiology are incomprehensible even more so when cell-to-cell functionality is implied.

Nonetheless, the establishment of mutational landscape databases with defining characteristics, in conjunction with the required systems biology and network analysis, has led to many insights in tumor dynamics. What has been lacking in cancer fundamentals are investigations addressing the origins of these vastly accrued DNA alterations.

Cancer hallmarks defined by Hanahan and Weinberg have more or less been universally agreed upon and now include "enabling hallmarks," those hallmarks that are not descriptive in nature but imply distinct contributions to neoplastic development [20]. One of these enabling hallmarks is referred to as genomic instability. A more apt description would be the connotation of mutator phenotype, originally described by Lawrence Loeb [21–23]. Briefly, the mutator phenotype is a trait shared by all cancer cells that endow cancer cells with the ability to create or enhance new and constant DNA alterations. This hallmark gives neoplastic cells, a constant source of new mutations allowing the genetic background to become widely disparate. Such cellular genetic diversity in turn allows for extreme selection processes to dictate tumoral evolution; selection processes are multiple: microenvironment on tumor cells, tumor cells on the microenvironment, and tumor cells on other tumor cells.

http://dx.doi.org/10.5772/64392

The origins of tumor DNA alterations are indeed critical. Therefore, it is hard to imagine that a tumor and tumor evolution can exist without any DNA alterations. Mutational load directly impacts tumor aggressiveness and metastatic potential. Understanding the origins of somatic DNA alterations is now fundamental to the understanding of tumor initiation and evolution, and the extent of DNA alterations is most likely more critical than the actual single definition and characterization of specific DNA alterations given the tremendous heterogeneity that exists.

2. Somatic mutations and prostate cancer

Prostate cancer (CaP) in many ways is unique. It is extremely common; as much as 50% of men will have CaP above the age of 55 and increases in incidence afterwards [24]. It is for the most part slow growing and only in a small percentage can develop advanced and life-threatening disease but still represents a significant number of individuals. However, due to the high incidence rates for CaP and the highly variable and unpredictable effects on morbidity and mortality, CaP is extremely vulnerable to over diagnosis (as aided by screening advocates) and thus overtreatment [25, 26]. Treatment regimens have been extremely controversial with the no clear benefits of endocrine manipulation in early disease; most likely, the era of anti-androgens or androgen deprivation therapy (ADT) in early disease will not be adhered to, the treatment of which may have provoked more aggressive disease and linked to selecting out very worrisome gain-of-function androgen receptor (AR) mutations [27–29]. Surgical prostatectomy remains the only curative procedure if the disease was localized to the prostate at the time of surgery.

CaP is universally multifocal and is uniformly associated with hypertrophy or hyperplasia. Its pathological scoring (Gleason) is based on the fact that multiple lesions coexist and, by itself, is solely used to assess overall staging [30]. Multifocal cancers are typically genetic in nature, associated with DNA repair deficiencies and somatic loss of heterozygosity. The best example of endocrine genetic cancers is MEN2 syndrome that has been now well studied in all age groups and dramatically displays the hypertrophy to hyperplasia to frank carcinoma evolution [31]. There is no obvious related gene candidate in multifocal CaP.

2.1. Androgen receptor

The X-linked AR protein is a member of the nuclear receptor superfamily [32, 33]. It is a ligand-inducible protein containing a polymorphic N-terminal region, a central DNA-binding domain (DBD), and a C-terminal ligand-binding domain (LBD) [34–36]. Although the AR gene is classically not associated with direct DNA maintenance, it is a single allele (loss of heterozygosity is not a prerequisite) and remains the most prominent candidate directing CaP initiation and evolutions. Hypogonadal individuals with low levels of 17C steroids or with elements of androgen receptor (AR) deficiency, CaP, are extremely rare. Most if not all molecular endocrinological studies of CaP implement the AR g as being a pivotal player in CaP. In all CaP, AR is highly mutated (androgendb.mcgill.ca) [37–42]. The most recent CaP mutational landscape is very comprehensive and is the new reference for mutational analysis of genes in both initial disease and more advanced disease [39]. In this study, AR remains the most consistent altered gene and is the earliest gene to be altered in localized diseases: AR gene amplifications is then followed by AR splice variants and AR missense mutations, but these alterations are hard pressed to explain multifocality. Other somatic mutations found include AR-associated proteins (ETS fusions, FOXA1, ZBTB16, NCOR1, NCOR2); PIK3 pathway PIK3CA, (PIK3CB, PIK3R1, AKT1); DNA repair (APC, BRCA2); and WNT signaling (RNF43); Cell cycle (RB1) [39].

2.2. AR and the CAG polymorphic tract

The AR gene has an extremely rare attribute. A polymorphic pure uninterrupted CAG tract in exon 1 is present coding for a polyglutamine tract in the N-terminus of the AR. This tract varies in length in individuals (n = 12–31), and tract length also varies racially [43–49]. This tract also has small but very important effect on AR functionality: smaller length polyglutamine tract ARs have more transcriptionally prowess [50]. The fundamental explanation for the presence of the AR polyglutamine tract within the AR protein itself is not known.

AR CAG tracts are unique to primates and are uninterrupted in almost all species (the exception being mice). It is interesting that humans vs. other primates have the longest tract and thus are the most unstable.

AR CAG tracts are unique to mammals and are uninterrupted in almost all species (the exception being mice) [34, 51]. Another trait related to all trinucleotide repeats is their inherent inability to remain stable; thus, AR CAG tract lengths are known to change in length somatically in various tissues including primary gonadal tissue [52, 53]. It is interesting that humans vs. other primates have the longest tract and thus are the most unstable. The instability exists at two levels: at cell division with DNA replication and more importantly with AR transcription by the transcription excision repair machinery. Instability is usually biased toward expansion rather than contraction (2:1).

In a study of CaP and AR CAG tract instability, AR CAG tract instability existed in normal tissue to a certain degree but was very much enhanced in adjacent CaP tissue [52, 54]. The CAG tract lengths varied from one foci of CaP to another foci of CaP in the same patient. The instability of the AR CAG tract is many orders of magnitude more than stable random DNA sequence and approaches error rates seen in DNA repair deficiency states. It thus remains a solid candidate for the gene that accounts for the multifocality of CaP. In brief, those cells that undergo the largest AR CAG tract contraction are the most active AR. These cells in turn through overactive AR pathways will provoke new DNA alterations and thus are ordained as a mutator phenotype.

2.3. AR somatic mutations

It has clear involvement in distinct diseases due to due well-characterized inherited loss-of-function or somatic acquired gain-of-function mutations. The one same protein with diverse-heterogeneous mutations, each with clear phenotypes, offers unique complementary structure-functional studies. Exploiting the AR mutational properties found in individuals with androgen resistance syndromes (loss-of-function AR) or CaP (gain-of-function AR), in conjunction with receptor kinetic studies, molecular biology, advanced dynamic structural modeling, and proteomic-coupled network analyses studies, has described many fundamental and new processes to account for disease processes [55–59].

Given the central role that AR has in prostate biology, it is not unexpected that somatic *AR* mutations may be selected for, adding to the CaP repertoire powerful new functions provoking neoplastic advancement [52, 54, 60, 61] (**Figure 1**). Recent studies in support of initial studies have again demonstrated that although most advanced prostatic cancers are uniformly androgen independent, the AR is still a very important contributor to the more progressive fatal disorder [62, 63]. Nearly, all "androgen-independent" or "castrate-resistant" prostatic tumors express high levels of AR, and levels are predictive of progressive disease [64, 65]. Indeed, as many as one-third of tumors exhibit AR gene amplification [66] and AR somatic prostate missense mutations and splice variants are well documented [38, 67, 68]. A number of somatic CaP AR (e.g., T877A) mutants have unique gain-of-function properties; they can bind several classes of steroids promiscuously with subsequent transactivation, be hyperactivated by normal ligands [69, 70] or be constitutively active without ligand [71]. Even more surprising is that anti-androgen treatments [e.g., flutamide, cyproterone acetate (CPA) or bicalutamide, and even the latest generation of anti-androgens (enzalutamide)] have selected out specific somatic AR gene (*AR*) mutations [72–75]. Missense mutations also have other related gain of functions beyond their relaxed ligand-binding parameters; normally ligand-binding promotes a dramatic conformation change inducing helix 12 movement creating a new co-activator interacting site. In T877A, helix 12 is slightly misplaced and alters the co-activator binding where co-activator binding motifs preferences are changed. As well another gain of function property is manipulated that is AR N-C-terminal interactions are favored.

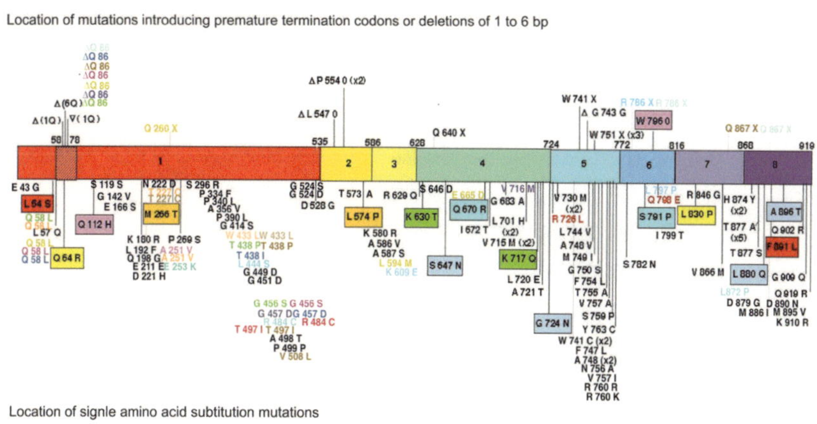

Figure 1. Schematic illustration of cataloged AR Somatic Mutations from the androgen receptor database. Mutations illustrated with the same color were present in the same cancer specimen. Mutations in red were found in the germline (image is courtesy of http://www.androgenbd.mcgill.ca">www.androgenbd.mcgill.ca, with permission from Dr. Mark Trifiro) [37].

Thus, any somatic mutated AR most likely will inherit multiple new functions, which can affect the whole AR complex itself.

In advanced CaP, new AR variants have been found (**Figure 2**). AR-V7 and ARv567es splice variants have an intact NTD and DBD. The AR-V7 splice variant excludes exon 4 through 8, resulting in a deletion of the LBD and the hinge regions, whereas ARv567es excludes exons 5 through 7 creating a LBD deletion; thus, these variants display "constitutive" ligand-independent transcriptional activity. It has been observed for many years that steroid receptor C-terminal truncated variants have constitutive activity; thus, in full-length steroid receptors, the presence of the C-terminal domains acts as a functional repressor whereupon ligand binding alleviates C-terminal repression.

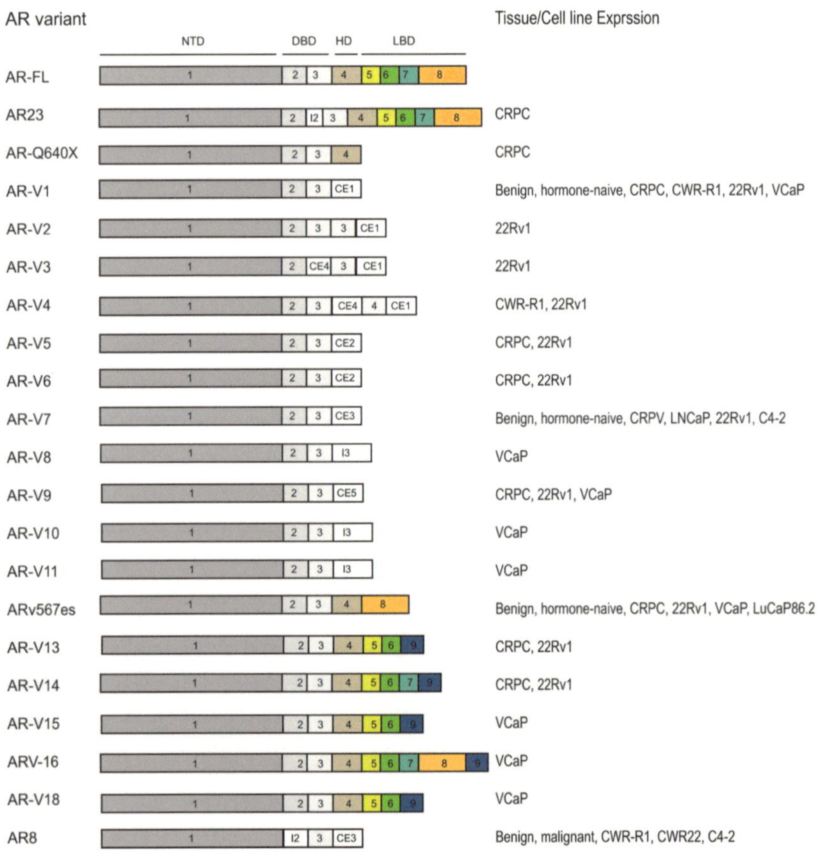

Figure 2. Schematic illustration of AR truncated and splice variants.

The repressive AR splice variants differ significantly from full-length AR in their transcriptional programs and subcellular localization [76, 77], implying different potential functions from wild-type AR (AR-WT). In an analysis of 46 castration-resistant prostate cancers (CRPCs), 80% expressed full-length AR, 73% expressed ARv567es and AR-V7; furthermore, 20% of metastatic cases expressed ARv567es solely [78]. Western blot analysis appears to reveal that AR splice variants are also expressed in a number of different prostatic cancer cell lines [79]; however, it is not quite clear whether these variants are actually active or possess any of the attributed "constitutive" activity. Attention has also been given to the molecular mechanism by which these splice variants may arise. One hypothesis asserts that genomic rearrangements is one mechanism [80, 81], which maybe a valid means for established and immortalized cells lines, but more difficult to account for in a progressive disorder. Such a precise process for DNA deletion/rearrangement to independently and exactly occur so many times to result in the expression of these variants is very unlikely. Most recently, a more valid mechanism has been put forward that involved the overexpression of specific RNA splicing factors, U2AF65 and ASF/SF2, influenced the expression of AR-V7 splice variant in CaP cell lines [82]. Alternative RNA splicing has been shown to change during disease progression, and thus, the expression of specific RNA splicing factors during different stages of disease could more adequately account for the both frequency and temporal incidences of these AR variants. Alternative RNA splicing can also be considered another degree of added genetic heterogeneity to evolving neoplasias [83–86].

These gain of functions can extend to other facets of AR activity, namely the ability to attract different interactors or interplay with other pathways and possibly target different genes; these diverse gain-of-function attributes are likely to be manifested by a changed constitution of mutant AR complexes, which may well be cell and ligand specific and lend to the molecular pathological processes. Thus, cumulative analysis still supports the AR as a pivotal role player in prostate cell tumor biology, as it plays a fundamental and decisive role in prostate cell biology including very important prostate cell metabolism; what is left to be assessed is what aspect of wt or mutant AR functionality promotes directly or indirectly the mutator phenotype.

3. AR protein complexes: contributors to CaP progression

Somatic gain-of-function mutations allow neoplastic cells to acquire new properties that can aid the cancerous cells in finding new avenues for progression to more advanced disease. A multitude of AR gain-of-function attributes are likely to exist and most probably reflected in the composition of the AR interactome. As such, many proteins have been identified that interact with the AR and collaborate with it to execute its transcriptional program [87–89]. These observations suggest that the interplay between the AR, its associated interactors, and specific transcription factors can be selective and very dynamic [37, 58, 59, 87, 89]. All together, these findings also point to the complexity of the AR-interacting protein unit, suggesting that many functions of the AR are beyond our current understanding. Furthermore, the great functional diversity of the components of AR complexes exemplifies the intricate nature of protein–protein interactions associated with generating the appropriate AR biological output, and that mutant CaP ARs may have a their own unique ability to define new interactions. Therefore, the functional effect of AR needs to be investigated and show that certain AR properties, through protein–protein interactions can confer a growth advantage to cells. To do so, one would need to take into consideration a number of factors: (1) mutational status of the protein; (2) ligand status; (3) an amendable technology to assess protein–protein interactions; and (4) an encompassing process by which to analyze the data that would provide information on ontological function and most importantly clinical relevancy.

3.1. AR protein isolation methodology

To date, several techniques have been employed to isolate AR protein complexes including two-hybrid screens and GST pull-downs; however, several limitations have been an obstacle to isolating complexes in their natural cellular environment. First, previous approaches have either used yeast or bacterial systems [90–92]. One shortcoming of these systems is that full-length AR cannot be expressed; therefore, only N- or C-terminal portions or specific AR domains have only been used. Second, within these systems, the use of a truncated AR, folding, and post-translationally modifications issues arise. Finally, the single most critical aspect of charactering any protein complex, for AR maintaining ligand binding, to the receptor during the isolation process, ensures an "active" complex is isolated. Therefore, our laboratory has developed a mammalian tissue cell culture expression and purification system that retains the ability of AR to maintain its ligand-binding activity [93, 94]. The purification method employed by the following methodology ensures up to 90% of labeled-androgen ligand is still bound to the AR following fractionation. We therefore have the ability to capture both cytoplasmic and nuclear ARs under physiological conditions, with excellent recovery, that demonstrate measurable hormone binding even in *in vitro* conditions. We then have undertaken the process of purifying a number of AR complexes: (1) 0CAG-AR, T877A-AR, WT-AR, in the presence or absence of the synthetic androgen mibolerone (MB) [59]; (2) T877A-AR, in the presence of a panel of hormone ligands (DHT, MB, testosterone, R1881, estradiol, dexamethasone, progesterone, and cyproterone acetate) [58]; (3) AR-V7 and ARv567es (Paliouras and Trifiro, unpublished data). We have been able to confirm the purification of our complexes by assessing known AR interactors [59]. However, to truly define the spectrum of proteins in the AR complexes, a more robust methodology and platform was needed, and as such, mass spectrometry approach was employed. Data generated by mass spectrometry were then analyzed using a sophisticated network analysis methodology.

3.2. Proteomic-coupled network analysis

Our ability to capture both liganded and unliganded AR complexes by affinity chromatography under physiological conditions allowed us to pursue a proteomics approach to characterize the components of AR complexes. This can be done by subjecting such complexes to tryptic digestion followed by MS to assign protein identification [95–97]. To our MS data, a label-free quantitative method was also applied for the comparison of peptide abundance across the different experimental paradigms [98, 99].

Therefore, to highlight potentially novel gain-of-function properties associated with mutant CaP ARs, comparative proteomic characterization studies of AR complexes were done in different experimental backgrounds. To do so, we performed network analysis on individual AR-interacting protein lists derived from our proteomic studies and pursued comparative studies to analyze changes in protein composition based on stimulation condition. We have compiled a human protein interaction data from diverse data resources and annotation databases, such as Biomolecular Interaction Network Database (BIND) [100], the Database of Interacting Proteins (DIP) [101], Human Protein Reference Database (HPRD) [102], IntAct [103], and Molecular INTeraction database (MINT) [104], most of which contain curated interaction data and high-throughput data, consisting of 4000 proteins and 22,000 signaling relations/protein interactions.

Quantitative MS data, between stimulation conditions, were used to discern protein abundances. These values were then incorporated into the protein interaction network mapping, to represent a "strength of interaction" coefficient. Between the different experimental conditions, a comparative network analysis was applied [105–108], which was different between our stimulation-specific networks, that is, hierarchical clustering. Immediately what was clear that specific AR protein complexes can be distinguished by the presence or absence of androgen [59]. Analysis of the T877A-AR promiscuous mutant, under different hormone stimulations, showed that although each hormone is able to induce androgen-dependent gene activation [e.g., prostate-specific antigen (PSA)], the proteome profile of each hormone is different. Moreover, although four different androgens were used (DHT, testosterone, MB, and R1881), the proteomic profiles of these androgen ligands do not segregate together. In our hierarchical clustering, we observed that progesterone and dexamethasone AR complexes have proteomic profiles that look like R1881 and MB, respectively [58]. Most recently, analysis of ARv567es protein interactome is very different from androgen stimulated full-length AR (unpublished data), even though ARv567es variant has been characterized as a "constitutively" active receptor [76, 77].

From the each AR variant protein interaction network, specific network modules (a set of interacting proteins constituting a subnetwork) are delineated by number of linked interacting proteins interactions and ontological function. The association of subnetwork modules based on biological processes may suggest pathways involved in either tumorigenesis or tumor metastasis. Therefore, to establish statistically significant biological functions, we also implemented the incorporation of Gene Ontological (GO) terms onto each protein the network. We extracted subnetworks in which GO-term-mapped-nodes were directly linked and highlighted subnetworks and pathways to identify gene enrichment of the proteins/genes from a set of clinical prostatic microarray datasets (http://www.ncbi.nlm.nih.gov/geo/) [109, 110] and RNA sequencing (https://tcga-data.nci.nih.gov/tcga/) [8, 111]. Results show that expression levels of the interacting partners/GO-terms were able to discern normal vs. cancer and correlated with patient survival. More intriguing, different AR protein interaction clusters could differentiate prostatic disease between White (non-Hispanic) vs. African-American males [58]. Nor could we find a gene set that was shared between the two diverse and genetically distinct groups of men. This would suggest that there are AR functional classes that can be used to predict prostatic disease between genetically diverse groups and presumably determine therapeutic modalities. However, the underlining mechanism for these results is not known at this time, although differential population-specific AR activity and disease susceptibility have been very well described clinically [112–115]. Although there have been numerous studies employing microarrays, and recent proteomic screens [116, 117], simple single gene or protein analysis is inadequate to the study of complexity of disease processes, if conclusions toward clinical outcomes wish to be made. Although several "single" genes and proteins have been identified in these studies that are involved with distinct tumor progression and survival profiles and are proposed as prognostic markers; however, once these genes begin to be analyzed as a combined "cluster" model, they do not to translate into statistically significant results related to clinical specimens. The lack of understanding how these genes and proteins act within their functional context and how these components are integrated into signaling pathways and exist as dynamic complexes to execute distinct programs may be responsible for their failure to predict disease progression.

3.3. AR: More than a transcription factor

The above-mentioned work now strongly suggests that the AR functionality extends beyond its classical role as a transcription factor and includes the novel properties of alternative RNA splicing, DNA methylation, proteasomal interaction, and RNA translation at polyribosomes [58, 59], with evidence now suggesting that the ARv567es variant may also participate in glucose metabolism (Paliouras and Trifiro, unpublished data). A number of novel AR-interacting partners have been characterized, with the majority having been identified in the proteomic screen. These proteins include, heat-shock protein 27 (HSP27) [118], DDX5 [119], SAM68 [120], deleted in breast cancer 1 (DBC1) [121], minichromosome maintenance 7 (MCM7) [122], α-actinin 4 (ACTN4) [116], peroxiredin 1 (PRDX1) [123], DEAD-box polypeptide 17 (DDX17) [124], nucleophosim (NPM1) [125], and Ying Yang 1 (YY1) [126]. Furthermore, these findings point to the complexity of the AR-interacting protein unit and suggest it is involved in a number of different pathways that could function as part of a group of interconnected pathways, whose individual compositions alter depending on AR mutational and stimulation status, to generate the appropriate AR biological output.

4. Animal models for CaP

The impact of animal models, especially mouse models, has contributed tremendously to our understanding of tumorigenesis, disease etiology, and drug development. However, one of the difficulties with animals is recapitulating the heterogeneousness of the human cancer. Although mice and other animals do share a high degree of genetic similarity and protein homology, there are still some stark differences in trying to mimic human disease. For use of genetically engineered mouse models (GEMMs), several outstanding issues have arisen for the study of CaP and include the following: animal life span and correlating disease onset and stages of disease progression to human counterparts; the dissimilarities in prostate organs; diet and nutrition; and assessing clinical relevancy to disease pathology, etiology, and outcomes. For CaP researchers, along with GEMMs, a number of other animal model approaches can also be utilized, including a number of spontaneous non-murine CaP models, will also be discussed. Moreover, throughout the discussion of assessing CaP animal models, attempts will be made discuss the role AR continues to make.

http://dx.doi.org/10.5772/64392

4.1. Spontaneous non-murine models

One of the first animal models to study CaP was in rats. Rats are one of the few animals that develop spontaneous CaP disease [127, 128]. The best studied rat model is the Dunning rat model, which develops slow-growing, well-differentiated, and non-metastatic tumors. Some of the outstanding issues that arise are the rarity of tumors and the variability in the phenotypes. There is also a long latency period in tumor development and a lack of metastasis. However, tumors from Dunning rats are initially androgen dependent and eventually becoming androgen independent. Further refinement of Dunning rats has produced animals that are able to develop highly metastatic tumors that spread to lymph nodes and the lungs [129].

CaP also spontaneously occurs in dogs and most closely resembles humans in terms of disease characteristics [130]. CaP in dogs is age dependent, which ideally allows for the study of disease progression, and, in 24% of cases, is able to metastasize to bone. DPC-1, CaP cells derived from dogs, have also been observed to potentially display a number of molecular characteristics including androgen-dependent gene profiling with positive prostate-specific antigen (PSA) and prostate-specific membrane antigen (PMSA) expression [131, 132]. The expression of the progressive disease PMSA marker in DPC-1 cells have allowed for the development of directed radiolabeled-PMSA monoclonal antibodies for SPECT/CT imaging [133]. Another dog model, using cells derived from bone metastasis and injected into dogs, could similarly be used for PET imaging [134]. However, tumors do not regress in castrated dogs and thus are androgen independent. As with rats, there is also a relatively long period for tumor development in dogs. However, the high costs, the gestation period, and the difficulty to genetic manipulate the animals make dogs a very difficult model to use experimentally.

4.2. Genetically engineered mouse models (GEMM) for prostate cancer

Murine models are also not without their limitations, especially as there has not been a single reported case of mice spontaneously developing CaP [135]. Mice have the similar limitations as all other animal models that they are significantly thousands of time smaller and live 30–50 times shorter than humans [136]. As such, a great deal of time and effort has been put into genetically manipulating mice so that they do develop CaP and accurately represent the human disease. However, the human prostate is anatomical different from its mouse counterpart, as the mouse prostate has a lobular structure consisting of four lobes (anterior/coagulating, ventral, dorsal, and lateral) [137], the human prostate organ is a single lobe divided into three zones (central, transitional, and peripheral), and whether the stroma cells surrounding the mouse lobes is similar in comparison with the human stroma cells. The majority of human CaP is also found in the peripheral zone. In mice, the dorsal/lateral lobes have been best described as most similar to the human peripheral zone [135, 138]. On closer assessment, human and mouse prostates become more similar, with stroma cells surrounding epithelial cells. The epithelial cell compartment is also comprised by two cell layers (basal and terminally differentiated luminal cells); also, there are populations of epithelial cell precursors and neuroendocrine cells. In mice, basal cells differentiate into luminal and neuroendocrine cells during prostate development [135, 139].

From the first GEMM for prostate cancer (CaP) developed by Greenberg et al., 1994 [140], to the most recent AR splice variant model by Liu et al. [141], no single model accurately encompasses the entire spectrum of human CaP progression. As CaP is late onset and slowly developing disease, it would be counterintuitive to experimental design. Thus, criteria need to be considered when using mouse models: (1) should reproducibly recapitulate one or more stages of disease progression; (2) should originate within epithelial cells of the prostate; (3) although ideally progression to invasive adenocarcinoma would be desired, but prostatic intraepithelial neoplasia (PIN) should be observed and display associated pathological criteria such as increased inflammation; (4) should display the molecular pathology observed in human CaP tumors, this would include gene and protein expression profile changes that are indicative of an androgen responsive tumor; (5) tumor should respond to ADT or castration. Often times in humans, failure to respond to ADT is linked with the emergence of CRPC and is usually associated with increased expression and nuclear localization of AR since CRPC remains dependent on AR signaling [142]; (6) tumors should achieve bone metastasis (common sites of metastasis observed in human patients). Although rare bone metastasis has been observed in some GEMM, visceral (lung and liver) metastasis appears to be most common.

4.2.1. AR targeted models

Several attempts have been undertaken to produce a GEMM that targets AR signaling and function. The mouse AR (mAR) shares over 90% homology with its human ortholog; however, mAR interestingly lacks an expanded CAG-polyglutamine tract, instead mice possess a mixed CAG/CAC-glutamine/histidine tract. One of the first AR-targeted mouse models was to target the overexpression of mAR to the prostate secretory epithelium, using the prostate-specific and androgen-responsive mouse probasin (Pb) promoter [143]. By 52 weeks, mice developed high-grade prostatic intraepithelial neoplasia (HGPIN) by 52 weeks. Mice also showed increased proliferation in dorsal/lateral and ventral lobes as marked by increased expression of Ki67 proliferation marker. Even with the increased expression/activity of the mAR, it was insufficient to progress prostatic pathology to CaP.

Another group of investigators opted to take into consideration the differences in the genetic polymorphism of the polyglutamine tract between mice and humans and replace exon 1 of the mAR with exon 1 of the human AR [144]. Three transgenic whole knock-in "humanized" AR mice expressing three different polyglutamine tract lengths (12Q, 21Q, and 48Q) were created. As the length of the polyglutamine tract is linked to AR activity and risk for CaP [34, 51], the reasoning behind the three mice was to differentiated disease progression with AR activity. All mice appear to maintain androgen-dependent gene expression, however, do not develop any prostatic pathology, even with the short 12Q tract mouse. However, when these mice were crossed to TRAMP mice (see below), the length of the polyglutamine tract was linked to the initiation of prostatic tumors, with shorter having higher incidence of tumors vs. longer tracts, which appear to offer a degree of protection in tumor initiation. Of note, researchers also assessed AR mutations of tumors from their 21Q humanized AR crossed to TRAMP mice under a number of different conditions (intact, intact/bicalutamide, intact/flutamide, and castrated). Along with assessing specific somatic mutations (missense, non-sense, small indolent insertion/deletions), they also assessed changes in the length of polyglutamine tract. They found an average mutation rate of 4.0/10,000 bp of AR coding sequence, with missense mutations accounting for 54.1% of putative mutations, with a majority of mutations identified in one or two clones per tumor [145]. Half of the mutations identified also were found in the LBD region, as has often been shown to be responsible for promiscuous ligand-binding gain-of-function properties of the receptor [68, 146]. Contraction of the polyglutamine tract was also assessed, as it is also commonly observed in disease initiation; however, it was not observed. Although this AR mutation rate is higher than reported in clinical samples [39], it does highlight the mutational sensitivity of AR correlated to disease progression.

Recently, a GEMM was created to study the role of the AR splice variant, ARv567es, in CaP development [141]. ARv567es clone was cloned downstream of androgen responsive Pb promoter, where endogenous mAR would initially drive expression of the ARv567es, then upon castration of the animals, an adequate expression of ARv567es would then continue to expand its own expression. Thus, the investigators would be able to study the influence of ARv567es on the progression of CaP in castrate-resistant state. The coordinate expression of full-length AR and ARv567es variants were able to illicit epithelial hyperplasia by 16 weeks and invasive adenocarcinoma by 52 weeks. Upon castration at 16 weeks, mice were able to maintain nuclear localization of ARv567es and able to develop more aggressive neoplasias than sham controls. Gene expression profiling of tumors from ARv567es castrated mice also suggested that there is an enrichment of oncogenic pathways, including Wnt/β-catenin, NFkB, and K-Ras signaling, that have been linked to aggressive CaP.

4.2.2. TRAMP and LADY

The first murine prostate cancer models took advantage of some recent advances in the areas of oncogenetics and steroid hormone receptor functionality. As such, the viral SV40 early region, comprised of the large T antigen (Tag) and small t antigen, was cloned downstream of the androgen hormone responsive rat Pb promoter. After selection of lines of animals with higher expression of SV40 early region in the ventral and dorsal lobes, it yielded the transgenic adenocarcinoma mouse prostate (TRAMP) model [140, 147]. TRAMP mice develop progressive forms of CaP, even distant site metastasis. They are characterized with rapid development of PIN by 12 weeks with adenocarcinoma, predominantly in the dorsal/lateral lobes, arising by 24 weeks of age. The mice can also display castrate-resistant disease, where mice castrated at 12 weeks did not affect primary tumor development or metastasis in the majority of mice with 100% in the lymph and 67% lung metastasis [148].

The LADY CaP model is similar to the TRAMP model, in that it utilizes, rather than the entire SV40 early region, only the large T antigen under the control of the long 12-kb Pb promoter [149]. These mice also lead to the development of hyperplasia and PIN by 10 weeks, followed by high-grade epithelial dysplasia and adenocarcinoma by 20 weeks. By 33 weeks of age, the mice display metastatic disease to the liver, lung, and bone with a 90% penetrance [150]. The metastatic tumors are all neuroendocrine type cancers, similar to TRAMP metastatic tumors [151].

TRAMP and LADY models also have been used for a number of preclinical drug studies [152–161]; however, questions arise Whether a model that develops localized primary prostatic disease between 20 and 24 weeks is a proper representation of human disease evolution? Furthermore, these models can be referred to as "brutish" with the utilization of the SV40 T antigen region; as such a genetic element has never been implicated in human CaP. However, the T antigen has been identified to bind and inhibit TP53 and RB tumor suppressors, the molecular chaperone DNAJ, and complement p300/CBP, while small t antigen has been shown to bind to the phosphatase PP2A and a number of proteins known to contribute to CaP and other neoplasias [162]. Loss-of-function/deletion mutations TP53 [163–166] and RB [167–172] have been linked to CaP progression, and together, DNAJ [173–175] and p300/CBP [87, 176] have also been describe as AR protein complex proteins and shown to be involved in mediating AR signaling [37, 59, 87]. However, even if the TRAMP/LADY models can be considered feed-forward models, because of their dependency on AR signaling, to both drive expression of SV40 through the Pb promoter and simultaneously potentially contribute to a favorable cellular environment for AR function; the other questions to arise are Whether the molecular pathology of TRAMP/LADY mice share concordance with expression profiles (genes/proteins) found in clinical CaP specimens from representative disease stages? Currently, the analysis has not been performed.

4.2.3. PTEN deficiency

Phosphatase and tensin homolog (PTEN) is an important regulator of the PI3K/AKT signaling pathway and is frequently deleted/mutated in a number of human cancers [177–182]. In CaP, PTEN deletions occur in approximately 23% of HGPIN, 68% of localized primary tumors [183], and 86% of CRPC [184] and thus has become a candidate for developing into a mouse model. Although homozygous knock-out (KO) Pten mice are embryonic lethal, heterozygous $Pten^{+/-}$ mice develop a number of neoplasias, including lymphomas, dysplastic intestinal polyps, endometrial complex atypical hyperplasia, and thyroid neoplasia [185]. However, common human tumors, such as brain, breast, and skin, associated with PTEN deletion are absent from mice. $Pten^{+/-}$ mice also have a spectrum of prostatic phenotypes, with 70% of mice displaying hyperplasia and dysplasia between 6 and 30 weeks [186]. Using a reduced activity of hypomorphic Pten allele, it has been shown that $Pten^{+/hyp}$ mice can promote progression from hyperplasia to PIN between 6 and 22 weeks of age between 25 and 37.5% of the time, however, with only a single case of adenocarcinoma observed [185, 187, 188].

Due to the latency of prostatic disease development in $Pten^{+/-}$ mice, researchers have undertaken to cross these mice with other genes associated with CaP with the objective to accelerate disease progression. This has included crosses to $p27^{Kip1}$ and Nkx3.1 loss-of-function allele mouse strains. In 13–22 weeks, $Pten^{+/-}$, $p27Kip1^{-/-}$ mice develop PIN with 100% penetrance and about 25% of mice develop invasive CaP [189]. Alone, Nkx3.1 loss-of-function mice do not develop PIN or CaP in mice; however, in combination with $Pten^{+/-}$ mice, they show an accelerated incidence and progression to HGPIN/early carcinoma at 26 weeks, with 100% penetrance of HGPIN at 52 weeks [190]. By allowing the $Pten^{+/-}$; $Nkx3.1^{+/-}$ mice to age more than 52 weeks, allows HGPIN lesions to progress to invasive adenocarcinoma. Furthermore,

http://dx.doi.org/10.5772/64392

surgical castration at 24 weeks, of these animals, resulted in partial regression of the prostatic lesions and decreased expression of AR [191].

In 2003, Wang et al., generated a mouse model that specifically deleted exon 5 of Pten in the prostate [192]. These mice developed hyperplasia in 4 weeks, PIN at 6 weeks, and frank adenocarcinoma with 100% penetrance between 9 and 24 weeks. The mice also respond to surgical castration with an observed increase in apoptosis and extended survival time vs. non-castrated animals. However, castrated animals still maintained prostates 5- to 10-fold larger than WT counterparts and reduced AR expression. Although reduced AR expression is consistent with other Pten deficiency mice, this is not what is observable in human CaP [193]. Additionally, metastasis to the lymph nodes and lungs at 12–29 weeks was observed in 45% of animals.

Currently, there are a number of prostate-specific conditional Pten KO mice that have been developed that employ alternative promoters. A PSA-promoter-driven Pten KO resulted in 100% penetrance of adenocarcinoma and carcinoma by 56 weeks [194]. However, by simultaneously knocking out, Pten and Nkx3.1, coupled with tamoxifen inductions, slowly developed HGPIN with microinvasion [195]. Tumors regress in castrated mice, but then continue to progress to microinvasive adenocarcinoma while maintaining nuclear AR expression, suggesting that AR signaling remains active in the mice following castration. Combinatorial ADT and inhibition of AKT (MK2206) and mTOR (MK8669) function significantly reduced tumor burden [196].

5. Cell metabolism, ROS, DNA damage, and the AR

The AR has long been known to have dramatic effects on the prostate gland. The acute withdrawal of androgens lead to severe atrophy of the prostate gland in short time frames originally referred to as involution, which in currently acknowledged as a programmed cell death event [197]. The AR also has significant effects on the overall anabolic and intermediary metabolism, promoting glucose uptake, and pursuing through both the glycolytic, TCA cycle and fatty acid metabolism.

A number of non-genomic influences have been associated with specific risks to the development of CaP, one of these risk factors has been nutrition and diet, especially Western (high-fat/low-carbohydrate) vs. non-Western (low fat/high carbohydrate) has been extensively reviewed [198–200]. Likewise, GEMM also have been shown to be influenced by high-fat diets. TRAMP mice given a Western-type diet containing 21.2% fat and 0.2% cholesterol vs. regular chow diet (4.5% fat and 0.002% cholesterol), with 33% of mice showing large and very pronounced tumors at 28 weeks, with increased tumor size and weight and hyperplasia [201]. Western-type fed TRAMP mice also showed increased expression of cell cycle-related (cyclin D1) and proliferation (proliferating cell nuclear antigen—PCNA) markers. There was also an increase in lung metastasis with an average of 3 ± 1.04 foci vs. 0.43 ± 0.2 foci, in Western-type vs. regular chow-fed mice. Another group also observed similar results with a high-fat diet fed TRAMP mouse [202]. Along with seeing an increase in tumor size and increase prostatic hyperplasia, they also observed a decrease in the expression of glutathione peroxidase 3 (GPx3). GPx3 is an important antioxidant enzyme responsible for detoxifying cells of reactive oxygen species (ROS). Increased ROS levels in one of the consequences on high-fat diets and has been shown to interfere with a number of cellular processes, including damaging DNA [203]. GPx3 levels have been shown to be downregulated in CaP [204, 205]. The combinatorial observation that high-fat fed TRAMP mice have larger tumors with cellular changes (increased ROS levels, reduced GPx3 expression) suggests a potential mechanism for a role of cellular metabolism in CaP progression. Increased cellular metabolism and downstream effects of increased ROS levels and DNA damage create the scenario for tumor cells to incur more mutations that may lead to more aggressive tumor growth and drug resistance.

The AR thus has an intrinsic ingrained property of promoting prostatic cellular metabolism. It is not unreasonable that in CaP initiation and evolution, alterations in AR allowing further enhanced metabolism may be the fundamental mechanisms allowing for new mutations to be created. Heightened metabolism has a direct effect on reactive oxygen species generation (ROS) as hypermetabolism can result in exaggerated mitochondria fluxes [206–211]. It is now well appreciated that cancer metabolism is unique many times demonstrating heightened glucose uptake and abnormal mitochondrial pathways including glutamine lysis and reverse carboxylation. These metabolic properties are not reflective of energy needs and can be considered in conjunction with fatty acid oxidations as a metabolic phenotype-supporting ROS leading to DNA alterations, in essence a powerful mutator phenotype.

Author details

Miltiadis Paliouras[1,2*], Carlos Alvarado[1,2] and Mark Trifiro[1,2]

*Address all correspondence to: miltiadis.paliouras@mcgill.ca

1 Lady Davis Institute for Medical Research, Jewish General Hospital, Montreal, QC, Canada

2 Department of Medicine, McGill University, Montreal, QC, Canada

References

[1] Forbes SA, Beare D, Gunasekaran P, et al. COSMIC: exploring the world's knowledge of somatic mutations in human cancer. Nucleic Acids Res 2015;43:D805–11.

[2] Forbes SA, Bindal N, Bamford S, et al. COSMIC: mining complete cancer genomes in the Catalogue of Somatic Mutations in Cancer. Nucleic Acids Res 2011;39:D945–50.

[3] Forbes SA, Tang G, Bindal N, et al. COSMIC (the Catalogue of Somatic Mutations in Cancer): a resource to investigate acquired mutations in human cancer. Nucleic Acids Res 2010;38:D652–7.

[4] Forbes SA, Bhamra G, Bamford S, et al. The Catalogue of Somatic Mutations in Cancer (COSMIC). Current protocols in human genetics / editorial board, Jonathan L Haines [et al] 2008;Chapter 10:10.11.1-.10.11.26.

[5] Forbes S, Clements J, Dawson E, et al. Cosmic 2005. Br J Cancer 2006;94:318–22.

[6] Bamford S, Dawson E, Forbes S, et al. The COSMIC (Catalogue of Somatic Mutations in Cancer) database and website. Br J Cancer 2004;91:355–8.

[7] Wu TJ, Schriml LM, Chen QR, et al. Generating a focused view of disease ontology cancer terms for pan-cancer data integration and analysis. Database (Oxford) 2015;2015:bav032.

[8] Tomczak K, Czerwinska P, Wiznerowicz M. The Cancer Genome Atlas (TCGA): an immeasurable source of knowledge. Contemp Oncol (Pozn) 2015;19:A68–77.

[9] Wu TJ, Shamsaddini A, Pan Y, et al. A framework for organizing cancer-related variations from existing databases, publications and NGS data using a high-performance Integrated Virtual Environment (HIVE). Database (Oxford) 2014;2014:bau022.

[10] Kandoth C, McLellan MD, Vandin F, et al. Mutational landscape and significance across 12 major cancer types. Nature 2013;502:333–9.

[11] Nishant KT, Singh ND, Alani E. Genomic mutation rates: what high-throughput methods can tell us. BioEssays 2009;31:912–20.

[12] Korneliussen TS, Albrechtsen A, Nielsen R. ANGSD: analysis of next generation sequencing data. BMC Bioinformatics 2014;15:356.

[13] Lawrence MS, Stojanov P, Mermel CH, et al. Discovery and saturation analysis of cancer genes across 21 tumour types. Nature 2014;505:495–501.

[14] Pleasance ED, Cheetham RK, Stephens PJ, et al. A comprehensive catalogue of somatic mutations from a human cancer genome. Nature 2010;463:191–6.

[15] Gawad C, Koh W, Quake SR. Single-cell genome sequencing: current state of the science. Nat Rev 2016;17:175–88.

[16] Li SC, Tachiki LM, Kabeer MH, Dethlefs BA, Anthony MJ, Loudon WG. Cancer genomic research at the crossroads: realizing the changing genetic landscape as intratumoral spatial and temporal heterogeneity becomes a confounding factor. Cancer Cell Int 2014;14:115.

[17] Gottlieb B, Alvarado C, Wang C, et al. Making sense of intratumor genetic heterogeneity: altered frequency of androgen receptor CAG repeat length variants in breast cancer tissues. Human Mutat 2013;34:610–8.

[18] Swanton C. Intratumor heterogeneity: evolution through space and time. Cancer Res 2012;72:4875–82.

[19] Fox EJ, Prindle MJ, Loeb LA. Do mutator mutations fuel tumorigenesis? Cancer Metastasis Rev 2013;32:353–61.

[20] Hanahan D, Weinberg RA. Hallmarks of cancer: the next generation. Cell 2011;144:646–74.

[21] Loeb LA. A mutator phenotype in cancer. Cancer Res 2001;61:3230–9.

[22] Loeb LA. Cancer cells exhibit a mutator phenotype. Adv Cancer Res 1998;72:25–56.

[23] Aizawa S, Ohashi M, Loeb LA, Martin GM. Multipotent mutator strain of mouse teratocarcinoma cells. Somat Cell Mol Genet 1985;11:211–6.

[24] Prostate Cancer. In: American Cancer Society; 2012. www.cancer.org/Cancer/ProstateCancer/DetailedGuide/prostate-cancer-what-causes

[25] Draisma G, Etzioni R, Tsodikov A, et al. Lead time and overdiagnosis in prostate-specific antigen screening: importance of methods and context. J Nat Cancer I 2009;101:374–83.

[26] Andriole GL, Crawford ED, Grubb RL, 3rd, et al. Mortality results from a randomized prostate-cancer screening trial. N Eng J Med 2009;360:1310–9.

[27] Andriole GL, Bostwick DG, Brawley OW, et al. Effect of dutasteride on the risk of prostate cancer. N Eng J Med 2010;362:1192–202.

[28] Guyader C, Ceraline J, Gravier E, et al. Risk of hormone escape in a human prostate cancer model depends on therapy modalities and can be reduced by tyrosine kinase inhibitors. PLoS One 2012;7:e42252.

[29] Linja MJ, Visakorpi T. Alterations of androgen receptor in prostate cancer. J Steroid Biochem Mol Biol 2004;92:255–64.

[30] Brimo F, Xu B, Scarlata E, et al. Biopsy characteristics in men with a preoperative diagnosis of prostatic adenocarcinoma with high Gleason score (8–10) predict pathologic outcome in radical prostatectomy. Hum Pathol 2014;45:2006–13.

[31] Marquard J, Eng C. Multiple endocrine Neoplasia type 2. In: Pagon RA, Adam MP, Ardinger HH, et al., eds. GeneReviews(R). Seattle, WA: University of Washington, 1993.

[32] Steinmetz AC, Renaud JP, Moras D. Binding of ligands and activation of transcription by nuclear receptors. Ann Rev Biophys Biomol Struct 2001;30:329–59.

[33] Whitfield GK, Jurutka PW, Haussler CA, Haussler MR. Steroid hormone receptors: evolution, ligands, and molecular basis of biologic function. J Cell Biochem 1999;(Suppl 32–33):110–22.

[34] Casella R, Maduro MR, Lipshultz LI, Lamb DJ. Significance of the polyglutamine tract polymorphism in the androgen receptor. Urology 2001;58:651–6.

[35] Gao W, Bohl CE, Dalton JT. Chemistry and structural biology of androgen receptor. Chem Rev 2005;105:3352–70.

[36] Gobinet J, Poujol N, Sultan C. Molecular action of androgens. Mol Cell Endocrinol 2002;198:15–24.

[37] Gottlieb B, Beitel LK, Nadarajah A, Paliouras M, Trifiro M. The androgen receptor gene mutations database: 2012 update. Human Mutat 2012;33:887–94.

[38] Gottlieb B, Beitel LK, Wu JH, Trifiro M. The androgen receptor gene mutations database (ARDB): 2004 update. Human Mutat 2004;23:527–33.

[39] Robinson D, Van Allen EM, Wu YM, et al. Integrative clinical genomics of advanced prostate cancer. Cell 2015;161:1215–28.

[40] Cooper CS, Eeles R, Wedge DC, et al. Analysis of the genetic phylogeny of multifocal prostate cancer identifies multiple independent clonal expansions in neoplastic and morphologically normal prostate tissue. Nat Genet 2015;47:367–72.

[41] Boutros PC, Fraser M, Harding NJ, et al. Spatial genomic heterogeneity within localized, multifocal prostate cancer. Nat Genet 2015;47:736–45.

[42] Wu C, Wyatt AW, Lapuk AV, et al. Integrated genome and transcriptome sequencing identifies a novel form of hybrid and aggressive prostate cancer. J Pathol 2012;227:53–61.

[43] Yu MW, Yang YC, Yang SY, et al. Androgen receptor exon 1 CAG repeat length and risk of hepatocellular carcinoma in women. Hepatology 2002;36:156–63.

[44] Ferro P, Catalano MG, Dell'Eva R, Fortunati N, Pfeffer U. The androgen receptor CAG repeat: a modifier of carcinogenesis? Mol Cell Endocrinol 2002;193:109–20.

[45] Bennett CL, Price DK, Kim S, et al. Racial variation in CAG repeat lengths within the androgen receptor gene among prostate cancer patients of lower socioeconomic status. J Clin Oncol 2002;20:3599–604.

[46] Yu MW, Cheng SW, Lin MW, et al. Androgen-receptor gene CAG repeats, plasma testosterone levels, and risk of hepatitis B-related hepatocellular carcinoma. J Nat Cancer Inst 2000;92:2023–8.

[47] Ferro P, Catalano MG, Raineri M, et al. Somatic alterations of the androgen receptor CAG repeat in human colon cancer delineate a novel mutation pathway independent of microsatellite instability. Cancer Genet Cytogenet 2000;123:35–40.

[48] Giovannucci E, Platz EA, Stampfer MJ, et al. The CAG repeat within the androgen receptor gene and benign prostatic hyperplasia. Urology 1999;53:121–5.

[49] Giovannucci E, Stampfer MJ, Krithivas K, et al. The CAG repeat within the androgen receptor gene and its relationship to prostate cancer. Proc Nat Acad Sci USA 1997;94:3320–3.

[50] Southwell J, Chowdhury SF, Gottlieb B, et al. An investigation into CAG repeat length variation and N/C terminal interactions in the T877A mutant androgen receptor found in prostate cancer. J Steroid Biochem Mol Biol 2008;111:138–46.

[51] Palazzolo I, Gliozzi A, Rusmini P, et al. The role of the polyglutamine tract in androgen receptor. J Steroid Biochem Mol Biol 2008;108:245–53.

[52] Sircar K, Gottlieb B, Alvarado C, et al. Androgen receptor CAG repeat length contraction in diseased and non-diseased prostatic tissues. Prostate Cancer Prostatic Dis 2007;10:360–8.

[53] Zhang L, Leeflang EP, Yu J, Arnheim N. Studying human mutations by sperm typing: instability of CAG trinucleotide repeats in the human androgen receptor gene. Nat Genet 1994;7:531–5.

[54] Alvarado C, Beitel LK, Sircar K, Aprikian A, Trifiro M, Gottlieb B. Somatic mosaicism and cancer: a micro-genetic examination into the role of the androgen receptor gene in prostate cancer. Cancer Res 2005;65:8514–8.

[55] Elhaji YA, Stoica I, Dennis S, Purisima EO, Trifiro MA. Impaired helix 12 dynamics due to proline 892 substitutions in the androgen receptor are associated with complete androgen insensitivity. Human Mol Genet 2006;15:921–31.

[56] Nguyen D, Steinberg SV, Rouault E, et al. A G577R mutation in the human AR P box results in selective decreases in DNA binding and in partial androgen insensitivity syndrome. Mol Endocrinol (Baltimore, Md) 2001;15:1790–802.

[57] Beitel LK, Prior L, Vasiliou DM, et al. Complete androgen insensitivity due to mutations in the probable alpha-helical segments of the DNA-binding domain in the human androgen receptor. Human Mol Genet 1994;3:21–7.

[58] Zaman N, Giannopoulos PN, Chowdhury S, et al. Proteomic-coupled-network analysis of T877A-androgen receptor interactomes can predict clinical prostate cancer outcomes between White (non-Hispanic) and African-American groups. PLoS One 2014;9:e113190.

[59] Paliouras M, Zaman N, Lumbroso R, et al. Dynamic rewiring of the androgen receptor protein interaction network correlates with prostate cancer clinical outcomes. Integr Biol 2011;10:1020–32.

[60] Bielas JH, Loeb KR, Rubin BP, True LD, Loeb LA. Human cancers express a mutator phenotype. Proc Nat Acad Sci USA 2006;103:18238–42.

[61] Venkatesan RN, Bielas JH, Loeb LA. Generation of mutator mutants during carcinogenesis. DNA Repair (Amst) 2006;5:294–302.

[62] Isaacs JT, Isaacs WB. Androgen receptor outwits prostate cancer drugs. Nat Med 2004;10:26–7.

[63] Taplin ME, Balk SP. Androgen receptor: a key molecule in the progression of prostate cancer to hormone independence. J Cell Biochem 2004;91:483–90.

[64] Culig Z, Hobisch A, Bartsch G, Klocker H. Androgen receptor—an update of mechanisms of action in prostate cancer. Urol Res 2000;28:211–9.

[65] Hobisch A, Culig Z, Radmayr C, Bartsch G, Klocker H, Hittmair A. Distant metastases from prostatic carcinoma express androgen receptor protein. Cancer Res 1995;55:3068–72.

[66] Koivisto P, Kononen J, Palmberg C, et al. Androgen receptor gene amplification: a possible molecular mechanism for androgen deprivation therapy failure in prostate cancer. Cancer Res 1997;57:314–9.

[67] Chang CY, McDonnell DP. Evaluation of ligand-dependent changes in AR structure using peptide probes. Mol Endocrinol (Baltimore, Md) 2002;16:647–60.

[68] Veldscholte J, Ris-Stalpers C, Kuiper GG, et al. A mutation in the ligand binding domain of the androgen receptor of human LNCaP cells affects steroid binding characteristics and response to anti-androgens. Biochemical and biophysical research communications 1990;173:534–40.

[69] Duff J, McEwan IJ. Mutation of histidine 874 in the androgen receptor ligand-binding domain leads to promiscuous ligand activation and altered p160 coactivator interactions. Mol Endocrinol (Baltimore, Md) 2005;19:2943–54.

[70] Vogelstein B, Kinzler KW. The Genetic Basis of Human Cancer. 2nd ed. New York: McGraw-Hill, Medical Publication Division; 2002.

[71] Ceraline J, Cruchant MD, Erdmann E, et al. Constitutive activation of the androgen receptor by a point mutation in the hinge region: a new mechanism for androgen-independent growth in prostate cancer. Int J Cancer 2004;108:152–7.

[72] Taplin ME, Bubley GJ, Ko YJ, et al. Selection for androgen receptor mutations in prostate cancers treated with androgen antagonist. Cancer Res 1999;59:2511–5.

[73] Taplin ME, Bubley GJ, Shuster TD, et al. Mutation of the androgen-receptor gene in metastatic androgen-independent prostate cancer. N Eng J Med 1995;332:1393–8.

[74] Taplin ME, Rajeshkumar B, Halabi S, et al. Androgen receptor mutations in androgen-independent prostate cancer: cancer and Leukemia Group B study 9663. J Clin Oncol 2003;21:2673–8.

[75] Korpal M, Korn JM, Gao X, et al. An F876L mutation in androgen receptor confers genetic and phenotypic resistance to MDV3100 (enzalutamide). Cancer Discov 2013;3:1030–43.

[76] Hu R, Lu C, Mostaghel EA, et al. Distinct transcriptional programs mediated by the ligand-dependent full-length androgen receptor and its splice variants in castration-resistant prostate cancer. Cancer Res 2012;72:3457–62.

[77] Watson PA, Chen YF, Balbas MD, et al. Constitutively active androgen receptor splice variants expressed in castration-resistant prostate cancer require full-length androgen receptor. Proc Nat Acad Sci USA 2010;107:16759–65.

[78] Sun S, Sprenger CC, Vessella RL, et al. Castration resistance in human prostate cancer is conferred by a frequently occurring androgen receptor splice variant. J Clin Invest 2010;120:2715–30.

[79] Li Y, Hwang TH, Oseth LA, et al. AR intragenic deletions linked to androgen receptor splice variant expression and activity in models of prostate cancer progression. Oncogene 2012;31:4759–67.

[80] Brand LJ, Dehm SM. Androgen receptor gene rearrangements: new perspectives on prostate cancer progression. Curr Drug Targets 2013;14:441–9.

[81] Li Y, Alsagabi M, Fan D, Bova GS, Tewfik AH, Dehm SM. Intragenic rearrangement and altered RNA splicing of the androgen receptor in a cell-based model of prostate cancer progression. Cancer Res 2011;71:2108–17.

[82] Liu LL, Xie N, Sun S, Plymate S, Mostaghel E, Dong X. Mechanisms of the androgen receptor splicing in prostate cancer cells. Oncogene 2014;33:3140–50.

[83] Lu ZX, Huang Q, Park JW, et al. Transcriptome-wide landscape of pre-mRNA alternative splicing associated with metastatic colonization. Mol Cancer Res 2015;13:305–18.

[84] Carpenter RL, Lo HW. Identification, functional characterization, and pathobiological significance of GLI1 isoforms in human cancers. Vitamins Horm 2012;88:115–40.

[85] Rajan P, Elliott DJ, Robson CN, Leung HY. Alternative splicing and biological heterogeneity in prostate cancer. Nat Rev Urol 2009;6:454–60.

[86] Venables JP. Aberrant and alternative splicing in cancer. Cancer Res 2004;64:7647–54.

[87] Heemers HV, Tindall DJ. Androgen receptor (AR) coregulators: a diversity of functions converging on and regulating the AR transcriptional complex. Endocr Rev 2007;28:778–808.

[88] Paliouras M, Diamandis EP. An AKT activity threshold regulates androgen-dependent and androgen-independent PSA expression in prostate cancer cell lines. Biol Chem 2008;389:773–80.

[89] Paliouras M, Diamandis EP. Intracellular signaling pathways regulate hormone-dependent kallikrein gene expression. Tumour Biol 2008;29:63–75.

[90] Doesburg P, Kuil CW, Berrevoets CA, et al. Functional *in vivo* interaction between the amino-terminal, transactivation domain and the ligand binding domain of the androgen receptor. Biochemistry 1997;36:1052–64.

[91] Rao J, Lee P, Benzeno S, et al. Functional interaction of human Cdc37 with the androgen receptor but not with the glucocorticoid receptor. J Biol Chem 2001;276:5814–20.

[92] Sharma M, Zarnegar M, Li X, Lim B, Sun Z. Androgen receptor interacts with a novel MYST protein, HBO1. J Biol Chem 2000;275:35200–8.

[93] Beitel LK, Sabbaghian N, Alarifi A, Alvarado C, Pinsky L, Trifiro M. Characterization of normal and point-mutated human androgen receptors expressed in the baculovirus system. J Mol Endocr 1995;15:117–28.

[94] Panet-Raymond V, Gottlieb B, Beitel LK, et al. Characterization of intracellular aggregates using fluorescently-tagged polyglutamine-expanded androgen receptor. Neurotoxicity Res 2001;3:259–75.

[95] Mann M, Hendrickson RC, Pandey A. Analysis of proteins and proteomes by mass spectrometry. Annu Rev Biochem 2001;70:437–73.

[96] Parker CE, Warren MR, Loiselle DR, Dicheva NN, Scarlett CO, Borchers CH. Identification of components of protein complexes. Methods Mol Biol 2005;301:117–51.

[97] Kaboord B, Perr M. Isolation of proteins and protein complexes by immunoprecipitation. Methods Mol Biol 2008;424:349–64.

[98] Saba J, Bonneil E, Pomies C, Eng K, Thibault P. Enhanced sensitivity in proteomics experiments using FAIMS coupled with a hybrid linear ion trap/orbitrap mass spectrometer. J Proteome Res 2009;8:3355–66.

[99] Kearney P, Thibault P. Bioinformatics meets proteomics—bridging the gap between mass spectrometry data analysis and cell biology. J Bioinform Comput Biol 2003;1:183–200.

[100] Alfarano C, Andrade CE, Anthony K, et al. The biomolecular interaction network database and related tools 2005 update. Nucleic Acids Res 2005;33:D418–24.

[101] Salwinski L, Miller CS, Smith AJ, Pettit FK, Bowie JU, Eisenberg D. The database of interacting proteins: 2004 update. Nucleic Acids Res 2004;32:D449–51.

[102] Peri S, Navarro JD, Amanchy R, et al. Development of human protein reference database as an initial platform for approaching systems biology in humans. Genome Res 2003;13:2363–71.

[103] Hermjakob H, Montecchi-Palazzi L, Lewington C, et al. IntAct: an open source molecular interaction database. Nucleic Acids Res 2004;32:D452–5.

[104] Zanzoni A, Montecchi-Palazzi L, Quondam M, Ausiello G, Helmer-Citterich M, Cesareni G. MINT: a molecular INTeraction database. FEBS Lett 2002;513:135–40.

[105] Awan A, Bari H, Yan F, et al. Regulatory network motifs and hotspots of cancer genes in a mammalian cellular signalling network. IET Syst Biol 2007;1:292–7.

[106] Cui Q, Ma Y, Jaramillo M, et al. A map of human cancer signaling. Mol Syst Biol 2007;3:152.

[107] Cui Q, Yu Z, Purisima EO, Wang E. Principles of microRNA regulation of a human cellular signaling network. Mol Syst Biol 2006;2:46.

[108] Kelley BP, Yuan B, Lewitter F, Sharan R, Stockwell BR, Ideker T. PathBLAST: a tool for alignment of protein interaction networks. Nucleic Acids Res 2004;32:W83–8.

[109] Clough E, Barrett T. The gene expression omnibus database. Methods Mol Biol 2016;1418:93–110.

[110] Barrett T, Wilhite SE, Ledoux P, et al. NCBI GEO: archive for functional genomics data sets—update. Nucleic Acids Res 2013;41:D991–5.

[111] Chin L, Andersen JN, Futreal PA. Cancer genomics: from discovery science to personalized medicine. Nat Med 2011;17:297–303.

[112] Abern MR, Bassett MR, Tsivian M, et al. Race is associated with discontinuation of active surveillance of low-risk prostate cancer: Results from the Duke Prostate Center. Prostate cancer and prostatic diseases 2012;16:85–90.

[113] Fukagai T, Namiki T, Carlile RG, Namiki M. Racial differences in clinical outcome after prostate cancer treatment. Methods Mol Biol 2009;472:455–66.

[114] Penson DF, Albertsen PC. Lessons learnt about early prostate cancer from large scale databases: population-based pearls of wisdom. Surg Oncol 2002;11:3–11.

[115] Powell IJ. Prostate cancer in the African American: is this a different disease? Semin Urol Oncol 1998;16:221–6.

[116] Jasavala R, Martinez H, Thumar J, et al. Identification of putative androgen receptor interaction protein modules: cytoskeleton and endosomes modulate androgen receptor signaling in prostate cancer cells. Mol Cell Proteomics 2007;6:252–71.

[117] Garbis SD, Tyritzis SI, Roumeliotis T, et al. Search for potential markers for prostate cancer diagnosis, prognosis and treatment in clinical tissue specimens using amine-specific isobaric tagging (iTRAQ) with two-dimensional liquid chromatography and tandem mass spectrometry. J Proteome Res 2008;7:3146–58.

[118] Zoubeidi A, Zardan A, Beraldi E, et al. Cooperative interactions between androgen receptor (AR) and heat-shock protein 27 facilitate AR transcriptional activity. Cancer Res 2007;67:10455–65.

[119] Clark EL, Coulson A, Dalgliesh C, et al. The RNA helicase p68 is a novel androgen receptor coactivator involved in splicing and is overexpressed in prostate cancer. Cancer Res 2008;68:7938–46.

[120] Rajan P, Gaughan L, Dalgliesh C, et al. The RNA-binding and adaptor protein Sam68 modulates signal-dependent splicing and transcriptional activity of the androgen receptor. J Pathol 2008;215:67–77.

[121] Fu J, Jiang J, Li J, et al. The deleted in breast cancer 1 (DBC-1): A novel AR coactivator that promotes AR DNA binding activity. The Journal of biological chemistry 2009;284:6832–40.

[122] Shi YK, Yu YP, Zhu ZH, et al. MCM7 interacts with androgen receptor. Am J Pathol 2008;173:1758–67.

[123] Park SY, Yu X, Ip C, Mohler JL, Bogner PN, Park YM. Peroxiredoxin 1 interacts with androgen receptor and enhances its transactivation. Cancer Res 2007;67:9294–303.

[124] Wong HY, Demmers JA, Bezstarosti K, Grootegoed JA, Brinkmann AO. DNA dependent recruitment of DDX17 and other interacting proteins by the human androgen receptor. Biochimica et Biophysica Acta 2009;1794:193–8.

[125] Leotoing L, Meunier L, Manin M, et al. Influence of nucleophosmin/B23 on DNA binding and transcriptional activity of the androgen receptor in prostate cancer cell. Oncogene 2008;27:2858–67.

[126] Deng Z, Wan M, Cao P, Rao A, Cramer SD, Sui G. Yin Yang 1 regulates the transcriptional activity of androgen receptor. Oncogene 2009;28:3746–57.

[127] Pollard M. Spontaneous prostate adenocarcinomas in aged germfree Wistar rats. J Nat Cancer I 1973;51:1235–41.

[128] Dunning WF. Prostate cancer in the rat. Nat Cancer Inst Monogr 1963;12:351–69.

[129] Isaacs JT, Weissman RM, Coffey DS, Scott WW. Concepts in prostatic cancer biology: dunning R-3327 H, HI, and AT tumors. Prog Clin Biol Res 1980;37:311–23.

[130] Leroy BE, Northrup N. Prostate cancer in dogs: comparative and clinical aspects. Vet J 2009;180:149–62.

[131] Anidjar M, Scarlata E, Cury FL, et al. Refining the orthotopic dog prostate cancer (DPC)-1 model to better bridge the gap between rodents and men. The Prostate 2012;72:752–61.

[132] Anidjar M, Villette JM, Devauchelle P, et al. *In vivo* model mimicking natural history of dog prostate cancer using DPC-1, a new canine prostate carcinoma cell line. The Prostate 2001;46:2–10.

[133] Chevalier S, Moffett S, Turcotte E, et al. The dog prostate cancer (DPC-1) model: a reliable tool for molecular imaging of prostate tumors and metastases. EJNMMI Res 2015;5:77.

[134] Keller JM, Schade GR, Ives K, et al. A novel canine model for prostate cancer. The Prostate 2013;73:952–9.

[135] Shappell SB, Thomas GV, Roberts RL, et al. Prostate pathology of genetically engineered mice: definitions and classification. The consensus report from the Bar Harbor meeting of the Mouse Models of Human Cancer Consortium Prostate Pathology Committee. Cancer Res 2004;64:2270–305.

[136] Rangarajan A, Weinberg RA. Opinion: Comparative biology of mouse versus human cells: modelling human cancer in mice. Nat Rev Cancer 2003;3:952–9.

[137] Abate-Shen C, Shen MM. Mouse models of prostate carcinogenesis. Trends Genet: TIG 2002;18:S1–5.

[138] Powell WC, Cardiff RD, Cohen MB, Miller GJ, Roy-Burman P. Mouse strains for prostate tumorigenesis based on genes altered in human prostate cancer. Curr Drug Targets 2003;4:263–79.

[139] Ousset M, Van Keymeulen A, Bouvencourt G, et al. Multipotent and unipotent progenitors contribute to prostate postnatal development. Nat Cell Biol 2012;14:1131–8.

[140] Greenberg NM, DeMayo FJ, Sheppard PC, et al. The rat probasin gene promoter directs hormonally and developmentally regulated expression of a heterologous gene specifically to the prostate in transgenic mice. Mol Endocrinol 1994;8:230–9.

[141] Liu G, Sprenger C, Sun S, et al. AR variant ARv567es induces carcinogenesis in a novel transgenic mouse model of prostate cancer. Neoplasia 2013;15:1009–17.

[142] Vis AN, Schroder FH. Key targets of hormonal treatment of prostate cancer. Part 1: the androgen receptor and steroidogenic pathways. BJU international 2009;104:438–48.

[143] Stanbrough M, Leav I, Kwan PW, Bubley GJ, Balk SP. Prostatic intraepithelial neoplasia in mice expressing an androgen receptor transgene in prostate epithelium. Proc Nat Acad Sci USA 2001;98:10823–8.

[144] Albertelli MA, Scheller A, Brogley M, Robins DM. Replacing the mouse androgen receptor with human alleles demonstrates glutamine tract length-dependent effects on physiology and tumorigenesis in mice. Mol Endocrinol (Baltimore, Md) 2006;20:1248–60.

[145] O'Mahony OA, Steinkamp MP, Albertelli MA, Brogley M, Rehman H, Robins DM. Profiling human androgen receptor mutations reveals treatment effects in a mouse model of prostate cancer. Mol Cancer Res: MCR 2008;6:1691–701.

[146] Thin TH, Wang L, Kim E, Collins LL, Basavappa R, Chang C. Isolation and characterization of androgen receptor mutant, AR(M749L), with hypersensitivity to 17-beta estradiol treatment. J Biol Chem 2003;278:7699–708.

[147] Greenberg NM, DeMayo F, Finegold MJ, et al. Prostate cancer in a transgenic mouse. Proc Nat Acad Sci USA 1995;92:3439–43.

[148] Gingrich JR, Barrios RJ, Morton RA, et al. Metastatic prostate cancer in a transgenic mouse. Cancer Res 1996;56:4096–102.

[149] Kasper S, Sheppard PC, Yan Y, et al. Development, progression, and androgen-dependence of prostate tumors in probasin-large T antigen transgenic mice: a model for prostate cancer. Lab Invest J Tech Methods Pathol 1998;78:i–xv.

[150] Klezovitch O, Chevillet J, Mirosevich J, Roberts RL, Matusik RJ, Vasioukhin V. Hepsin promotes prostate cancer progression and metastasis. Cancer Cell 2004;6:185–95.

[151] Chiaverotti T, Couto SS, Donjacour A, et al. Dissociation of epithelial and neuroendocrine carcinoma lineages in the transgenic adenocarcinoma of mouse prostate model of prostate cancer. Am J Pathol 2008;172:236–46.

[152] Wada S, Jackson CM, Yoshimura K, et al. Sequencing CTLA-4 blockade with cell-based immunotherapy for prostate cancer. J Transl Med 2013;11:89.

[153] Mueller M, Reichardt W, Koerner J, Groettrup M. Coencapsulation of tumor lysate and CpG-ODN in PLGA-microspheres enables successful immunotherapy of prostate carcinoma in TRAMP mice. J Control Release 2012;162:159–66.

[154] Kang BH, Tavecchio M, Goel HL, et al. Targeted inhibition of mitochondrial Hsp90 suppresses localised and metastatic prostate cancer growth in a genetic mouse model of disease. Br J Cancer 2011;104:629–34.

[155] Zierhut ML, Yen YF, Chen AP, et al. Kinetic modeling of hyperpolarized 13C1-pyruvate metabolism in normal rats and TRAMP mice. J Magn Reson 2010;202:85–92.

[156] Young JG, Green NK, Mautner V, Searle PF, Young LS, James ND. Combining gene and immunotherapy for prostate cancer. Prostate Cancer Prostatic Dis 2008;11:187–93.

[157] Qian DZ, Wei YF, Wang X, Kato Y, Cheng L, Pili R. Antitumor activity of the histone deacetylase inhibitor MS-275 in prostate cancer models. The Prostate 2007;67:1182–93.

[158] Bao Y, Peng W, Verbitsky A, et al. Human coxsackie adenovirus receptor (CAR) expression in transgenic mouse prostate tumors enhances adenoviral delivery of genes. The Prostate 2005;64:401–7.

[159] Huss WJ, Lai L, Barrios RJ, Hirschi KK, Greenberg NM. Retinoic acid slows progression and promotes apoptosis of spontaneous prostate cancer. The Prostate 2004;61:142–52.

[160] Martiniello-Wilks R, Dane A, Mortensen E, Jeyakumar G, Wang XY, Russell PJ. Application of the transgenic adenocarcinoma mouse prostate (TRAMP) model for pre-clinical therapeutic studies. Anticancer Res 2003;23:2633–42.

[161] Kaplan-Lefko PJ, Chen TM, Ittmann MM, et al. Pathobiology of autochthonous prostate cancer in a pre-clinical transgenic mouse model. The Prostate 2003;55:219–37.

[162] Ahuja D, Saenz-Robles MT, Pipas JM. SV40 large T antigen targets multiple cellular pathways to elicit cellular transformation. Oncogene 2005;24:7729–45.

[163] Eastham JA, Stapleton AM, Gousse AE, et al. Association of p53 mutations with metastatic prostate cancer. Clin Cancer Res: An Off J Am Assoc Cancer Res 1995;1:1111–8.

[164] Kallakury BV, Figge J, Ross JS, Fisher HA, Figge HL, Jennings TA. Association of p53 immunoreactivity with high gleason tumor grade in prostatic adenocarcinoma. Human Pathol 1994;25:92–7.

[165] Effert PJ, Neubauer A, Walther PJ, Liu ET. Alterations of the P53 gene are associated with the progression of a human prostate carcinoma. J Urol 1992;147:789–93.

[166] Meyers FJ, Gumerlock PH, Chi SG, Borchers H, Deitch AD, deVere White RW. Very frequent p53 mutations in metastatic prostate carcinoma and in matched primary tumors. Cancer 1998;83:2534–9.

[167] Jarrard DF, Sarkar S, Shi Y, et al. p16/pRb pathway alterations are required for bypassing senescence in human prostate epithelial cells. Cancer Res 1999;59:2957–64.

[168] Tan HL, Sood A, Rahimi HA, et al. Rb loss is characteristic of prostatic small cell neuroendocrine carcinoma. Clin Cancer Res: An Off J Am Assoc Cancer Res 2014;20:890–903.

[169] Tricoli JV, Gumerlock PH, Yao JL, et al. Alterations of the retinoblastoma gene in human prostate adenocarcinoma. Genes Chromosomes Cancer 1996;15:108–14.

[170] Kubota Y, Fujinami K, Uemura H, et al. Retinoblastoma gene mutations in primary human prostate cancer. The Prostate 1995;27:314–20.

[171] Brooks JD, Bova GS, Isaacs WB. Allelic loss of the retinoblastoma gene in primary human prostatic adenocarcinomas. The Prostate 1995;26:35–9.

[172] Bookstein R, Rio P, Madreperla SA, et al. Promoter deletion and loss of retinoblastoma gene expression in human prostate carcinoma. Proc Nat Acad Sci USA 1990;87:7762–6.

[173] Fliss AE, Rao J, Melville MW, Cheetham ME, Caplan AJ. Domain requirements of DnaJ-like (Hsp40) molecular chaperones in the activation of a steroid hormone receptor. J Biol Chem 1999;274:34045–52.

[174] Terada K, Yomogida K, Imai T, et al. A type I DnaJ homolog, DjA1, regulates androgen receptor signaling and spermatogenesis. EMBO J 2005;24:611–22.

[175] Caplan AJ, Langley E, Wilson EM, Vidal J. Hormone-dependent transactivation by the human androgen receptor is regulated by a dnaJ protein. J Biol Chem 1995;270:5251–7.

[176] Heemers HV, Sebo TJ, Debes JD, et al. Androgen deprivation increases p300 expression in prostate cancer cells. Cancer Res 2007;67:3422–30.

[177] Xi Y, Chen Y. Oncogenic and therapeutic targeting of PTEN loss in bone malignancies. J Cell Biochem 2015;116:1837–47.

[178] Dean JL, Knudsen KE. The role of tumor suppressor dysregulation in prostate cancer progression. Curr Drug Targets 2013;14:460–71.

[179] Nardella C, Carracedo A, Alimonti A, et al. Differential requirement of mTOR in postmitotic tissues and tumorigenesis. Sci Signal 2009;2:ra2.

[180] Lei Q, Jiao J, Xin L, et al. NKX3.1 stabilizes p53, inhibits AKT activation, and blocks prostate cancer initiation caused by PTEN loss. Cancer Cell 2006;9:367–78.

[181] Zhao H, Dupont J, Yakar S, Karas M, LeRoith D. PTEN inhibits cell proliferation and induces apoptosis by downregulating cell surface IGF-IR expression in prostate cancer cells. Oncogene 2004;23:786–94.

[182] Wu X, Senechal K, Neshat MS, Whang YE, Sawyers CL. The PTEN/MMAC1 tumor suppressor phosphatase functions as a negative regulator of the phosphoinositide 3-kinase/Akt pathway. Proc Nat Acad Sci USA 1998;95:15587–91.

[183] Yoshimoto M, Cutz JC, Nuin PA, et al. Interphase FISH analysis of PTEN in histologic sections shows genomic deletions in 68% of primary prostate cancer and 23% of high-grade prostatic intra-epithelial neoplasias. Cancer Genet Cytogenet 2006;169:128–37.

[184] Holcomb IN, Young JM, Coleman IM, et al. Comparative analyses of chromosome alterations in soft-tissue metastases within and across patients with castration-resistant prostate cancer. Cancer Res 2009;69:7793–802.

[185] Podsypanina K, Ellenson LH, Nemes A, et al. Mutation of Pten/Mmac1 in mice causes neoplasia in multiple organ systems. Proc Nat Acad Sci USA 1999;96:1563–8.

[186] Di Cristofano A, Pesce B, Cordon-Cardo C, Pandolfi PP. Pten is essential for embryonic development and tumour suppression. Nat Genet 1998;19:348–55.

[187] Backman SA, Ghazarian D, So K, et al. Early onset of neoplasia in the prostate and skin of mice with tissue-specific deletion of Pten. Proc Nat Acad Sci USA 2004;101:1725–30.

[188] Stambolic V, Tsao MS, Macpherson D, Suzuki A, Chapman WB, Mak TW. High incidence of breast and endometrial neoplasia resembling human Cowden syndrome in pten$^{+/-}$ mice. Cancer Res 2000;60:3605–11.

[189] Di Cristofano A, De Acetis M, Koff A, Cordon-Cardo C, Pandolfi PP. Pten and p27KIP1 cooperate in prostate cancer tumor suppression in the mouse. Nat Genet 2001;27:222–4.

[190] Kim MJ, Cardiff RD, Desai N, et al. Cooperativity of Nkx3.1 and Pten loss of function in a mouse model of prostate carcinogenesis. Proc Nat Acad Sci USA 2002;99:2884–9.

[191] Abate-Shen C, Banach-Petrosky WA, Sun X, et al. Nkx3.1; Pten mutant mice develop invasive prostate adenocarcinoma and lymph node metastases. Cancer Res 2003;63:3886–90.

[192] Wang S, Gao J, Lei Q, et al. Prostate-specific deletion of the murine Pten tumor suppressor gene leads to metastatic prostate cancer. Cancer Cell 2003;4:209–21.

[193] Zhang W, Zhu J, Efferson CL, et al. Inhibition of tumor growth progression by antiandrogens and mTOR inhibitor in a Pten-deficient mouse model of prostate cancer. Cancer Res 2009;69:7466–72.

[194] Ma X, Ziel-van der Made AC, Autar B, et al. Targeted biallelic inactivation of Pten in the mouse prostate leads to prostate cancer accompanied by increased epithelial cell proliferation but not by reduced apoptosis. Cancer Res 2005;65:5730–9.

[195] Ratnacaram CK, Teletin M, Jiang M, Meng X, Chambon P, Metzger D. Temporally controlled ablation of PTEN in adult mouse prostate epithelium generates a model of invasive prostatic adenocarcinoma. Proc Nat Acad Sci USA 2008;105:2521–6.

[196] Floc'h N, Kinkade CW, Kobayashi T, et al. Dual targeting of the Akt/mTOR signaling pathway inhibits castration-resistant prostate cancer in a genetically engineered mouse model. Cancer Res 2012;72:4483–93.

[197] Moore RA. The evolution and involution of the prostate gland. Am J Pathol 1936;12:599–624.

[198] Lin PH, Aronson W, Freedland SJ. Nutrition, dietary interventions and prostate cancer: the latest evidence. BMC Med 2015;13:3.

[199] Cowey S, Hardy RW. The metabolic syndrome: a high-risk state for cancer? Am J Pathol 2006;169:1505–22.

[200] McMillan DC, Sattar N, McArdle CS. ABC of obesity. Obes Cancer. BMJ 2006;333:1109–11.

[201] Llaverias G, Danilo C, Wang Y, et al. A Western-type diet accelerates tumor progression in an autochthonous mouse model of prostate cancer. Am J Pathol 2010;177:3180–91.

[202] Chang SN, Han J, Abdelkader TS, et al. High animal fat intake enhances prostate cancer progression and reduces glutathione peroxidase 3 expression in early stages of TRAMP mice. The Prostate 2014;74:1266–77.

[203] Venkateswaran V, Klotz LH. Diet and prostate cancer: mechanisms of action and implications for chemoprevention. Nat Rev Urol 2010;7:442–53.

[204] Khandrika L, Kumar B, Koul S, Maroni P, Koul HK. Oxidative stress in prostate cancer. Cancer Lett 2009;282:125–36.

[205] Yu YP, Yu G, Tseng G, et al. Glutathione peroxidase 3, deleted or methylated in prostate cancer, suppresses prostate cancer growth and metastasis. Cancer Res 2007;67:8043–50.

[206] Zhang S, Yang C, Yang Z, et al. Homeostasis of redox status derived from glucose metabolic pathway could be the key to understanding the Warburg effect. Am J Cancer Res 2015;5:928–44.

[207] Paschos A, Pandya R, Duivenvoorden WC, Pinthus JH. Oxidative stress in prostate cancer: changing research concepts towards a novel paradigm for prevention and therapeutics. Prostate Cancer Prostatic Dis 2013;16:217–25.

[208] Chetram MA, Bethea DA, Odero-Marah VA, Don-Salu-Hewage AS, Jones KJ, Hinton CV. ROS-mediated activation of AKT induces apoptosis via pVHL in prostate cancer cells. Mol Cell Biochem 2013;376:63–71.

[209] Weinberg F, Hamanaka R, Wheaton WW, et al. Mitochondrial metabolism and ROS generation are essential for Kras-mediated tumorigenicity. Proc Nat Acad Sci USA 2010;107:8788–93.

[210] Yang S, Chintapalli J, Sodagum L, et al. Activated IGF-1R inhibits hyperglycemia-induced DNA damage and promotes DNA repair by homologous recombination. Am J Physiol Renal Phys 2005;289:F1144–52.

[211] Feig DI, Loeb LA. Mechanisms of mutation by oxidative DNA damage: reduced fidelity of mammalian DNA polymerase beta. Biochemistry 1993;32:4466–73.

Chapter 9

Reconsideration of Hormonal Therapy in the Era of Next-Generation Hormonal Therapy

Yasuyoshi Miyata, Yohei Shida, Tomohiro Matsuo,
Tomoaki Hakariya and Hideki Sakai

Additional information is available at the end of the chapter

http://dx.doi.org/10.5772/63282

Abstract

Hormonal therapy is a major and effective tool in the treatment of prostate cancer patients. This is especially true for patients in the advanced stages of disease. Unfortunately, almost all prostate cancer cells will develop into castration-resistant prostate cancer (CRPC) despite continued therapy and suppression of testosterone levels. Up until 5–6 years ago, there was little effective therapy for the treatment of CRPC patients. However, recently, a variety of methodologies and drugs such as cabazitaxel and sipuleucel-T have been approved globally for the treatment of CRPC. Two novel drugs, abiraterone acetate and enzartamide, have also become available as potential treatment options. However, the anticancer effects of these two drugs are not always satisfactory in terms of prolonging survival. These drugs are also associated with adverse events and are expensive when compared with the costs of previously used anticancer drugs. In this section, we pay particular attention to hormonal therapies that do not include the use of abiraterone acetate or enzartamide. We believe that a detailed understanding of the range of currently available hormonal therapies, including their associated benefits and limitations, is important for supporting the prolongation of survival in patients with advanced prostate cancer. Therefore, this section offers a valuable discussion on the treatment strategies for prostate cancer including CRPC.

Keywords: steroidal antiandrogens, nonsteroidal anti-androgens, estrogens, steroids, castration-resistant prostate cancer

1. Introduction

Prostate cancer is one of the most common malignancies diagnosed worldwide in men. At present, prostate cancer patients with organ-confined disease can obtain an excellent oncological outcome through radical operation and radiotherapy. On the other hand, a variety of hormonal therapies are often necessitated for patients with advanced prostate cancer. Because the malignant aggressiveness of prostate cancer has been known to be suppressed by orchiectomy since the 1940s, androgen deprivation therapy (ADT) has been commonly administered. This is associated with the fact that the prostate is an androgen-dependent organ and that androgen receptor (AR) signaling plays an important role in the growth and progression of prostate cancer cells. In fact, as a first-line therapy, surgical castration, chemical castration, and anti-androgen treatment are usually used in the treatment of patients with metastatic prostate cancer [1]. Anti-androgens are broadly divided into two chemical types, steroidal and nonsteroidal. As a part of hormone therapy, estrogen and estrogen-containing agents can also be administered to patients with prostate cancer. A variety of glucocorticoids is also commonly used.

However, most hormone-naive prostate cancer patients will develop castration-resistant prostate cancer (CRPC) despite therapeutic suppression of testosterone levels and even though continued therapy can proceed without adverse effects. Furthermore, CRPC has a high malignant potential and aggressiveness. This is due to the number of heterogeneous types of cancer cells that develop a variety of abnormal signal pathways as a means to survive in the castration environment. In fact, the prognosis of patients with CRPC is often poor and no therapy that had high efficacy and high compliance had been available until the middle of the 2000s. In 2004, two clinical trials with large study populations and sophisticated methodologies demonstrated that the anticancer effects of docetaxel-based chemotherapy are superior to those of mitoxantrone and prednisolone treatments [2, 3]. Based on these facts, docetaxel has become a standard therapy for the treatment of CRPC. However, prolongation of survival by docetaxel chemotherapy is less than six months [4]. Additionally, docetaxel has major problems related to multiple and severe adverse events [3, 5]. Consequently, many urologists, physicians, and investigators have focused on the development of new therapeutic strategies to prolong survival in CRPC patients.

During the past 5–6 years, a variety of treatment methods and drugs for CRPC have been approved in many countries. Approved drugs include cabazitaxel and sipuleucel-T [6, 7]. In addition, ADT options for patients with CRPC have also changed during the past few years as the novel drugs, abiraterone acetate and enzartamide (termed as next-generation anti-androgens) have become available [8, 9]. Abiraterone is a specific steroidogenic inhibitor that irreversibly inhibits CYP17A1 [10]. Enzalutamide is an anti-androgen-receptor inhibitor that has been shown to improve prognosis in patients with CRPC [11]. Thus, many urologists and medical oncologists agree that treatment strategies for patients with CRPC are developing remarkably well [12]. However, the anticancer effects, including prolongation of patient survival, associated with these new treatments are not always adequate. For example, CRPC develops resistance to these second-generation agents quickly and thus the anticancer effects of abiraterone acetate and enzartamide can be decreased [13, 14].

Thus, although a variety of new anticancer agents have been developed, their anticancer effects in CRPC patients are not always satisfactory, particularly in terms of prolonging patient survival. In addition, CRPC patients often have many comorbidities due to past treatments and aging. Therefore, in discussions on treatment strategies for prostate cancer patients, it is essential to assess information regarding drug adverse reactions and safety. In addition, special attention must be paid to the cost of therapies as treatment periods are usually lengthy, and recently developed anticancer agents, including next-generation anti-androgens, are expensive. Based on these facts, we present in this chapter, the clinical benefits, safety, and caution points of hormonal therapies that do not involve next-generation antiandrogens. In other words, we will re-evaluate hormonal therapy for treatment of prostate cancer patients in the era of next-generation antiandrogen agents.

2. Antiandrogen agents

As mentioned earlier, prostate cancer cells are, in the majority of cases, androgen-dependent. Testosterone, of testicular origin, comprises 95% of androgen content. Androgens stimulate cell proliferation and tumor growth by binding to AR in the cancer cells. Therefore, the first-line of treatment for advanced prostate cancer has been androgen deprivation by medical castration through administration of luteinizing hormone-releasing hormone agonist/antagonists or by surgical castration with bilateral orchiectomy. Antiandrogens are AR receptor antagonists that compete with dihydroteststerone for AR binding. Upon binding, the antiandrogens act to inhibit the tumor growth in patients with prostate cancer. This section reviews first-generation antiandrogens used in the treatment of prostate cancer including CRPC.

2.1. Steroidal antiandrogens

Antiandrogens can be classified based on their chemical structure into two types, steroidal and nonsteroidal. The steroidal antiandrogens, cyproterone acetate, spironolactone, synthetic progestins, and chlormadinone acetate are well known in oncology. We first discuss the steroidal antiandrogens, progesterone analogue mifepristone (RU-486), cyproterone acetate, and the mineralocorticoid analogue, spironolactone. However, it should be noted that these agents are rarely used in clinical situations because of their partial androgenic agonistic–antagonistic activity.

RU-486 is a progesterone analogue best known as a progesterone receptor (PR) antagonist. It was developed in France as a medical approach to terminating pregnancy [15]. RU-486 also inhibits glucocorticoid receptor (GR) function and has been used for treating Cushing syndrome [16]. More importantly, RU-486 is also an AR antagonist. Binding studies indicate that it has a higher affinity for AR than either hydroxyflutamide or bicalutamide [17]. However, a Phase II study of RU-486 demonstrated limited activity in patients with CRPC. In that study,

RU-486 also stimulated a marked increase in the levels of adrenal androgens, testosterone, and dihydrotestosterone (DHT) [18].

Cyproterone acetate is nonspecific and can activate the mineralocorticoid receptor (MR), GR, and PR. A meta-analysis of randomized trials showed that combined androgen blockade (CAB) with nonsteroidal antiandrogens, including nilutamide and flutamide, appeared slightly favorable to cancer patient survival when compared with the effects of androgen suppression (AS) monotherapy. On the other hand, CAB with cyproterone acetate was associated with an inferior survival rate [19].

Spironolactone is an MR antagonist that is used to treat side effects related to mineralocorticoid excess. Richards et al. [20] showed that spironolactone significantly activates both wild type and mutant AR and that it should be avoided in the treatment of all patients with CRPC. As a result, CAB with steroidal antiandrogens has been recognized as an inferior treatment to the use of nonsteroidal antiandrogens and is considered unsuitable for prostate cancer treatment.

2.1.1. Steroidal antiandrogens in Japan

Cyproterone acetate, RU-486, and nilutamide are not approved in Japan for use in the treatment of patients with prostate cancer. On the other hand, chlormadinone acetate is approved in Japan but is not used in other countries. Evaluation of the relative efficacy and safety of these agents globally is therefore difficult. However, chlormadinone acetate has been reported to have advantages in terms of causing fewer adverse events. We therefore present information regarding chlormadinone acetate in this section.

Several Japanese groups have reported on the efficacy of chlormadinone acetate as an alternative antiandrogen therapy in the treatment of men with relapsed prostate cancer following first- or second-line hormonal therapy [21–23]. Steroidal antiandrogens including cyproterone acetate and chlormadinone acetate have also proven efficacious in the treatment of prostate cancer patients who suffer from hot flushes [24, 25]. However, Igawa et al. [26] reported that CAB therapy using chlormadinone acetate led to a significantly poorer survival outcome versus the use of bicalutamide. Nevertheless, because this survival trend was not observed in M0 cases, they concluded that chlormadinone acetate might still be an option for CAB therapy, depending on the clinical stage and the severity of adverse effects including hot flushes [26].

2.1.2. Clinical study and basic research

Ongoing clinical studies and basic research using chlormadinone are presented in **Table 1**. There has been at least one evaluation on whether low-dose chlormadinone has an effect on continued active surveillance (**Table 1**, No.1; UMIN000012284). Another study has evaluated whether chlormadinone has a more favorable effect on lipid and bone metabolism than that of bicalutamide (No.2; UMIN000018478). In terms of basic research, Koike et al. [27] have reported on the effects of chlormadinone acetate on the development and progression of prostate cancer in their *PTEN*-deficient mouse model (**Table 1**, No. 3). They demonstrated that chlormadinone acetate treatment suppressed the proliferation of cancer cells but did not decrease the development of prostatic intraepithelial neoplasia (PIN). This means that chlormadinone did not act to prevent prostate cancer onset. The findings from this study suggest that inhibiting androgen signaling is effective in preventing the proliferation of prostate cancer caused by PTEN dysfunction. It has also been suggested that androgen plays an important role at the early stages of prostate cancer development in this mouse model [27].

	Clinical study	
No	**Concept and outline**	**Objectives**
1	Multicenter, randomized, double blind, placebo-controlled parallel group comparative study to evaluate the effect of low-dose chlormadinone acetate on the rate of continued active surveillance of patients with low-risk prostate cancer	To evaluate the effect of chlormadinone acetate on the rate of continued active surveillance by administration of low-dose chlormadinone acetate or placebo to patients with low-risk prostate cancer
2	Impact of endocrine therapy on lipid metabolism and bone metabolism of prostate cancer patients Comparison with chlormadinone acetate and bicalutamide	To investigate the effect of chlormadinone acetate and GnRH agonist combination therapy or bicalutamide and GnRH agonist combination therapy for prostate cancer men on lipid metabolism and bone metabolism
Basic research		
3	Conditional *PTEN*-deficient Mice as a Prostate Cancer Chemoprevention Model [27]	The potential of *PTEN*-deficient mice was examined by evaluating the chemopreventive efficacy of the anti-androgen, chlormadinone acetate

Table 1. Clinical studies and basic research on chlorm.

2.2. Nonsteroidal antiandrogens

The nonsteroidal antiandrogens, flutamide and bicalutamide, are well known in oncology and are major therapeutic tools in the treatment of prostate cancer patients. Therefore, information on their anticancer effects, including causation of decreases in serum prostate-specific antigen (PSA) levels and enhanced survival rates, has been presented in numerous reviews. There is also a corresponding amount of literature on their adverse effects. Here, we introduce the clinical benefits and limitations of nonsteroidal antiandrogens in the treatment of CRPC patients.

2.2.1. Optional treatment for castration-resistant prostate cancer

Bicalutamide is the most common used steroidal antiandrogen due to its good curative effects and limited adverse effects. It is combined with luteinizing hormone-releasing hormone agonist/antagonist therapy to treat CRPC. Some researchers have indicated that dose elevation of antiandrogen agents may enhance their efficacy. For example, the routine dose of bicalutamide is 50 mg/day but evidence suggests that higher doses might be more effective [28]. Klotz et al. [29] reported that 22% of the patients showed a ≥50% decline in serum PSA levels following an increase in the dose of bicalutamide from 50 mg/day to 150 mg/day. Lodde et al. [30] reported the palliative benefits of 150 mg/day bicalutamide therapy in 44.7% of 38 CRPC nonmetastasis patients. These studies therefore demonstrate that a high proportion of CRPC patients could benefit from treatments involving elevated doses of steroidal antiandrogens. Available data also indicate that bicalutamide at a dose of much greater than 50 mg (at least 150 mg) daily in combination with castration may increase efficacy against CRPC progression. However, in all these studies earlier, either the median response duration is brief or the evaluation indices are limited.

Meanwhile, potential predictive factors for improved responses to high-dose (150 mg) bicalutamide therapy have been discussed. Qian et al. [28] suggested that secondary hormonal therapy with 150 mg bicalutamide daily was effective in patients with CRPC. Patients with a lower Gleason score, lower serum PSA concentrations, and who were using flutamide as a first-line nonsteroidal antiandrogen achieved more benefits when treated with bicalutamide 150 mg therapy. Patients with PSA decreases ≥85% had improved times of response to bicalutamide 150 mg therapy. Moreover, when compared with the common side effects of androgen-deprivation therapy, the adverse effects of bicalutamide 150 mg therapy were well-tolerated.

2.2.2. Combination with molecular target drugs

Angiogenesis, mediated by the vascular endothelial growth factor receptor (VEGFR) pathway, may be a good target for treatment of prostate cancer; it has been implicated in both the development and progression of the disease [31–33]. Studies have found that median levels of plasma VEGF are significantly higher in patients with metastatic prostate cancer when compared with those with localized cancer and that elevated plasma and urine levels of VEGF may be independent negative prognostic factors [34–36]. These findings suggest that inhibiting the VEGFR pathway might be an effective approach in prostate cancer.

In addition, the mammalian target-of-rapamycin (mTOR) is a critical molecule in controlling the proliferation of tumor cells. It can be activated by mutation or activation of signaling molecules such as PI3K or Akt. Alterations in the PI3K/Akt/mTOR pathway play an important role in prostate cancer, and it is estimated that upregulation occurs in 30–50% of prostate cancer

http://dx.doi.org/10.5772/63282

cases [37]. Recently, clinical trials on the efficacy and tolerability of antiandrogen and molecular target combination therapy have been conducted (**Table 2**), but these have included only a small number of patients. Results have shown that neither the PSA-response rate nor the PSA-progression free survival is fully satisfactory. In addition, peculiar adverse events have been associated with molecular target agents. Hence, these therapies are not currently in practical use.

Year	Molecular target therapy	N	Phase	PSA-RR	PSA-PFS	Ref
2012	Everolimus: 10 mg	36	II	5.6%	8.7 wks.	[33]
2012	Sorafenib: 400 mg	39	II			[38]
2013	Ridaforolimus: 30 mg	12	–	36%	–	[39]
2014	Vandetanib: 300 mg	19	II	18%	3.16 mos.	[40]
2015	Pazopanib: 800 mg	13	II	17%	–	[41]

N, number of patients; PSA, prostate specific antigen; RR, response rates; Ref, references; wks, weeks; mos, months.

*PSA response was defined as ≥ 50% decline.

**PSA response was defined as ≥ 30% decline.

Table 2. Combination therapy of bicalutamide and molecular target therapy for castration-resistant prostate cancer.

3. Estrogens and estrogen-based therapy

It is well-known that estrogens carry a significant risk for cardiovascular events. Androgen deprivation therapy is therefore the first choice as primary therapy for advanced prostate cancer. However, many authors have now investigated the anticancer effects of diethylstilbestrol [42], transdermal estradiol [43], and more recently, oral ethinylestradiol [44, 45] in the treatment of CRPC as well as in the treatment of hormone-naive prostate cancer. These authors have concluded that estrogen therapy is still relevant and can induce PSA response (50% PSA decline) rates as high as 69.6% in CRPC patients. Moreover, estrogen therapy is associated with fewer of the toxicities associated with ADT. It can maintain bone mineral density, suppress hot flushes, and improve cognitive function and lipo-metabolism in castrated men.

Estrogens inhibit the hypothalamic–pituitary–testicular axis through negative feedback mechanisms. Moreover, estrogen administration can induce a decrease in the levels of adrenal androgens and testosterone produced by the Leydig cells of the testes [46]. A direct cytotoxic effect of estrogens on prostate cancer cells has not been fully investigated. However, there are some reports on their cytotoxic effects on *in vivo* and *in vitro* castrate xenograft models [47, 48].

3.1. Diethylstilbestrol

Diethylstilbestrol (DES) is a synthetic estrogen. In the 1940s, Huggins and Hodges [49] reported that DES suppressed the progression of prostate cancer. DES was then used as a first-line hormonal therapy for over 10 years in the treatment of prostate cancer patients. However, in 1970, increased mortality from cardiovascular and thromboembolic events associated with DES was reported in a prospective randomized controlled trial (VACURG study) [50]. Briefly, of the 1103 patients treated with DES (5 mg/daily) with no anticoagulation therapy, 17% of the patients died due to cardiovascular events (the mortality associated with cardiovascular event in the placebo group was 11.7%). Therefore, to suppress the risk of adverse events including cardiovascular disease, administration of lower doses of DES was investigated in clinical trials. However, although this approach significantly reduced cardiovascular morbidity, it was still higher than that associated with castration. For example, in the EORTC 30805 study, the cardiovascular mortality of the DES (1 mg/daily) and orchidectomy-alone groups was 14.8% and 8.3%, respectively [51]. Meanwhile, the cardiovascular toxicity of DES was significantly decreased by the use of anticoagulants such as warfarin or aspirin [52, 53]. From these facts, we note that DES treatment has a relatively high risk of cardiovascular events and that it must be used with anticoagulation therapy. On the other hand, we also understand that DES is one of the most effective and useful therapeutic options for prostate cancer patients as it can suppress cancer progression.

In terms of PSA response (>50% decline from baseline) to DES treatment in CRPC patients, approximately 40% patients were reported to be PSA responders [42, 54]. More recently, Wilkins et al. [55] disclosed results from a larger CRPC cohort (231 patients) treated with DES at a dose of 1–3 mg daily and with aspirin at 75 mg. They reported that the PSA response rate was 28.9% and that the median time to PSA progression was 4.6 months. These results cannot be considered satisfactory in terms of cancer control. However, interestingly, Wilkins et al. also reported that 18% of the patients showed an improvement in bone pain. Other investigators have also observed an improvement in certain types of pain in CRPC patients treated with DES [56]. Overall, DES remains a reasonable palliative option for patients with symptomatic CRPC even though its survival benefits may be limited. However, careful informed consent from the patients who are fully apprised of the cardiovascular risks associated with DES should be required.

3.2. Transdermal estradiol

As mentioned earlier, cardiovascular disease and thrombosis are the most dangerous adverse events associated with estrogen-based agents. In contrast to oral estrogens, parenterally administered estrogens do not increase liver protein synthesis and may be less prothrombotic [43]. In fact, in women who receive estrogen replacement therapy, the risk of cardiovascular events is increased with oral, but not transdermal, estradiol. There have been several informative studies about safety, potential side effects, and efficacy in the use of transdermal estradiol in the treatment of CRPC patients [43, 57]. In a Phase II study, CRPC patients suffering continued disease progression after primary hormonal therapy were treated with transdermal estradiol (0.6 mg per 24 h) [43]. Toxicity associated with the transdermal estradiol application was modest and no cardiovascular events occurred. In terms of cancer control, three of the 24 patients (12.5%) showed a PSA response. Another study analyzed the safety and efficacy of transdermal estradiol patch in the treatment of CRPC patients after ADT and chemotherapy

[57]. This study showed a PSA response rate of 10%. No cardiovascular events were observed. Thus, transdermal estrogen therapy was well-tolerated in the CRPC patients, and there were no significant cardiovascular complications. However, as with oral estradiol, the anticancer effects of transdermal estradiol appear to offer very limited survival benefit.

3.3. Ethinylestradiol

Treatment with ethinylestradiol was used in the 1980s as palliative therapy in patients with advanced prostate cancer. However, ethinylestradiol treatment has become less common since the development of newer treatment forms such as ADT [58]. On the other hand, one advantage of ethinylestradiol is that it is inexpensive. This is an important consideration in assessing treatment strategies. At present, ethinylestradiol is not used as a first-line hormonal therapy. However, it is still used as a second-line or a later option for CRPC patients [59]. Several investigators have reported on the efficacy and adverse events of ethinylestradiol in treatments of CRPC patients. For example, Onita et al. [60] reported that a decrease in serum PSA levels was seen in all 15 tested CRPC; 11 patients (73.3%) showed decreases of more than 50% without severe side effects. Other investigators have performed ethinylestradiol monotherapy at a dose of 1.5 mg/day for CRPC patients for whom more than one salvage therapy had not been effective [45]. In this retrospective study, the PSA response rate was 69.6%, and the median progression-free survival was estimated as 300 days. On the other hand, adverse events occurred in 3 of the 23 patients (13%). These adverse effects included elevation of liver enzymes, anorexia, and heart failure. Recently, results of a larger prospective study of ethinylestradiol monotherapy were reported [44]. In this study, 116 patients with metastatic CRPC were administered ethinylestradiol at a daily dose of 1 mg and with aspirin at a daily dose of 100 mg. A PSA response was observed in 79 patients (70.5%). PSA levels lower than 4 ng/mL in serum were observed in 24 patients (21.4%). Toxic adverse effects that required

	Year	N	Daily dose (mg)	PSA-RR (%)	PSA-PFS	Ref
Diethylstilbestrol	1998	21	1.0	42.9	–	[42]
Diethylstilbestrol	2000	34	1.0	NA	6 mos.	[54]
Diethylstilbestrol	2012	243	1.0–3.0	28.9	137 days	[55]
Trans. estradiol	2005	24	0.6	12.5	12 wks.	[56]
Trans. estradiol	2012	20	0.4	10.0	–	[57]
Ethinylestradiol	2003	10	1.0	90.0	12.0 mos	[59]
Ethinylestradiol	2009	18	1.0–3.0	73.3	15.0 mos	[60]
Ethinylestradiol	2010	24	1.5	69.6	300 days	[45]
Ethinylestradiol	2015	116	1.0	70.5	15.1 mos	[44]

N, number of patients; PSA, prostate specific antigen; RR, response rates; PFS, progression-free survival; Ref, references; mos, months; NA, not available; wks., weeks; Trans, transdermal.

*PSA response was defined as ≥50% decline.

Table 3. Summary of the anticancer effects in the studies of estrogens.

treatment cessation were described for 26 patients (23.2%). The main adverse effect requiring treatment cessation was thromboembolism (18 patients). Overall, however, no patient died as a result of treatment toxicity.

In addition to monotherapy, several clinical studies on combination therapies that include ethinylestradiol have been conducted. For example, in one small study, administration of 1 mg oral ethinylestradiol combined with lanreotide acetate (somatostatin analog) resulted in a decline in serum PSA levels of >50% in 9 out of the 10 CRPC patients (90%) [59]. Overall, administration of ethinylestradiol in CRPC cases resulted in a high percentage of PSA responses. The potential for cardiovascular toxicity could be managed through appropriate patient selection and concomitant anticoagulation therapy. A summary of the anticancer effects of estrogens is shown in **Table 3**.

4. Corticosteroids

Corticosteroids suppress the production of androgens from the adrenal gland through the regulation of the pituitary–adrenal axis. Consequently, corticosteroids can inhibit the malignant behavior and survival of prostate cancer cells. In addition to this indirect role, they are known to inhibit the growth of prostate cancer cells by interfering directly with a variety of cancer-related factors [61]. Recognizing this, corticosteroids have been used in cancer therapy for decades. They have been administered to prostate cancer patients both as a mono-therapy and in combination with other anticancer agents. Unfortunately, its anticancer effects, including prolongation of survival, are limited when used as a single agent [62]. In this section, we discuss corticosteroids in terms of their efficacy when used in combination therapy for the treatment of CRPC.

4.1. Which types of glucocorticoids are better?

A variety of glucocorticoids, including prednisone, prednisolone, hydrocortisone, and dexamethasone, have anticancer effects and associated clinical benefits for prostate cancer patients [63–65]. However, many investigators have suggested that their anticancer effects differ from each other. For example, the PSA response rates of prednisolone (5 mg × 2 =10 mg daily) and hydrocortisone (40 mg daily) administered to CRPC patients were reported to be 26% and 22%, respectively [66, 67]. In the case of prednisone, 34% of the patients had a decrease in PSA levels of more than 50% [64]. In the previous reports, PSA response rates associated with prednisone, prednisolone, and hydrocortisone treatments have ranged from 9 to 33% [68]. On the other hand, in the case of dexamethasone, decreases in PSA levels of ≥50% were detected in 50 of 102 (49%) of the CRPC patients treated at a dose of 0.5 mg daily [68]. Other investigators also reported a similar decrease in PSA levels in 61% of CRPC patients treated with dexamethasone at a dose of 1.5 mg or 2.25 mg daily [69]. Based on these reports, dexamethasone appears to have a significantly greater anticancer effect than other glucocorticoids [70]. However, one report indicated that dexamethasone at a dose of 1.5 mg daily showed a reduction of PSA levels of ≥50% in only 28% of the CRPC patients [70]. Thus, there is no general agreement on what specific glucocorticoid should be recommended for the treatment of CRPC patients. Recently, the first head-to-head clinical comparison of prednisolone versus dexamethasone as monotherapies in the treatment of CRPC patients was conducted [68]. In this study, patients were randomized, in a 1:1:1 ratio, between administration of intermittent dexamethasone (8 mg twice daily for 3 days every 3 weeks), daily dexamethasone (0.5 mg once daily), and prednisolone (5 mg twice daily). The intermittent dexamethasone treatment was terminated mid-study due to a lack of observed antitumor activity. Thus, comparisons of anticancer effects were conducted only between the daily dexamethasone and prednisolone treatments. A decrease in PSA levels of ≥50% was detected in 16 of 39 (41%) of the dexamethasone-treated patients and in 8 of 36 (22%) prednisolone-treated patients. Although this difference did not approach statistical significance, the investigators concluded that dexamethasone might be a more effective treatment than prednisolone. Other investigators have supported this conclusion [70].

4.2. Combination with next-generation antiandrogens

One clinical study evaluated the anticancer effects and safety profile of abiraterone acetate when used in combination with prednisone as a means to suppress secondary mineralocorticoid excess [71]. Another study reported a reduction in the PSA levels >50% in CRPC patients treated with dexamethasone in addition to abiraterone acetate [71]. This report also demonstrated that the anticancer effects of combination therapy of abiraterone acetate and prednisone were detected regardless of prior dexamethasone exposure [71]. Furthermore, the PSA response rates, defined as a 50% or more reduction in PSA levels associated with dexamethasone and prednisolone were reported to be 47% and 24% ($P = 0.05$), respectively, in CRPC patients during a randomized Phase II trial [67]. Based on this, a hypothesis that a "steroid switch" from prednisone to dexamethasone would be effective in the treatment of CRPC patients with disease progression under abiraterone and prednisone treatment has been suggested [72]. In fact, one retrospective study of 30 CRPC patients who underwent such a "steroid switch" while abiraterone was administered, showed that durable PSA responses occurred in up to 40% of the patients [72]. In this study, the dosage of prednisolone or dexamethasone was 5 mg b.i.d and 0.5–1.0 mg daily.

4.3. Combination with immunotherapy

Sipuleucel-T is the recognized leading immunotherapeutic cancer vaccine (dendritic cell vaccine therapy). A variety of additional immunotherapeutic agents that can be used singly or combination therapy is currently under development. In fact, based on results from clinical trials, personalized peptide vaccination strategies that use multiple anticancer peptides has been reported to be effective and safe in CRPC patients [73, 74]. Several reports have also demonstrated that low-dose dexamethasone is a useful partner for personalized peptide vaccination in the treatment of CRPC. This is because dexamethasone does not suppress the immune system. Dexamethasone also exerts its anticancer effects in a direct manner as well as by reducing AR signaling [5, 75]. Recently, Phase II randomized controlled trials have demonstrated that immunotherapy that comprised personalized peptide vaccination and low-dose dexamethasone was well-tolerated in chemotherapy-naive CRPC patients and yielded a better outcome when compared to the effects of dexamethasone alone [76]. In short, progression-free survival periods, as evaluated by serum PSA responses, with peptide vaccine + dexamethasone (n = 37) and dexamethasone alone (n = 35) were 22.0 and 7.0 months (P = 0.076), respectively. In addition, the median overall survival in patients treated with peptide vaccine + dexamethasone (73.9 months) was significantly longer (P = 0.00084) than those treated with dexamethasone alone (34.9 month)

4.4. Modulatory approach for castration-resistant prostate cancer

Dexamethasone is often used as a component of modular therapy approaches in the treatment of CRPC. The aim of the modulatory approach is to inhibit the malignant activities of cancer and stroma cells through regulation of a variety of different pathological features including cancer-related molecules, angiogenesis, inflammation, and altered immune responses.

The effect of a modular therapy consisting of capecitabine, pioglitazone (PPARα/γ receptor agonist), refecoxib (or etoricoxib, a cyclooxygenase (COX)-2 inhibitor), and dexamethasone on 36 patients with metastatic CRPC was analyzed [77]. One half of treated patients (n = 18) showed a biochemical response defined as a ≥25% PSA decrease. Median periods of progression-free and overall survival were 4 and 14.4 months, respectively [77]. Results from a study on a modulatory therapy comprising imatinib (a platelet derived growth factor receptor (PDGFR) inhibitor), pioglitazone, etoricoxib, dexamethasone, and low-dose treosulfan have also been reported [78]. In that Phase II study, the anticancer effects and adverse events of the modular therapy were assessed in 61 CRPC patients. A total of the 23 patients (37.7%) were reported as PSA responders. Median progression-free survival period was approximately 15 months. However, all the patients experienced one or more adverse events and 27 patients (41.5%) had serious events. The most frequent adverse event was peripheral edema (56.9%). Nausea (38.5%), fatigue (35.4%), and dyspnea (35.4%) were also common occurrences. One of key characteristics of CRPC is its heterogeneity. Therefore, a variety of different approaches is essential in controlling tumor growth and progression. Based on this, modulatory therapy would appear to be a useful strategy. However, in general, this approach has been associated with a relatively high frequency of adverse events. In this section, we emphasized the importance of dexamethasone because of its anticancer effects as a GR agonist and its suppression of a variety of adverse events.

Author details

Yasuyoshi Miyata*, Yohei Shida, Tomohiro Matsuo, Tomoaki Hakariya and Hideki Sakai

*Address all correspondence to: int.doc.miya@m3.dion.ne.jp

Department of Urology, Nagasaki University Graduate School of Biomedical Sciences, Sakamoto, Nagasaki, Japan

References

[1] Singer EA, Golijanin DJ, Miyamoto H, Messing EM: Androgen deprivation therapy for prostate cancer. Opin Pharmacother. 2008;9:211–228. DOI: 10.1517/14656566.9.2.211 .

[2] Petrylak DP, Tangen CM, Hussain MH, Lara PN Jr, Jones JA, Taplin ME, Burch PA, Berry D, Moinpour C, Kohli M, Benson MC, Small EJ, Raghavan D, Crawford ED: Docetaxel and estramustine compared with mitoxantrone and prednisone for advanced refractory prostate cancer. N Engl J Med. 2004;351:1513–1520.

[3] Tannock IF, de Wit R, Berry WR, Horti J, Pluzanska A, Chi KN, Oudard S, Théodore C, James ND, Turesson I, Rosenthal MA, Eisenberger MA; TAX 327 Investigators: Docetaxel plus prednisone or mitoxantrone plus prednisone for advanced prostate cancer. N Engl J Med. 2004;351:1502–1512.

[4] Oudard S, Banu E, Beuzeboc P, Voog E, Dourthe LM, Hardy-Bessard AC, Linassier C, Scotté F, Banu A, Coscas Y, Guinet F, Poupon MF, Andrieu JM: Multicenter randomized phase II study of two schedules of docetaxel, estramustine, and prednisone versus mitoxantrone plus prednisone in patients with metastatic hormone-refractory prostate cancer. J Clin Oncol. 2005;23:3343–3351.

[5] Naito S, Tsukamoto T, Koga H, Harabayashi T, Sumiyoshi Y, Hoshi S, Akaza H: Docetaxel plus prednisolone for the treatment of metastatic hormone-refractory prostate cancer: a multicenter Phase II trial in Japan. Jpn J Clin Oncol. 2008;38:365–372. DOI: 10.1093/jjco/hyn029

[6] De Bono JS, Oudard S, Ozguroglu M, Hansen S, Machiels JP, Kocak I, Gravis G, Bodrogi I, Mackenzie MJ, Shen L, Roessner M, Gupta S, Sartor AO; TROPIC Investigators: Prednisone plus cabazitaxel or mitoxantrone for metastatic castration-resistant prostate cancer progressing after docetaxel treatment: a randomised open-label trial. Lancet. 2010;376:1147–1154. DOI: 10.1016/S0140-6736(10)61389-X.

[7] Kantoff PW, Halabi S, Conaway M, Picus J, Kirshner J, Hars V, Trump D, Winer EP, Vogelzang NJ: Hydrocortisone with or without mitoxantrone in men with hormone-refractory prostate cancer: results of the cancer and leukemia group B 9182 study. J Clin Oncol. 1999;17:2506–2513.

[8] Ryan CJ, Smith MR, de Bono JS, Molina A, Logothetis CJ, de Souza P, Fizazi K, Mainwaring P, Piulats JM, Ng S, Carles J, Mulders PF, Basch E, Small EJ, Saad F, Schrijvers D, Van Poppel H, Mukherjee SD, Suttmann H, Gerritsen WR, Flaig TW, George DJ, Yu EY, Efstathiou E, Pantuck A, Winquist E, Higano CS, Taplin ME, Park Y, Kheoh T, Griffin T, Scher HI, Rathkopf DE; COU-AA-302 Investigators: Abiraterone in metastatic prostate cancer without previous chemotherapy. N Engl J Med. 2013;368:138–148. DOI: 10.1016/S1470-2045(14)71205-7.

[9] Scher HI, Fizazi K, Saad F, Taplin ME, Sternberg CN, Miller K, de Wit R, Mulders P, Chi KN, Shore ND, Armstrong AJ, Flaig TW, Fléchon A, Mainwaring P, Fleming M,

Hainsworth JD, Hirmand M, Selby B, Seely L, de Bono JS; AFFIRM Investigators: Increased survival with enzalutamide in prostate cancer after chemotherapy. N Engl J Med. 2012;367:1187–1197.

[10] Jarman M, Barrie SE, Llera JM: The 16,17-double bond is needed for irreversible inhibition of human cytochrome p45017alpha by abiraterone (17-(3-pyridyl)androsta-5, 16-dien-3beta-ol) and related steroidal inhibitors. J Med Chem. 1998;41:5375–5381.

[11] Ramadan WH, Kabbara WK, Al Basiouni Al Masri HS: Enzalutamide for patients with metastatic castration-resistant prostate cancer. Onco Targets Ther. 2015;8:871–876. DOI: 10.2147/OTT.S80488.

[12] Recine F, Sternberg CN: Hormonal therapy and chemotherapy in hormone-naive and castration resistant prostate cancer. Transl Androl Urol 2015;4:355–364. DOI: 10.3978/j.issn.2223-4683.2015.04.11.

[13] Loriot Y, Bianchini D, Ileana E, Sandhu S, Patrikidou A, Pezaro C, Albiges L, Attard G, Fizazi K, De Bono JS, Massard C: Antitumour activity of abiraterone acetate against metastatic castration-resistant prostate cancer progressing after docetaxel and enzalutamide (MDV3100). Ann Oncol. 2013;24:1807–1812. DOI: 10.1093/annonc/mdt136.

[14] Schrader AJ, Boegemann M, Ohlmann CH, Schnoeller TJ, Krabbe LM, Hajili T, Jentzmik F, Stoeckle M, Schrader M, Herrmann E, Cronauer MV: Enzalutamide in castration-resistant prostate cancer patients progressing after docetaxel and abiraterone. Eur Urol. 2014;65:30–6. DOI: 10.1016/j.eururo.2013.06.042.

[15] Cadepond F, Ulmann A, Baulieu E: RU86 (Mifepristone): Mechanisms of action and clinical uses. Annual Review of Medicine. 1997;48:129–156. DOI: 10.1146/annurev.med.48.1.129.

[16] Chu J, Matthias D, Belanoff J et al. Successful long-term treatment of refractory Cushing's disease with high dose mifepristone (RU-46). J Clin Endocrinol Metab. 2001;86:3568–3573. DOI: http://dx.doi.org/10.1210/jcem.86.8.7740

[17] Song L, Coghlan M, Gelmann E. Antiandrogen effects of mifepristone on coactivator and corepressor interactions with the androgen receptor. Mol Endocrinol. 2004;18:70–85. DOI: http://dx.doi.org/10.1210/me.2003-0189.

[18] Taplin ME, Manola J, Oh WK et al. A phase II study of mifepristone (RU-486) in castration-resistant prostate cancer, with a correlative assessment of androgen-related hormones. BJU Int. 2008;101(9):1084–1089. DOI: 10.1111/j.1464-410X.2008.07509.x

[19] Prostate Cancer Trialists' Collaborative Group. Maximum androgen blockade in advanced prostate cancer: an overview of the randomised trials. THE LANCET. 2000;355(9214):1491–1498. DOI: 10.1016/S0140-6736(00)02163-2.

[20] Richards J, Lim AC, Hay CW et al. Interactions of abiraterone, eplerenone, and prednisolone with wild-type and mutant androgen receptor: a rationale for increasing

abiraterone exposure or combining with MDV3100. Cancer Res. 2012;72(9):2176–2182. DOI: 10.1158/0008-5472.CAN-11-3980.

[21] Kojima S, Suzuki H, Akakura K et al. Alternative antiandrogens to treat prostate cancer relapse after initial hormone therapy. J Urol. 2004;171:679–683. DOI: 10.1097/01.ju.0000106190.32540.6c

[22] Okihara K, Ukimura O, Kanemitsu N et al. Clinical efficacy of alternative antiandrogen therapy in Japanese men with relapsed prostate cancer after first-line hormonal therapy. Int Urol. 2007;14:128–132. DOI: 10.1111/j.1442-2042.2007.01698.x.

[23] Okegawa, T, Nutahara K, Higashihara E. Alternative antiandrogen therapy in patients with castration-resistant prostate cancer: a single-center experience. Int J Urol. 2010;17:950–955. DOI: 10.1111/j.1442-2042.2010.02620.x

[24] Sakai H, Igawa T, Tsurusaki T et al. Hot flashes during androgen deprivation therapy with luteinizing hormone-releasing hormone agonist combined with steroidal or nonsteroidal antiandrogen for prostate cancer. Urology. 2009;73(3):635–640. DOI: 10.1016/j.urology.2008.09.013

[25] Koike H, Morikawa Y, Matsui H et al. Chlormadinone acetate is effective for hot flush during androgen deprivation therapy. Prostate Int. 2013;1(3):113–116. DOI: http://dx.doi.org/10.12954/PI.12010

[26] Igawa T, Tsurusaki T, Nomata K et al. Oncological outcomes of hormonal therapy with a gonadotropin-releasing hormone agonist combined with a steroidal or non-steroidal antiandrogen in patients with prostate cancer. Anticancer Res. 2014; 34(4):1983–1988.

[27] Koike H, Nozawa M, De Velasco MA et al. Conditional *PTEN*-deficient mice as a prostate cancer chemoprevention model. Asian Pac J Cancer P. 2015;16:1827–1831. DOI: 10.7314/APJCP.2015.16.5.1827.

[28] Qian SB, Shen HB, Cao QF, Zhang L, Chen YF, Qi J. Bicalutamide 150 mg as secondary hormonal therapy for castration-resistant prostate cancer. Int Urol Nephrol. 2015;47:479–484. DOI: 10.1007/s11255-015-0919-y.

[29] Klotz L, Drachenberg D, Singal R, Aprikian A, Fradet Y, Kebabdjian M *et al.* An open-label, phase 2 trial of bicalutamide dose escalation from 50 mg to 150 mg in men with CAB and castration resistance. A Canadian Urology Research Consortium Study. Prostate Cancer Prostatic Dis. 2014;17:320–324.DOI: 10.1038.

[30] Lodde M, Lacombe L, Fradet Y. Salvage therapy with bicalutamide 150 mg in nonmetastatic castration-resistant prostate cancer. Urology. 2010;76:1189–1193. DOI: 10.1016.

[31] Ferrer FA, Miller LJ, Lindquist R, Kowalczyk P, Laudone VP, Albertsen PC *et al.* Expression of vascular endothelial growth factor receptors in human prostate cancer. Urology 1999;54:567–572. PubMed PMID: 10475375.

[32] Weidner N, Carroll PR, Flax J, Blumenfeld W, Folkman J. Tumor angiogenesis correlates with metastasis in invasive prostate carcinoma. Am J Pathol 1993; 143: 401–409. PubMed PMID: 7688183; PubMed Central PMCID: PMC1887042.

[33] Nakabayashi M, Werner L, Courtney KD, Buckle G, Oh WK, Bubley GJ *et al.* Phase II trial of RAD001 and bicalutamide for castration-resistant prostate cancer. BJU Int. 2012;110:1729–1735. doi: 10.1111/j.1464-410X.2012.11456.x

[34] Duque JL, Loughlin KR, Adam RM, Kantoff PW, Zurakowski D, Freeman MR. Plasma levels of vascular endothelial growth factor are increased in patients with metastatic prostate cancer. Urology 1999; 54:523–527. PubMed PMID: 10475365.

[35] George DJ, Halabi S, Shepard TF, Vogelzang NJ, Hayes DF, Small EJ *et al*. Prognostic significance of plasma vascularendothelial growth factor levels in patients with hormone-refractory prostate cancer treated on Cancer and Leukemia Group B 9480. Clin Cancer Res 2001;7:1932–1936. PubMed PMID: 11448906.

[36] Bok RA, Halabi S, Fei DT, Rodriquez CR, Hayes DF, Vogelzang NJ *et al.* Vascular endothelial growth factor and basic fibroblast growth factor urine levels as predictors of outcome in hormone-refractory prostate cancer patients: a Cancer and Leukemia Group B study. Cancer Res 2001;61:2533–2536. PubMed PMID: 11289126

[37] Morgan TM, Koreckij TD, Corey E. Targeted therapy for advanced prostate cancer: inhibition of the PI3K/Akt/mTOR pathway. Curr Cancer Drug Targets. 2009;9:237–249. PubMed PMID: 19275762; PubMed Central PMCID: PMC2921605.

[38] Beardsley EK, Hotte SJ, North S, Ellard SL, Winquist E, Kollmannsberger C *et al.* A phase II study of sorafenib in combination with bicalutamide in patients with chemotherapy-naive castration resistant prostate cancer. Invest New Drugs. 2012;30:1652–1659. doi:10.1007/s10637-011-9722-5.

[39] Meulenbeld HJ, de Bono JS, Tagawa ST, Whang YE, Li X, Heath KH *et al.* Tolerability, safety and pharmacokinetics of ridaforolimus in combination with bicalutamide in patients with asymptomatic, metastatic castration resistant prostate cancer (CRPC). Cancer Chemother Pharmacol. 2013;72:909–916. doi: 10.1007/s00280-013-2250-6.

[40] Azad AA, Beardsley EK, Hotte SJ, Ellard SL, Klotz L, Chin J *et al.* A randomized phase II efficacy and safety study of vandetanib (ZD6474) in combination with bicalutamide versus bicalutamide alone in patients with chemotherapy naïve castration-resistant prostate cancer. Invest New Drugs. 2014;32:746–752. doi: 10.1007/s10637-014-0091-8.

[41] Sridhar SS, Joshua AM, Gregg R, Booth CM, Murray N, Golubovic J *et al.* A phase II study of GW786034 (pazopanib) with or without bicalutamide in patients with castration-resistant prostate cancer. Clin Genitourin Cancer. 2015;13:124-129. doi: 10.1016/j.clgc.2014.06.001.

[42] Smith DC, Redman BG, Flaherty LE, Li L, Strawderman M and Pienta KJ: A phase II trial of oral diethylstilbestrol as a second-line hormonal agent in advanced prostate cancer. Urology 1998;52(2):257–260. DOI: 10.1016/S0090-4295(98)00173-3.

[43] Bland LB, Garzotto M, DeLoughery TG, Ryan CW, Schuff KG, Wersinger EM, Lemmon D and Beer TM: Phase II study of transdermal estradiol in androgen-independent prostate carcinoma. Cancer 2005;103(4):717–723. DOI: 10.1002/cncr.20857.

[44] Sciarra A, Gentile V, Cattarino S, Gentilucci A, Alfarone A, D'Eramo G and Salciccia S: Oral ethinylestradiol in castration-resistant prostate cancer: a 10-year experience. Int J Urol 2015;22:98–103. DOI: 10.1111/iju.12613.

[45] Izumi K, Kadono Y, Shima T, Konaka H, Mizokami A, Koh E and Namiki M: Ethinylestradiol improves prostate-specific antigen levels in pretreated castration-resistant prostate cancer patients. Anticancer Res 2010;30:5201–5206.

[46] Aggarwal R, Weinberg V, Small EJ, Oh W, Rushakoff R and Ryan CJ: The mechanism of action of estrogen in castration-resistant prostate cancer: clues from hormone levels. Clin Genitouri Cancer 2009;7(3):E71-E76. DOI: 10.3816/CGC.2009.n.027.

[47] Corey E, Quinn JE, Emond MJ, Buhler KR, Brown LG and Vessella RL: Inhibition of androgen-independent growth of prostate cancer xenografts by 17 beta-estradiol. Clin Cancer Res 2002;8:1003–1007.

[48] Montgomery B, Nelson PS, Vessalla R, Kalhorn T, Hess D and Corey E: Estradiol suppresses tissue androgens and prostate cancer growth in castration resistant prostate cancer. BMC Cancer 2010;10:1–7. DOI: 10.1186/1471-2407-10-244.

[49] Huggins CH and Hodges CV: Studies on prostate cancer. I. The effect of castration, of estrogen and of androgen injection on serum phosphatases in metastatic carcinoma of the prostate. Cancer Res 1941;1:293–297.

[50] Blackard CE , Doe RP , Mellinger GT and Byar DP: Incidence of cardiovascular disease and death in patients receiving diethylstilbestrol for carcinoma of the prostate. Cancer 1970;26:249–256. DOI: 10.1002/1097-0142(197008)26:2<249::AID-CNCR2820260202>3.0.CO;2-7

[51] Robinson MR , Smith PH , Richards B , Newling DW , de Pauw M and Sylvester R: The final analysis of the EORTC Genito-Urinary Tract Cancer Co-Operative Group phase III clinical trial (protocol 30805) comparing orchidectomy, orchidectomy plus cyproterone acetate and low dose stilboestrol in the management of metastatic carcinoma of the prostate. Eur Urol 1995;28(4):273–283.

[52] Klotz L , McNeill I and Fleshner N: A phase 1-2 trial of diethylstilbestrol plus low dose warfarin in advanced prostate carcinoma. J Urol 1999;161:169-172. DOI: 10.1016/S0022-5347(01)62089-5.

[53] Oh WK, Kantoff PW, Weinberg V et al: Prospective, multicenter, randomized phase II trial of the herbal supplement, PC-SPES, and diethylstilbestrol in patients with

androgen-independent prostate cancer. J Clin Oncol 2004;22:3705–3712. DOI: 10.1200/JCO.2004.10.195.

[54] Farrugia D , Ansell W , Singh M , Philp T , Chinegwundoh F , Oliver RT: Stilboestrol plus adrenal suppression as salvage treatment for patients failing treatment with luteinizing hormonereleasing hormone analogues and orchidectomy. BJU Int 2000;85: 1069–1073. DOI: 10.1046/j.1464-410x.2000.00673.x.

[55] Wilkins A, Shahidi M, Parker C, Gunapala R, Thomas K, Huddart R, Hoewich A and Dearnaley D: Diethylstilbestrol in castration-resistant prostate cancer. BJU Int 2012;110:727–735. DOI: 10.1111/j.1464-410X.2012.11546.x.

[56] Jazieh A , Munshi NC , Muirhead M and Ross SW: Clinical efficacy of diethylstilbestrol treatment in post orchidectomy progressive prostate cancer. Proc Am Assoc Cancer Res 1994;35:233. Abstract.

[57] Bland LB, Garzotto M, DeLoughery TG, Ryan CW, Schuff KG, Wersinger EM, Lemmon D and Beer TM: Phase II study of transdermal estradiol in androgen-independent prostate carcinoma. Cancer 2005;103(4):717–723. DOI: 10.1002/cncr.20857.

[58] Dörner G, Schnorr D, Stahl F and Rohde W: Successful treatment of prostatic cancer with the orally active depot estrogen ethinylestradiol sulfonate (Turisteron). Exp Clin Endocrinol 1985;86:190–196.

[59] Di Silverio F and Sciarra A: Combination therapy of ethinylestradiol and somatostatin analogue reintroduces objective clinical responses and decreases chromogranin A in patients with androgen ablation-refractory prostate cancer. J Urol 2003;170:1812–1816. DOI: 10.1097/01.ju.0000092480.71873.26.

[60] Onita T, Igawa T, Hisamatsu H, Sakai H and Kanetake H: Secondary endocrine therapy with oral estrogen for relapsed prostate cancer. Hinyokika Kiyo 2009;55:595–598.

[61] Yano A, Fujii Y, Iwai A, Kawakami S, Kageyama Y, Kihara K: Glucocorticoids suppress tumor lymphangiogenesis of prostate cancer cells. Clin Cancer Res. 2006;12(20 Pt 1): 6012–6017.

[62] Lam JS, Leppert JT, Vemulapalli SN, Shvarts O, Belldegrun AS: Secondary hormonal therapy for advanced prostate cancer. J Urol. 2006;175:27–34.

[63] Tannock I, Gospodarowicz M, Meakin W, Panzarella T, Stewart L, Rider W: Treatment of metastatic prostatic cancer with low-dose prednisone: evaluation of pain and quality of life as pragmatic indices of response. J Clin Oncol. 1989;7:590–597.

[64] Sartor O, Weinberger M, Moore A, Li A, Figg WD: Effect of prednisone on prostate-specific antigen in patients with hormone-refractory prostate cancer. Urology. 1998;52:252–256.

[65] Shamash J, Powles T, Sarker SJ, Protheroe A, Mithal N, Mills R, Beard R, Wilson P, Tranter N, O'Brien N, McFaul S, Oliver T: A multi-centre randomised phase III trial of Dexamethasone vs Dexamethasone and diethylstilbestrol in castration-resistant

prostate cancer: immediate vs deferred Diethylstilbestrol. Br J Cancer. 2011;104:620–628. DOI: 10.1038/bjc.2011.7.

[66] Fosså SD, Jacobsen AB, Ginman C, Jacobsen IN, Overn S, Iversen JR, Urnes T, Dahl AA, Veenstra M, Sandstad B: Weekly docetaxel and prednisolone versus prednisolone alone in androgen-independent prostate cancer: a randomized phase II study. Eur Urol. 2007;52:1691–1698.

[67] Venkitaraman R, Lorente D, Murthy V, Thomas K, Parker L, Ahiabor R, Dearnaley D, Huddart R, De Bono J, Parker C: A randomised phase 2 trial of dexamethasone versus prednisolone in castration-resistant prostate cancer. Eur Urol. 2015;67:673–679. DOI: 10.1016/j.eururo.2014.10.004.

[68] Storlie JA, Buckner JC, Wiseman GA, Burch PA, Hartmann LC, Richardson RL: Prostate specific antigen levels and clinical response to low dose dexamethasone for hormone-refractory metastatic prostate carcinoma. Cancer. 1995;76:96–100.

[69] Saika T, Kusaka N, Tsushima T, Yamato T, Ohashi T, Suyama B, Arata R, Nasu Y, Kumon H; Okayama Urological Cancer Collaborating Group: Treatment of androgen-independent prostate cancer with dexamethasone: a prospective study in stage D2 patients. Int J Urol. 2001 Jun;8(6):290–4.

[70] Holder SL, Drabick J, Zhu J, Joshi M: Dexamethasone may be the most efficacious corticosteroid for use as monotherapy in castration-resistant prostate cancer. Cancer Biol Ther. 2015;16: 207–209. DOI: 10.1080/15384047.2014.1002687.

[71] Attard G, Reid AH, A'Hern R, Parker C, Oommen NB, Folkerd E, Messiou C, Molife LR, Maier G, Thompson E, Olmos D, Sinha R, Lee G, Dowsett M, Kaye SB, Dearnaley D, Kheoh T, Molina A, de Bono JS: Selective inhibition of CYP17 with abiraterone acetate is highly active in the treatment of castration-resistant prostate cancer. J Clin Oncol. 2009;27:3742–3748. DOI: 10.1200/JCO.2008.20.0642.

[72] Lorente D, Omlin A, Ferraldeschi R, Pezaro C, Perez R, Mateo J, Altavilla A, Zafeirou Z, Tunariu N, Parker C, Dearnaley D, Gillessen S, de Bono J, Attard G: Tumour responses following a steroid switch from prednisone to dexamethasone in castration-resistant prostate cancer patients progressing on abiraterone. Br J Cancer. 2014;111:2248–2253. DOI: 10.1038/bjc.2014.531

[73] Uemura H, Fujimoto K, Mine T, Uejima S, de Velasco MA, Hirao Y, Komatsu N, Yamada A, Itoh K: Immunological evaluation of personalized peptide vaccination monotherapy in patients with castration-resistant prostate cancer. Cancer Sci. 2010;101:601–608. DOI: 10.1111/j.1349-7006.2009.01459.x

[74] Noguchi M, Kakuma T, Uemura H, Nasu Y, Kumon H, Hirao Y, Moriya F, Suekane S, Matsuoka K, Komatsu N, Shichijo S, Yamada A, Itoh K: A randomized phase II trial of personalized peptide vaccine plus low dose estramustine phosphate (EMP) versus standard dose EMP in patients with castration resistant prostate cancer. Cancer Immunol Immunother. 2010;59:1001–1009. DOI: 10.1007/s00262-010-0822-4.

[75] Nishimura K, Nonomura N, Satoh E, Harada Y, Nakayama M, Tokizane T, Fukui T, Ono Y, Inoue H, Shin M, Tsujimoto Y, Takayama H, Aozasa K, Okuyama A.: Potential mechanism for the effects of dexamethasone on growth of androgen-independent prostate cancer. J Natl Cancer Inst. 2001;93:1739–1746.

[76] Yoshimura K, Minami T, Nozawa M, Kimura T, Egawa S, Fujimoto H, Yamada A, Itoh K, Uemura H: A Phase 2 Randomized Controlled Trial of Personalized Peptide Vaccine Immunotherapy with Low-dose Dexamethasone Versus Dexamethasone Alone in Chemotherapy-naive Castration-resistant Prostate Cancer. Eur Urol. 2016, in press. DOI: 10.1016/j.eururo.2015.12.050

[77] Walter B, Rogenhofer S, Vogelhuber M, Berand A, Wieland WF, Andreesen R, Reichle A: Modular therapy approach in metastatic castration-refractory prostate cancer. World J Urol. 2010;28:745–750. DOI: 10.1007/s00345-010-0567-x.

[78] Vogelhuber M, Feyerabend S, Stenzl A, Suedhoff T, Schulze M, Huebner J, Oberneder R, Wieland W, Mueller S, Eichhorn F, Heinzer H, Schmidt K, Baier M, Ruebel A, Birkholz K, Bakhshandeh-Bath A, Andreesen R, Herr W, Reichle A: Biomodulatory Treatment of Patients with Castration-Resistant Prostate Cancer: A Phase II Study of Imatinib with Pioglitazone, Etoricoxib, Dexamethasone and Low-Dose Treosulfan. Cancer Microenviron. 2015;8:33–41. DOI: 10.1007/s12307-014-0161-7.

Chapter 10

Genetic Association Studies on Prostate Cancer

Zorana Nikolić, Dušanka Savić Pavićević and
Goran Brajušković

Additional information is available at the end of the chapter

http://dx.doi.org/10.5772/63280

Abstract

The modern research on molecular basis of prostate cancer (PCa) development includes studies aiming to identify potential genetic markers which could be used in diagnostics and/or monitoring of PCa. Genome-wide association studies (GWASs) have identified over 75 variants associated with PCa risk. One of the major PCa-related regions identified through GWASs is found to be a segment of 8q24. Other important PCa-susceptibility regions are 17q12, 17q24, 10q11, and 19q13. Candidate-gene based approach has also provided evidence of association between PCa risk and genetic variants located in functionally significant genes (both protein-coding and noncoding RNA genes) involved in normal prostatic cell growth, malignant transformation, or in the development of metastases. Nevertheless, the success of these studies is questionable, since numerous candidates for PCa-susceptibility variants were identified, but these results failed to replicate. The main aim of both types of genetic association studies on PCa is the identification of potential PCa genetic markers which could be used for constructing reliable algorithms for evaluating the risk for PCa development and/or PCa progression.

Keywords: prostate cancer, association study, GWAS, candidate gene, validation study, replication study

1. Introduction

Alarming statistics on prostate cancer (PCa) incidence and mortality, as well as the results of epidemiological studies, have led to focusing research efforts on discovering molecular mechanisms underlying its onset and progression [1]. Still, molecular basis of PCa pathogenesis remains largely unknown, while the results of studies in this area of research suggest that

PCa is one of the most genetically and molecularly heterogeneous malignant tumors [2]. Among PCa cases, most are sporadic, while a significantly smaller percent represents familial type, including hereditary cases. High-penetrability PCa-related loci are not common in populations and are found to be associated with hereditary PCa. Since PCa represents a multifactorial disease with polygenic basis, and sporadic cases are much more frequently diagnosed, most of the research in the area of PCa molecular genetics has focused on genetic variants with low penetrability [3].

The modern research on molecular basis of PCa development includes studies aiming to identify potential genetic markers which could be used in diagnostics and/or monitoring of PCa [1]. This is of utmost importance, since one of the major issues in clinical practice related to PCa is a large percent of latent PCa among newly diagnosed [4]. The overdiagnosis of PCa in early diagnosed cases, due to indolent forms, leads to unnecessary morbidity because of application of invasive therapeutic procedures [5]. This led to focusing the research efforts on discovering genetic markers that could be used for assessing the biological potential of early diagnosed PCa. Therefore, the use of these genetic markers, together with standard prognostic parameters of PCa progression, which include initial serum PSA level, Gleason score, and clinical stage, could greatly improve the current clinical protocols by being implemented in algorithms for evaluating the patient's risk of PCa and/or PCa aggressiveness [1].

Studies aiming to identify potential PCa-related loci are designed as case-control or case-only studies, which evaluate the differences in genotype distributions between cases and controls, as well as between different groups of patients, classified according to clinical characteristics. The most validated loci associated with PCa risk were identified through Genome-wide association studies (GWAS) [6]. Nevertheless, numerous PCa-related genetic variants were found in studies based on selected candidate genes [7].

2. Linkage analyses and high-penetrability loci

Linkage analyses have led to identification of the first high-penetrability PCa susceptibility loci [1]. These studies were based on analyses in hereditary PCa, which is a less frequent type of PCa, and yielded high or moderate-penetrability loci, such as HPC1 (eng. *Hereditary Prostate Cancer 1*, HPC1) mapped in chromosomal region 1q24-25 [8], PCAP (eng. *Predisposing for Cancer Prostate*, PCAP) mapped in 1q42.2-43 [9] and HPCX (eng. *Hereditary Prostate Cancer on X Chromosome*, HPCX) located in 1q42.2-43 [10]. Later on, additional linkage studies identified several other loci primarily associated with familial PCa and rarely found to be altered in sporadic type [1, 3]. Fine-mapping of these regions has led to identifying several candidate genes, such as *RNASEL* or *ELAC2* [11, 12]. Nevertheless, since the major percent of PCa is sporadic types, numerous studies have focused on identifying low-penetrability loci associated with not only sporadic PCa, but also potentially contributing to the risk of developing familial type of disease [3]. These studies were not designed as linkage, but instead as genetic association studies with case–control matched groups.

3. Genome-wide association studies

The *Human genome project* was critical for making high-throughput genome-wide analyses possible. Not only that this project yielded DNA sequence information but also provided basis for development of methodology, including high-throughput genotyping assays, as well as software tools for analyzing large amount of genetic data [13]. Therefore, sequencing of human DNA provided basis for GWASs, including those on PCa [14].

To date (February 2016), GWASs have identified over 75 variants associated with prostate cancer risk, predominantly in populations of European ancestry (**Figure 1**) [15, 16]. The first GWASs were conducted in 2007, for which a large collection of samples were obtained from PCa patients and healthy controls, as well as databases that included clinical data of patients were constructed [17–19]. The necessity of a large number of subjects for this type of study was obvious even in this early period of conducting GWASs.

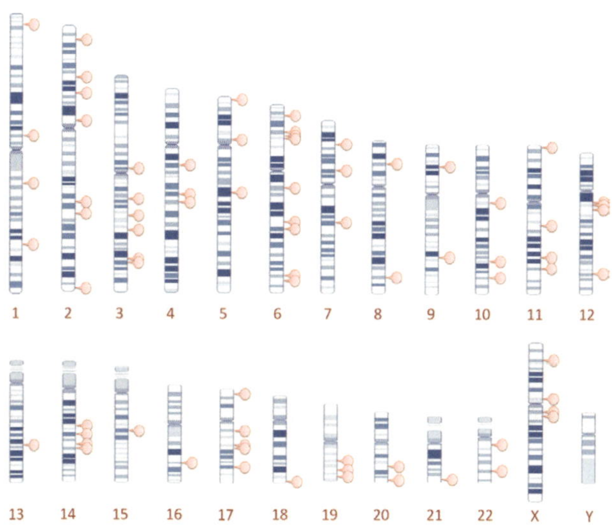

Figure 1. Ideograms of human chromosomes with marked PCa susceptibility loci identified through GWASs. Ideograms were obtained from NCBI Map Viewer, while GWAS hits were found in NHGRI-EBI GWAS catalog.

As in other complex diseases, PCa GWASs are usually designed in a multistage manner, with the whole set of tag-single nucleotide polymorphisms (tag-SNPs) being evaluated in the first phase, and only subsets of the most significant SNP being replicated in much larger groups of patients and controls in next phases [20, 21]. Thus, repeating the tests yields the most significant results [20].

The results of initial GWASs showed that most of the PCa-associated genetic variants are located in so-called "gene-deserts". The lack of protein-coding genes in these regions was explained by the supposed presence of regulatory sequences of major proto-oncogenes and tumor-suppressive genes [22, 23]. Today, another explanation is also the presence of genes encoding regulatory RNA molecules within PCa-risk regions [24].

3.1. 8q24 region

One of the major PCa-related regions was found to be 8q24. Within approximately 1 million base pairs segment of 8q24 reside multiple variants associated with PCa [25]. This region was first identified as associated with PCa susceptibility in a genome-wide linkage study conducted in Icelandic population [26]. Later on, the association of genetic variants within this region with PCa risk was shown in initial GWASs from 2007. Gudmunsson et al., Haiman et al. and Yeager et al. have shown the association between previously reported rs1447295 and PCa risk [17–19]. Also, these first GWASs identified other PCa susceptibility variants within 8q24, rs6983267, and rs16901979. Afterward, GWASs have provided evidence for association of other single-nucleotide genetic variants (SNVs) from 8q24 with PCa risk, such as rs4242382, rs7017300, and rs7837688 [27, 28]. In the recent years, by implementing clinical data and by using case-only design, both GWASs and validation studies have provided evidence for an association of several loci within 8q24 with PCa aggressiveness or survival [29–32].

PCa-susceptibility region within 8q24 was defined as *gene desert*, since no known protein-coding genes were located within it. Nevertheless, the possible biological explanation for the effect of genetic variants located in 8q24 on PCa risk was their influence on the regulation of the expression of nearby genes, mainly *C-MYC*. It was suggested that regulatory sequences controlling the transcription rate of *C-MYC* gene were located in 8q24, and that functional genetic variants which are in strong linkage disequilibrium (LD) with PCa susceptibility locus or several loci effect the sequence and therefore the function of regulatory elements [23]. Previous studies on molecular mechanisms of PCa pathogenesis have shown the functional significance of *C-MYC*, both by analyzing mutational signatures of malignant prostate tissue and by conducting functional analyses in cell cultures, which included stimulation or silencing of *C-MYC* expression [33]. Other than prostate cancer, several other malignancies were associated with 8q24, including breast and colorectal cancer. Some of the subregions of 8q24 associated with these cancers are found to overlap with those related to PCa, while others differ (**Figure 2**) [34].

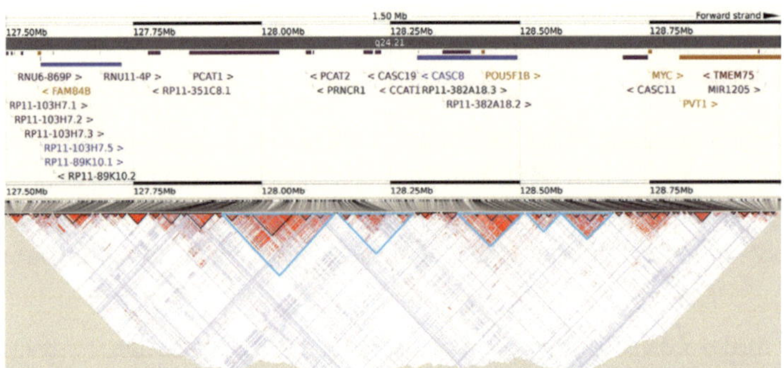

Figure 2. PCa risk-associated regions within 8q24. Lower part of the figure represents Haploview output for a segment of 8q24 (ch8:127500000..129000000) with marked subregions associated with PCa in GWASs. The upper part of the figure is a representation of genes located in the region of interest obtained from Ensembl genome browser (GRCh37).

3.2. 17q12

17q12 is another PCa susceptibility region identified through initial GWAS. Two of the genetic variants located in 17q12, rs7501939 and rs3760511, were found to be associated with the risk of developing PCa in the study by Gudmundsson et al. conducted in 2007 [35]. In this GWAS, minor alleles of these two single nucleotide genetic variants were found to confer the increased risk of PCa in cohorts of participants from Iceland, Netherlands, and the USA, while in the group of Hispanics this genetic association was not shown [35]. The results of this GWAS were further validated in multiple populations, mostly of European origin [36–43]. Validation studies were even conducted in Africans in which genetic association studies on PCa are scarce [37, 44–47]. The most recent meta-analysis of both GWASs and validation studies has also shown the association of these genetic variants with PCa risk [43].

SNVs rs7501939 and rs3760511 are located in the first intron of the hepatocyte nuclear factor 1 β(*HNF1β*) or transcription factor 2 (*TCF2*) which is a transcription factor showing tissue-specific expression pattern. Therefore, the association of genetic variants located in 17q12 with PCa risk could be explained by the effect of functional genetic variants on *HNF1β* function or expression [41].

3.3. 17q24

Another PCa-susceptibility region on chromosome 17 is 17q24. Genetic variants located within this region which were found to be associated with PCa are intergenic variants. Similar to 8q24 genetic variants, those located in 17q24 are found in a gene desert, probably harboring multiple regulatory sequences controlling the expression of surrounding genes [48]. One of the most proximal genes is *SOX9*, which is an important proto-oncogene in prostatic tissue. Recent findings have shown the location of PCa-associated genetic variants in an enhancer looping to *SOX9* gene [48]. Among these genetic variants is a tag-SNP previously identified through GWAS, as well as potentially functional genetic variants found by deep sequencing of PCa-susceptibility region [35, 48].

3.4. 10q11

Two out of the three GWASs, which were published in 2008 in the same issue of *Nature Genetics*, have identified PCa-associated genetic variants in the region 10q11 [27, 36]. Afterward, other studies have provided additional evidence to support the association between 10q11 and PCa susceptibility, including both GWASs and validation studies [49–55]. One of these PCa risk-associated genetic variants was located in the close proximity of the transcription start site of the gene Microseminoprotein B (*MSMB*) which encodes a tumor-suppressor, and was, therefore, even considered as potentially functional. For the risk allele of this genetic variant, it was further shown to affect the expression of *MSMB* gene in a negative manner [56, 57]. The other gene in proximity to this genetic variant is *Nuclear receptor coactivator 4* (*NCOA4*). NCOA4 protein interacts with androgen receptor (AR) and acts as corepressor of androgen-responding genes. Therefore, functional genetic variants in LD with GWAS hits could potentially contribute to PCa risk by affecting the expression of these two genes, or others in proximity [58].

3.5. 19q13

Region 19q13 harboring kallikrein genes *KLK2* and *KLK3* was found to be associated with PCa susceptibility through GWASs [59]. Several genetic variants associated with PCa risk were located in *KLK3* gene, such as missense SNV rs17632542 identified by fine-mapping of PCa-associated subregion 19q13.33. These genes encode serine-proteases, one of which is PSA, used for PCa diagnosis and disease monitoring. Therefore, the association of PCa-risk genetic variants with serum PSA level was evaluated, yielding statistically significant results for potentially functional SNV rs17632542 [15, 59].

Another subregion associated with PCa risk is 19q13.4 in which a GWASs hit is in strong LD in Chinese population with germline deletion affecting *LILRA3* gene, involved in inflammatory pathways [60].

4. Candidate gene-based approaches

Even before GWASs, the necessity of conducting association studies in order to identify low and moderate penetrability genetic variants that contribute to PCa risk was obvious. Therefore, numerous candidate genes were analyzed for genetic variants associated with PCa, with questionable success due to false discoveries and the lack of replication [61]. Candidates were selected based on their potential functional significance in normal prostatic cell growth, malignant transformation, or in the development of metastases. Therefore, among these candidate genes are those encoding proteins involved in androgen signaling, cell-cycle control mechanisms, major tumor-suppressors, or proto-oncogenes, as well as those involved in cellular adhesion or communication with surrounding cellular or matrix components of prostate epithelium [62, 63]. This implies the need for previous knowledge when designing case-control studies using candidate gene approach [64].

Even though these studies were common before GWASs, they are still conducted in numerous populations, aiming to confirm previously found associations, or to identify new ones by analyzing other candidates, selected by using modern research results, such as those involved in regulatory functions of non-coding RNAs [65].

4.1. Protein-coding genes

4.1.1. Androgen signaling

Since androgen signaling is essential for growth and survival of prostate epithelial cells, genes involved in androgen biosynthesis, signal reception and transduction, as well as in androgen metabolism have emerged as candidates for case–control studies [63]. Most of these studies involved Androgen receptor (AR), as the major component of androgen signaling and regulation of expression of androgen-responding genes. Among these studies, major percentage relied on analyzing the potential association of the length of CAG repeat string with exon 1 which encodes a poly-glutamine tract of AR with PCa risk [66]. This homopolymeric tract is located in N-terminal domain of AR, which possesses transactivational properties and its length is inversely correlated with transactivation function [67]. Even though initial results were promising, the supposed association was not confirmed in a large percentage of later studies, and the effect sizes were not large enough to support the substantial biological role. Therefore, the association of this genetic variant with PCa risk remains controversial [68–70].

Another three-nucleotide (GGN) repeat string, encoding polyglycine tract in AR, was analyzed for potential association between its length and PCa risk. This repeat string is also located in exon 1, but less studied than the CAG repeat tract, possibly due to technical problems in amplifying GC-rich DNA regions [71]. The effect of the length of GGN repeat string on transactivational properties of AR is still unclear, and the other proposed mechanism of potential functional significance is the effect on AR translation [72]. Studies on the potential association of this microsatellite on PCa risk and progression yielded contrasting results [73–79].

Mixed results were also found for *SRD5A2* (type II steroid 5α-reductase), which is the major enzyme converting testosterone to dihydrotestosterone. Similarly, studies analyzing genetic variants within *CYP17, CYP19A, HSD17B,* and *HSD3B* have shown initial promising results, lacking consistent validation [63, 80].

4.1.2. Carcinogen metabolism

Among genes involved in cell detoxification, those encoding glutathione-S-transferases have been mostly analyzed. Nevertheless, most of these studies yielded insignificant results on association with PCa risk [81]. Other frequently analyzed genes involved in metabolism of carcinogens are *PON1, CYP1A1, CYP1B1,* and *CYP3A4* [80, 82–85].

Two genetic variants within *PON1* have been analyzes in multiple populations, L55M and Q129R. The results to date are inconclusive, but the meta-analysis conducted in 2012 suggested the association of L55M missense variant with PCa risk [82]. Also, a recent meta-analysis on only three PCa studies and Q129R showed statistically significant association for several genetic models of association [83].

The most commonly analyzed SNVs in *CYP1A1* are missense variants rs1048943 (p.Ile462Val) and rs4646903, which are also called MspI polymorphisms, since they alter the recognition site for MspI restriction enzyme. Numerous studies and also the recent meta-analyses showed the association between these SNVs and PCa risk [84–86].

The results obtained for genetic variants in *CYP1B1* and *CYP3A4* are controversial, with the recent meta-analyses suggesting the association of L432V, N453S, and A119S polymorphisms of *CYP1B1* and A392G in *CYP3A4* with PCa susceptibility [87, 88].

4.1.3. DNA repair, cell cycle control, and apoptosis

Dysfunctions of DNA repair pathway, apoptosis regulation, and cell cycle control mechanisms alter the cells response to DNA damage and lead to uncontrolled proliferation, progression and metastasis of malignant diseases. Also, genetic variants in genes involved in these processes could potentially attribute to cancer susceptibility and/or progression risk [62].

Among the genes analyzed for association between genetic variants and prostate cancer risk or aggressiveness are *XRCC1* and *XRCC3* (X-ray repair cross-complementing proteins 1 and 3), *ERCC1* and *ERCC2* (Excision repair cross-complementing rodent repair deficiency, complementation group 1 and 2), *LIG4* (Ligase IV), *ATM* (Ataxia telangiectasia mutated), *XPD* (Xeroderma pigmentosum group D), *MDM2* (Human mouse double-minute 2 protein), *CDKN1A*, and *CDKN1B* (Cyclin-Dependent Kinase Inhibitors 1A, and 1B), *CCND1* (Cyclin D1) as well as *BCL2* (B-cell lymphoma 2) and *TP53* (tumor protein p53) [89–102]. Genetic variants within most of these genes were found to be associated with PCa aggressiveness or response to therapy. Nevertheless, these results were seldom replicated in multiple populations.

The most common SNVs in *XRCC1* studied in case–control studies on cancer risk are rs1799782 (p.Arg194Trp), rs25489 (p.Arg280His), and rs25487 (p.Arg399Gln) [89, 103]. These genetic variants were also analyzed for their potential association with PCa risk in numerous studies, but the obtained results were inconsistent [89, 90]. For rs25489, association with radiation-induced late toxicity in PCa patients was also shown [104]. Similarly, rs861539 (p.Thr241Met) in *XRCC3* was found to be associated with early adverse effects induced by radiotherapy, based on quantitative data synthesis of 6 studies [105].

A recent study conducted in Spain showed the association of rs11615 in *ERCC1* and rs17503908 in *ATM* with PCa aggressiveness [93]. Genetic variants in the same chromosomal region as *ERCC1* were previously analyzed in a large study that provided opposing results. Nevertheless, this previous study was designed as to include subjects from multiple populations, and its results could therefore be influenced by genetic backgrounds of study participants [93, 106].

Among genetic variants located in *MDM2*, missense variant SNP309 in the promoter region was most frequently analyzed. This SNV was found to be associated with both PCa risk and aggressiveness in multiple studies [107, 108]. The first study on this subject yielded no evidence of the supposed association [109]. Nevertheless, results obtained in several later studies suggested the association of SNP309 with the risk of PCa progression to the more advanced stage, or the statistical trend of significance was reached [108].

Numerous studies conducted on a potential association between *CCND1* genetic variant rs603965 (p.Ala870Gly) and PCa risk, yielding inconsistent results [99]. This SNV was found to affect alternative splicing and thus alter the C-terminal domain. Other genetic variants within this gene were shown to be associated with the risk of PCa biochemical reoccurrence after radical prostatectomy [110].

The most extensively analyzed SNV located in *TP53* gene is rs1042522 (p.Arg72Pro). This genetic variant was found to be associated with PCa risk, especially among Caucasians [102]. When it comes to *BCL2*, encoding the founding member of apoptosis regulatory proteins, promoter SNV c.-938C > A was associated with PCa risk, although lacking replication, as well as with disease-free survival and biochemical recurrence of PCa after radical prostatectomy [100, 101, 111].

4.1.4. Vitamin D signaling

Vitamin D signaling in PCa has stimulatory effect on apoptosis, as well as inhibitory effect on the progression of cell cycle. Therefore, multiple genetic variants within the gene encoding the receptor for vitamin D (*VDR*) were analyzed for their potential association with PCa risk and/or progression. Most of them are loci named FokI, BsmI, ApaI, and T I, according to restriction enzyme used for genotyping, Cdx2 in promoter region and polyA microsatellite, which were most frequently tested [112–114].

Even though the initial results on these loci were promising, in multiple populations, they were not replicated [113, 115]. The association of these genetic variants with PCa progression parameters and the disease outcome also remains inconclusive [113, 116].

4.1.5. Chronic inflammation and angiogenesis

Numerous genes involved in chronic inflammation have been studies for association of genetic variants that reside within them with PCa risk and/or progression [117]. Also, the importance of vascular support to cancer growth stimulated the association studies on PCa analyzing genetic variants located in angiogenesis-related genes [62]. Since these processes are codependent, numerous genes primarily found to be involved in chronic inflammation are also discussed as angiogenesis-related genes, and vice versa.

Among the most important factors of chronic inflammation are *TGF-β*, *COX2*, *TNF-α*, and *IL-1-β*, as well as *PPAR-γ*. To date, several SNVs in *TGF-β1* have been identified as PCa-susceptibility variants, some of them also associated with PCa aggressiveness [118–123]. The studies on the most of the chronic inflammation-related genes provided conflicting results [117].

There have been various PCa case–control studies involving *Vascular endothelial growth factor* (*VEGF*) gene, encoding the important proangiogenic growth factor, as well as genes encoding Interleukin 8 (IL-8) and Interleukin 10 (IL-10) [96, 124–128] for genetic variant rs1570360 [c.-1154G > A] located in the promoter region of *VEGF*, statistically significant association with PCa risk was shown in several studies [126]. Most other *VEGF* genetic variants analyzed for potential association with PCa risk and/or progression are also located in the promoter region [126, 129–131]. These SNVs could be associated with transcription rate of *VEGF* [132], which is positively correlated with tumor stage, Gleason score, as well as with shorter period of disease-free survival [133].

Candidates for this type of studies were also genes encoding transcription factors which regulate the expression of *VEGF*, such as Hypoxia inducible factor 1 (*HIF1A*), Epidermal growth factor (*EGF*), and Lymphotoxin α (*LTA*). Nevertheless, except for *HIF1A*, association of genetic variants within these genes with PCa risk was not shown, or was mostly found in small sample studies and poorly replicated [62, 125, 126, 134].

Some of the key regulators of angiogenesis are also fibroblast growth factors (*FGF*s). Therefore, receptor *FGFR4* gene has been analyzed for genetic variants associated with PCa risk and/or progression. The most commonly tested SNV is a missense variant rs351855 (p.Gly388Arg), found to be associated with PCa risk and aggressiveness in a relatively small number of studies [135].

Among the most extensively analyzed candidate genes in PCa-related case-control studies are *NOS3* and *NOS2A*, encoding nitric oxide synthases [136]. Both endothelial and inducible nitric oxide synthases, encoded by these genes, are enzymes that catalyze the production of NO from L-arginine and L-citrulline amino acids [137]. Being the major producer of NO in endothelial cells, eNOS, encoded by *NOS3*, is involved in the control of vascular tone and angiogenesis, which is essential for tumor growth and the development of metastases. Yet, the synthesis of NO is associated with apoptosis, which has the opposing effect on carcinogenesis [138]. Numerous genetic variants within these genes, especially *NOS3*, have been analyzed for potential association with PCa risk and/or progression [136]. Most commonly analyzed SNVs are -786 T > C (rs2070744) and 894G > T (rs1799983) [139–147], while several studies included insertion-deletion polymorphism 4a4b located in intron 4 of *NOS3* [140, 146, 148, 149]. For rs1799983, which is a missense genetic variant, it was hypothesized to affect NOS3 stability [150]. The other common SNV, rs2070744, affects promoter activity by allele C creating a binding site with validation protein 1A (RPA1) [151].

Angiogenesis process and tumor invasion also require degradation of extracellular matrix and basal membranes, which are catalyzed by matrix metalloproteinases. Among the genes encoding this class of enzymes, *MMP2* and *MMP9* are analyzed for genetic variants associated with PCa risk, and also for disease aggressiveness, due to their functional significance in tumor invasiveness [139, 152–156]. Commonly analyzed genetic variant in *MMP2* promoter is rs243865. For minor allele of this SNV it was shown to be associated with reduced transcription rate of *MMP2* [157].

4.1.6. Cellular adhesion

Among genes involved in cellular adhesion, *CDH1* encoding E-cadherin was the candidate gene for the most case-control studies on PCa. Since aberrant expression of this gene is correlated with the increased metastatic potential of PCa, genetic variants in its promoter region were analyzed for potential association with PCa risk and progression [158, 159]. Most extensively studied SNV−160C > A was found to affect *CDH1* expression and was identified as PCa susceptibility genetic variant in multiple populations [158, 160].

Only few studies also included genetic variants in genes encoding intercellular adhesion molecules (ICAMs), proteins involved in cellular adhesion and signaling. The analyzed genetic variants are those located in *ICAM-1*, *ICAM-4*, and *ICAM-5* genes and need a further evaluation for potential association with PCa risk and/or progression [161, 162].

4.2. Long noncoding RNA genes

The potential involvement of long noncoding RNAs (lncRNAs) in prostate carcinogenesis was suggested not only by the results of expression analyses that showed several known oncogenic and/or tumor-suppressive lcnRNAs to be aberrantly expressed in malignant prostatic tissue or plasma samples from patients with PCa but also by the identification of several PCa-specific lncRNAs [163, 164].

Several SNVs in lncRNA genes were identified as PCa susceptibility variants in case–control studies on PCa. In their study published in 2011, Jin et al. have stated that eight SNVs identified to that time through GWAS are located in lncRNA intervals [165]. They also identified a SNV in a putative lncRNA which was not later experimentally confirmed as a PCa-susceptibility variants [165]. In a study published in 2013, Xue et al. have shown the association between two tag-SNPs in Prostate cancer gene expression marker 1 (*PCGEM1*) and PCa risk in Chinese population [166]. Genetic variant in another PCa-specific gene, prostate cancer associated 3 (*PCA3*), was analyzed for the length of a TAAA repeat string in the promoter region. This genetic variant was also found to be associated with PCa risk [167]. In a GWAS published in 2014, Cook et al. have identified rs7918885 in *RP11-543 F8.2* gene as a PCa-susceptibility SNV in West African men, although GWAS statistical significance threshold was not reached [168]. Also, by using fine-mapping and resequencing of PCa-susceptibility subregion of 8q24, *lncRNA* gene prostate cancer noncoding RNA 1 (*PRNCR1*) was found to be located between the most significantly associated genetic variant [169].

4.3. *MicroRNA* genes

Dysregulation of diverse regulatory mechanisms based on microRNA activity has been implicated in prostate carcinogenesis. Therefore, possibly functional genetic variants located in *microRNA* genes emerged as potential PCa-associated loci. Among these genetic variants are those that potentially influence microRNA biogenesis, stability of mature microRNAs, efficiency of target gene regulation, as well as target specificity. By affecting these features of microRNA regulatory mechanisms, microRNA SNVs could be associated with aberrant expression of various important PCa-related oncogenes or tumor-suppressive genes [170–172].

MicroRNA genetic variants have been analyzed for their potential association with PCa in only a few studies conducted in Asian populations and in a single population of European origin. These studies have provided discordant results on the effects of genetic variants in rs2910164 in *hsa-miR-146a* [173–176], *hsa-miR-196a2* [174, 176, 177], and rs3746444 in *hsa-miR-499* gene on PCa risk [174, 177]. In a recent study, rs4705342 located in *hsa-miR-143* gene promoter was found to be associated with the risk of developing PCa [178]. Since the number of conducted studies is small, additional findings from multiple populations are needed in order to make further conclusions.

Another SNV, rs895819 located in a gene encoding miR-27a, which is androgen-regulated and stimulates the androgen signalization in a positive feedback loop, was found to be associated with PCa risk, as well as with the development of distant metastases. Nevertheless, these results are derived from a single study on PCa risk and rs895819 conducted relatively recent and needs further validation [177].

5. Replication, validation studies, and Meta-analyses

Differences in genetic backgrounds are an important issue in genetic association studies. Therefore, interpretation of data requires discussing the potential differences between populations. Therefore, in order to analyze such differences, multiple validation analyses are conducted in various population and ethnicities. These studies are designed so that they resemble as much as possible to the original study that yielded genetic associations, or the lack of it. The ratio for conducting such studies is the possible lack of association between identified PCa-susceptibility variants with PCa risk in certain populations, or the differences in effect sizes [179]. Replication studies, conducted in confirmation group of participants from the same population in which the initial results were found, is a method of checking reproducibility and evaluating possible false positives and effect overestimation [179, 180].

Currently, replications and validations are conducted for both GWASs results, as well as for results from candidate gene-based studies. Of utmost importance is conducting replication and validation analyses of hits from studies with relatively small sample sizes, as well as with poorly clinically characterized cases with the lack of data on possible confounders, or questionable recruitment of controls [180]. Also, an important issue in case–control studies on PCa is the type of control group, which is in some cases healthy controls, while in others group of patients with benign prostatic hyperplasia (BPH). Furthermore, classification systems for patients with PCa which are used for evaluating potential genetic associations with PCa progression differ between studies, which together with small sizes of patient groups, calls for replication of acquired statistically significant data.

All of these issues are a potential reason for the opposing results on the association of the most of genetic variants analyzed in multiple studies with PCa risk and progression. Therefore, in order to elucidate the effect of these genetic variants, meta-analyses of eligible studies are frequently conducted. Combining the results from smaller studies through data synthesis in meta-analysis could result in increased statistical power [181]. Therefore, meta-analyses could provide more precise estimations, as well as the insight in the potential effect of confounders [182], such as ethnicity, participant recruitment strategy, or study size.

6. Future perspectives

The main aim of genetic association studies on PCa is the identification of potential PCa genetic markers which could be used for constructing reliable algorithms for evaluating the risk for PCa development and/or PCa progression [1]. Therefore, it is important not only to identify these PCa-related genetic variants, but also to precisely characterize their effect sizes. In order to do that, ethnic differences need to be taken into account [179]. Other important issues in interpreting results of association studies are gene–gene and gene-environment interactions. Therefore, future research and designing such algorithms require integration of knowledge on genetic associations, cellular pathways, and statistical epistasis in which real biological interaction could be reflected.

Since the major problem in clinical practice related to PCa is the overdiagnosis and monitoring of patients [4], additional studies on PCa aggressiveness with clinically well characterized groups of PCa patients are needed to identify genetic variants associated with PCa progression risk. The later implementation of algorithms based on these genetic variants could greatly improve clinical protocols in monitoring and treating PCa.

7. Conclusion

The efforts for improving clinical protocols in PCa diagnostics, monitoring and treatment resulted in conducting genetic association studies on PCa. These studies aim to identify potential PCa genetic markers and characterize their association with PCa risk and/or progression through measuring effect sizes. The identified and validated genetic markers could then be used for constructing reliable algorithms for evaluating the risk for PCa development and, more importantly, for PCa progression. Implementing such algorithms in clinical practice is expected to improve the distinction between early diagnosed PCa cases that require aggressive treatment and latent PCa cases which remain indolent during patient's lifetime.

Author details

Zorana Nikolić, Dušanka Savić Pavićević and Goran Brajušković*

*Address all correspondence to: brajuskovic@bio.bg.ac.rs

Faculty of Biology, Centre for Human Molecular Genetics, University of Belgrade, Belgrade, Serbia

References

[1] Goh CL, Eeles RA. Germline genetic variants associated with prostate cancer and potential relevance to clinical practice. In: Cuzick J, Thorat MA, editors. Prostate Cancer Prevention. Heidelberg, Germany: Springer; 2014. pp. 9–26. (Recent Results in Cancer Research; vol 202).

[2] Boyd LK, Mao X, Lu YJ. The complexity of prostate cancer: genomic alterations and heterogeneity. Nat Rev Urol. 2012; 9(11):652–64. doi: 10.1038/nrurol.2012.185.

[3] Alberti C. Hereditary/familial versus sporadic prostate cancer: few indisputable genetic differences and many similar clinicopathological features. Eur Rev Med Pharmacol Sci. 2010; 14(1):31–41.

[4] Mühlberger N, Kurzthaler C, Iskandar R, Krahn MD, Bremner KE, Oberaigner W, et al. The ONCOTYROL Prostate Cancer Outcome and Policy Model: Effect of Prevalence Assumptions on the Benefit-Harm Balance of Screening. Med Decis Making. 2015; 35(6):758–72.

[5] Klotz L. Active surveillance for favorable-risk prostate cancer: background, patient selection, triggers for intervention, and outcomes. Curr Urol Rep. 2012;13(2):1539.

[6] Chen R, Ren S, Sun Y. Genome-wide association studies on prostate cancer: the end or the beginning? Protein Cell. 2013; 4(9):677–86.

[7] Cartwright R, Mangera A, Tikkinen KA, Rajan P, Pesonen J, Kirby AC, Thiagamoorthy G, Ambrose C, Gonzalez-Maffe J, Bennett PR, Palmer T, Walley A, Järvelin MR, Khullar V, Chapple C. Systematic review and meta-analysis of candidate gene association studies of lower urinary tract symptoms in men. Eur Urol. 2014 Oct;66(4):752–68. doi: 10.1016/j.eururo.2014.01.007.

[8] Smith JR, Freije D, Carpten JD, Grönberg H, Xu J, Isaacs SD, Brownstein MJ, Bova GS, Guo H, Bujnovszky P, Nusskern DR, Damber JE, Bergh A, Emanuelsson M, Kallioniemi OP, Walker-Daniels J, Bailey-Wilson JE, Beaty TH, Meyers DA, Walsh PC, Collins FS, Trent JM, Isaacs WB. Major susceptibility locus for prostate cancer on chromosome 1 suggested by a genome-wide search. Science. 1996; 274(5291):1371–4.

[9] Berthon P1, Valeri A, Cohen-Akenine A, Drelon E, Paiss T, Wöhr G, Latil A, Millasseau P, Mellah I, Cohen N, Blanché H, Bellané-Chantelot C, Demenais F, Teillac P, Le Duc A, de Petriconi R, Hautmann R, Chumakov I, Bachner L, Maitland NJ, Lidereau R, Vogel W, Fournier G, Mangin P, Cussenot O, et al. Predisposing gene for early-onset prostate cancer, localized on chromosome 1q42.2-43. Am J Hum Genet. 1998; 62(6): 1416–24.

[10] Xu J, Meyers D, Freije D, Isaacs S, Wiley K, Nusskern D, Ewing C, Wilkens E, Bujnovszky P, Bova GS, Walsh P, Isaacs W, Schleutker J, Matikainen M, Tammela T, Visakorpi T, Kallioniemi OP, Berry R, Schaid D, French A, McDonnell S, Schroeder J, Blute M, Thibodeau S, Grönberg H, Emanuelsson M, Damber JE, Bergh A, Jonsson BA, Smith J, Bailey-Wilson J, Carpten J, Stephan D, Gillanders E, Amundson I, Kainu T, Freas-Lutz D, Baffoe-Bonnie A, Van Aucken A, Sood R, Collins F, Brownstein M, Trent J. Evidence for a prostate cancer susceptibility locus on the X chromosome. Nat Genet. 1998; 20(2):175–9.

[11] Carpten J, Nupponen N, Isaacs S, Sood R, Robbins C, Xu J, Faruque M, Moses T, Ewing C, Gillanders E, Hu P, Bujnovszky P, Makalowska I, Baffoe-Bonnie A, Faith D, Smith J, Stephan D, Wiley K, Brownstein M, Gildea D, Kelly B, Jenkins R, Hostetter G, Matikainen M, Schleutker J, Klinger K, Connors T, Xiang Y, Wang Z, De Marzo A, Papadopoulos N, Kallioniemi OP, Burk R, Meyers D, Grönberg H, Meltzer P, Silverman

R, Bailey-Wilson J, Walsh P, Isaacs W, Trent J. Germline mutations in the ribonuclease L gene in families showing linkage with HPC1. Nat Genet. 2002; 30(2):181–4

[12] Tavtigian SV, Simard J, Teng DH, Abtin V, Baumgard M, Beck A, Camp NJ, Carillo AR, Chen Y, Dayananth P, Desrochers M, Dumont M, Farnham JM, Frank D, Frye C, Ghaffari S, Gupte JS, Hu R, Iliev D, Janecki T, Kort EN, Laity KE, Leavitt A, Leblanc G, McArthur-Morrison J, Pederson A, Penn B, Peterson KT, Reid JE, Richards S, Schroeder M, Smith R, Snyder SC, Swedlund B, Swensen J, Thomas A, Tranchant M, Woodland AM, Labrie F, Skolnick MH, Neuhausen S, Rommens J, Cannon-Albright LA. A candidate prostate cancer susceptibility gene at chromosome 17p. Nat Genet. 2001; 27(2):172–80.

[13] Hood L, Rowen L. The Human Genome Project: big science transforms biology and medicine. Genome Med. 2013; 5(9):79.

[14] Shen H. Progress of cancer genomics. Thorac Cancer. 2015; 6(5):557-60. doi: 10.1111/1759-7714.12281.

[15] Sullivan J, Kopp R, Stratton K, Manschreck C, Corines M, Rau-Murthy R, Hayes J, Lincon A, Ashraf A, Thomas T, Schrader K, Gallagher D, Hamilton R, Scher H, Lilja H, Scardino P, Eastham J, Offit K, Vijai J, Klein RJ. An analysis of the association between prostate cancer risk loci, PSA levels, disease aggressiveness and disease-specific mortality. Br J Cancer. 2015; 113(1):166-72. doi: 10.1038/bjc.2015.199.

[16] Al Olama AA, Kote-Jarai Z, Berndt SI, Conti DV, Schumacher F, Han Y, Benlloch S, Hazelett DJ, Wang Z, Saunders E, Leongamornlert D, Lindstrom S, Jugurnauth-Little S, Dadaev T, Tymrakiewicz M, Stram DO, Rand K, Wan P, Stram A, Sheng X, Pooler LC, Park K, Xia L, Tyrer J, Kolonel LN, Le Marchand L, Hoover RN, Machiela MJ, Yeager M, Burdette L, Chung CC, Hutchinson A, Yu K, Goh C, Ahmed M, Govindasami K, Guy M, Tammela TL, Auvinen A, Wahlfors T, Schleutker J, Visakorpi T, Leinonen KA, Xu J, Aly M, Donovan J, Travis RC, Key TJ, Siddiq A, Canzian F, Khaw KT, Takahashi A, Kubo M, Pharoah P, Pashayan N, Weischer M, Nordestgaard BG, Nielsen SF, Klarskov P, Røder MA, Iversen P, Thibodeau SN, McDonnell SK, Schaid DJ, Stanford JL, Kolb S, Holt S, Knudsen B, Coll AH, Gapstur SM, Diver WR, Stevens VL, Maier C, Luedeke M, Herkommer K, Rinckleb AE, Strom SS, Pettaway C, Yeboah ED, Tettey Y, Biritwum RB, Adjei AA, Tay E, Truelove A, Niwa S, Chokkalingam AP, Cannon-Albright L, Cybulski C, Wokołorczyk D, Kluźniak W, Park J, Sellers T, Lin HY, Isaacs WB, Partin AW, Brenner H, Dieffenbach AK, Stegmaier C, Chen C, Giovannucci EL, Ma J, Stampfer M, Penney KL, Mucci L, John EM, Ingles SA, Kittles RA, Murphy AB, Pandha H, Michael A, Kierzek AM, Blot W, Signorello LB, Zheng W, Albanes D, Virtamo J, Weinstein S, Nemesure B, Carpten J, Leske C, Wu SY, Hennis A, Kibel AS, Rybicki BA, Neslund-Dudas C, Hsing AW, Chu L, Goodman PJ, Klein EA, Zheng SL, Batra J, Clements J, Spurdle A, Teixeira MR, Paulo P, Maia S, Slavov C, Kaneva R, Mitev V, Witte JS, Casey G, Gillanders EM, Seminara D, Riboli E, Hamdy FC, Coetzee GA, Li Q, Freedman ML, Hunter DJ, Muir K, Gronberg H, Neal DE, Southey M, Giles GG, Severi G; Breast and Prostate Cancer Cohort Consortium (BPC3); PRACTICAL

(Prostate Cancer Association Group to Investigate Cancer-Associated Alterations in the Genome) Consortium; COGS (Collaborative Oncological Gene-environment Study) Consortium; GAME-ON/ELLIPSE Consortium, Cook MB, Nakagawa H, Wiklund F, Kraft P, Chanock SJ, Henderson BE, Easton DF, Eeles RA, Haiman CA. A meta-analysis of 87,040 individuals identifies 23 new susceptibility loci for prostate cancer. Nat Genet. 2014; 46(10):1103–9, doi: 10.1038/ng.3094.

[17] Gudmundsson J, Sulem P, Manolescu A, Amundadottir LT, Gudbjartsson D, Helgason A, Rafnar T, Bergthorsson JT, Agnarsson BA, Baker A, Sigurdsson A, Benediktsdottir KR, Jakobsdottir M, Xu J, Blondal T, Kostic J, Sun J, Ghosh S, Stacey SN, Mouy M, Saemundsdottir J, Backman VM, Kristjansson K, Tres A, Partin AW, Albers-Akkers MT, Godino-Ivan Marcos J, Walsh PC, Swinkels DW, Navarrete S, Isaacs SD, Aben KK, Graif T, Cashy J, Ruiz-Echarri M, Wiley KE, Suarez BK, Witjes JA, Frigge M, Ober C, Jonsson E, Einarsson GV, Mayordomo JI, Kiemeney LA, Isaacs WB, Catalona WJ, Barkardottir RB, Gulcher JR, Thorsteinsdottir U, Kong A, Stefansson K. Genome-wide association study identifies a second prostate cancer susceptibility variant at 8q24. Nat Genet. 2007; 39(5):631–7.

[18] Haiman CA, Patterson N, Freedman ML, Myers SR, Pike MC, Waliszewska A, Neubauer J, Tandon A, Schirmer C, McDonald GJ, Greenway SC, Stram DO, Le Marchand L, Kolonel LN, Frasco M, Wong D, Pooler LC, Ardlie K, Oakley-Girvan I, Whittemore AS, Cooney KA, John EM, Ingles SA, Altshuler D, Henderson BE, Reich D. Multiple regions within 8q24 independently affect risk for prostate cancer. Nat Genet. 2007; 39(5):638-44.

[19] Yeager M, Orr N, Hayes RB, Jacobs KB, Kraft P, Wacholder S, Minichiello MJ, Fearnhead P, Yu K, Chatterjee N, Wang Z, Welch R, Staats BJ, Calle EE, Feigelson HS, Thun MJ, Rodriguez C, Albanes D, Virtamo J, Weinstein S, Schumacher FR, Giovannucci E, Willett WC, Cancel-Tassin G, Cussenot O, Valeri A, Andriole GL, Gelmann EP, Tucker M, Gerhard DS, Fraumeni JF Jr, Hoover R, Hunter DJ, Chanock SJ, Thomas G. Genome-wide association study of prostate cancer identifies a second risk locus at 8q24. Nat Genet. 2007; 39(5):645-9.

[20] Witte JC. Genome-Wide Association Studies and Beyond. Annu Rev Public Health. 2010; 31:9-20. doi: 10.1146/annurev.publhealth.012809.103723.

[21] Lange EM, Salinas CA, Zuhlke KA, Ray AM, Wang Y, Lu Y, Ho LA, Luo J, Cooney KA. Early onset prostate cancer has a significant genetic component. Prostate. 2012; 72(2): 147-56. doi: 10.1002/pros.21414. Epub 2011 May 2. PubMed PMID: 21538423; PubMed Central PMCID: PMC3784829.

[22] Schierding W, Cutfield WS, O'Sullivan JM. The missing story behind Genome Wide Association Studies: single nucleotide polymorphisms in gene deserts have a story to tell. Front Genet. 2014; 5:39. doi: 10.3389/fgene.2014.00039.

[23] Wasserman NF, Aneas I, Nobrega MA. An 8q24 gene desert variant associated with prostate cancer risk confers differential in vivo activity to a MYC enhancer. Genome Res. 2010; 20(9):1191-7. doi: 10.1101/gr.105361.110.

[24] Huppi K, Pitt JJ, Wahlberg BM, Caplen NJ. The 8q24 gene desert: an oasis of non-coding transcriptional activity. Front Genet. 2012; 3:69. doi: 10.3389/fgene.2012.00069.

[25] Li Q, Liu X, Hua RX, Wang F, An H, Zhang W, Zhu JH. Association of three 8q24 polymorphisms with prostate cancer susceptibility: evidence from a meta-analysis with 50,854 subjects. Sci Rep. 2015; 5:12069. doi: 10.1038/srep12069.

[26] Amundadottir LT, Sulem P, Gudmundsson J, Helgason A, Baker A, Agnarsson BA, Sigurdsson A, Benediktsdottir KR, Cazier JB, Sainz J, Jakobsdottir M, Kostic J, Magnusdottir DN, Ghosh S, Agnarsson K, Birgisdottir B, Le Roux L, Olafsdottir A, Blondal T, Andresdottir M, Gretarsdottir OS, Bergthorsson JT, Gudbjartsson D, Gylfason A, Thorleifsson G, Manolescu A, Kristjansson K, Geirsson G, Isaksson H, Douglas J, Johansson JE, Bälter K, Wiklund F, Montie JE, Yu X, Suarez BK, Ober C, Cooney KA, Gronberg H, Catalona WJ, Einarsson GV, Barkardottir RB, Gulcher JR, Kong A, Thorsteinsdottir U, Stefansson K. A common variant associated with prostate cancer in European and African populations. Nat Genet. 2006; 38(6):652–8.

[27] Thomas G, Jacobs KB, Yeager M, Kraft P, Wacholder S, Orr N, Yu K, Chatterjee N, Welch R, Hutchinson A, Crenshaw A, Cancel-Tassin G, Staats BJ, Wang Z, Gonzalez-Bosquet J, Fang J, Deng X, Berndt SI, Calle EE, Feigelson HS, Thun MJ, Rodriguez C, Albanes D, Virtamo J, Weinstein S, Schumacher FR, Giovannucci E, Willett WC, Cussenot O, Valeri A, Andriole GL, Crawford ED, Tucker M, Gerhard DS, Fraumeni JF Jr, Hoover R, Hayes RB, Hunter DJ, Chanock SJ. Multiple loci identified in a genome-wide association study of prostate cancer. Nat Genet. 2008; 40(3):310–5. doi: 10.1038/ng.91.

[28] Zheng SL, Sun J, Cheng Y, Li G, Hsu FC, Zhu Y, Chang BL, Liu W, Kim JW, Turner AR, Gielzak M, Yan G, Isaacs SD, Wiley KE, Sauvageot J, Chen HS, Gurganus R, Mangold LA, Trock BJ, Gronberg H, Duggan D, Carpten JD, Partin AW, Walsh PC, Xu J, Isaacs WB. Association between two unlinked loci at 8q24 and prostate cancer risk among European Americans. J Natl Cancer Inst. 2007; 99(20):1525–33.

[29] Cussenot O, Azzouzi AR, Bantsimba-Malanda G, Gaffory C, Mangin P, Cormier L, Fournier G, Valeri A, Jouffe L, Roupret M, Fromont G, Sibony M, Comperat E, Cancel-Tassin G. Effect of genetic variability within 8q24 on aggressiveness patterns at diagnosis and familial status of prostate cancer. Clin Cancer Res. 2008; 14(17):5635–9. doi: 10.1158/1078-0432.CCR-07-4999.

[30] Suzuki M, Liu M, Kurosaki T, Suzuki M, Arai T, Sawabe M, Kasuya Y, Kato M, Fujimura T, Fukuhara H, Enomoto Y, Nishimatsu H, Ishikawa A, Kume H, Homma Y, Kitamura T. Association of rs6983561 polymorphism at 8q24 with prostate cancer mortality in a Japanese population. Clin Genitourin Cancer. 2011; 9(1):46–52. doi: 10.1016/j.clgc.2011.04.004.

[31] Bensen JT, Xu Z, Smith GJ, Mohler JL, Fontham ET, Taylor JA. Genetic polymorphism and prostate cancer aggressiveness: a case-only study of 1,536 GWAS and candidate SNPs in African-Americans and European-Americans. Prostate. 2013; 73(1):11–22. doi: 10.1002/pros.22532.

[32] Grin B, Loeb S, Roehl K, Cooper PR, Catalona WJ, Helfand BT. A rare 8q24 single nucleotide polymorphism (SNP) predisposes North American men to prostate cancer and possibly more aggressive disease. BJU Int. 2015; 115(1):101–5. doi: 10.1111/bju.12847.

[33] Koh CM, Bieberich CJ, Dang CV, Nelson WG, Yegnasubramanian S, De Marzo AM. MYC and Prostate Cancer. Genes Cancer. 2010; 1(6):617–28. doi: 10.1177/1947601910379132.

[34] Ahmadiyeh N, Pomerantz MM, Grisanzio C, Herman P, Jia L, Almendro V, He HH, Brown M, Liu XS, Davis M, Caswell JL, Beckwith CA, Hills A, Macconaill L, Coetzee GA, Regan MM, Freedman ML. 8q24 prostate, breast, and colon cancer risk loci show tissue-specific long-range interaction with MYC. Proc Natl Acad Sci U S A. 2010; 107(21):9742–6. doi: 10.1073/pnas.0910668107.

[35] Gudmundsson J, Sulem P, Steinthorsdottir V, Bergthorsson JT, Thorleifsson G, Manolescu A, Rafnar T, Gudbjartsson D, Agnarsson BA, Baker A, Sigurdsson A, Benediktsdottir KR, Jakobsdottir M, Blondal T, Stacey SN, Helgason A, Gunnarsdottir S, Olafsdottir A, Kristinsson KT, Birgisdottir B, Ghosh S, Thorlacius S, Magnusdottir D, Stefansdottir G, Kristjansson K, Bagger Y, Wilensky RL, Reilly MP, Morris AD, Kimber CH, Adeyemo A, Chen Y, Zhou J, So WY, Tong PC, Ng MC, Hansen T, Andersen G, Borch-Johnsen K, Jorgensen T, Tres A, Fuertes F, Ruiz-Echarri M, Asin L, Saez B, van Boven E, Klaver S, Swinkels DW, Aben KK, Graif T, Cashy J, Suarez BK, van Vierssen Trip O, Frigge ML, Ober C, Hofker MH, Wijmenga C, Christiansen C, Rader DJ, Palmer CN, Rotimi C, Chan JC, Pedersen O, Sigurdsson G, Benediktsson R, Jonsson E, Einarsson GV, Mayordomo JI, Catalona WJ, Kiemeney LA, Barkardottir RB, Gulcher JR, Thorsteinsdottir U, Kong A, Stefansson K. Two variants on chromosome 17 confer prostate cancer risk, and the one in TCF2 protects against type 2 diabetes. Nat Genet. 2007 Aug; 39(8):977–83.

[36] Eeles RA, Kote-Jarai Z, Giles GG, Olama AA, Guy M, Jugurnauth SK, Mulholland S, Leongamornlert DA, Edwards SM, Morrison J, Field HI, Southey MC, Severi G, Donovan JL, Hamdy FC, Dearnaley DP, Muir KR, Smith C, Bagnato M, Ardern-Jones AT, Hall AL, O'Brien LT, Gehr-Swain BN, Wilkinson RA, Cox A, Lewis S, Brown PM, Jhavar SG, Tymrakiewicz M, Lophatananon A, Bryant SL; UK Genetic Prostate Cancer Study Collaborators; British Association of Urological Surgeons' Section of Oncology; UK ProtecT Study Collaborators, Horwich A, Huddart RA, Khoo VS, Parker CC, Woodhouse CJ, Thompson A, Christmas T, Ogden C, Fisher C, Jamieson C, Cooper CS, English DR, Hopper JL, Neal DE, Easton DF. Multiple newly identified loci associated with prostate cancer susceptibility. Nat Genet. 2008; 40(3):316–21. doi: 10.1038/ng.90.

[37] Sun J, Purcell L, Gao Z, Isaacs SD, Wiley KE, Hsu FC, Liu W, Duggan D, Carpten JD, Grönberg H, Xu J, Chang BL, Partin AW, Walsh PC, Isaacs WB, Zheng SL. Association between sequence variants at 17q12 and 17q24.3 and prostate cancer risk in European and African Americans. Prostate. 2008; 68(7):691–7. doi:10.1002/pros.20754.

[38] Zheng SL, Sun J, Wiklund F, Smith S, Stattin P, Li G, Adami HO, Hsu FC, Zhu Y, Bälter K, Kader AK, Turner AR, Liu W, Bleecker ER, Meyers DA, Duggan D, Carpten JD, Chang BL, Isaacs WB, Xu J, Grönberg H. Cumulative association of five genetic variants with prostate cancer. N Engl J Med. 2008; 358(9):910–9. doi:10.1056/NEJMoa075819.

[39] Levin AM, Machiela MJ, Zuhlke KA, Ray AM, Cooney KA, Douglas JA. Chromosome 17q12 variants contribute to risk of early-onset prostate cancer. Cancer Res. 2008; 68(16): 6492–5. doi: 10.1158/0008-5472.CAN-08-0348.

[40] Stevens VL, Ahn J, Sun J, Jacobs EJ, Moore SC, Patel AV, Berndt SI, Albanes D, Hayes RB. HNF1B and JAZF1 genes, diabetes, and prostate cancer risk. Prostate. 2010; 70(6): 601–7. doi: 10.1002/pros.21094.

[41] Berndt SI, Sampson J , Yeager M, Jacobs KB, Wang Z, Hutchinson A, Chung C, Orr N, Wacholder S, Chatterjee N, Yu K, Kraft P, Feigelson HS, Thun MJ, Diver WR, Albanes D, Virtamo J, Weinstein S, Schumacher FR, Cancel-Tassin G, Cussenot O, Valeri A, Andriole GL, Crawford ED, Haiman C, HendersonB, Kolonel L, Le Marchand L, Siddiq A, Riboli E, Travis RC, KaaksR, Isaacs W, Isaacs S, Wiley KE, Gronberg H, Wiklund F, Stattin P, Xu J, Zheng SL, Sun J, Vatten LJ, Hveem K, Njølstad I, Gerhard DS, Tucker M, Hayes RB, Hoover RN, Fraumeni JF Jr, Hunter DJ, Thomas G, Chanock SJ. Large-scale fine mapping of the HNF1B locus and prostate cancer risk. Hum Mol Genet. 2011; 20(16):3322–9. doi: 10.1093/hmg/ddr213.

[42] Kim HJ, Bae JS, Lee J, Chang IH, Kim KD, Shin HD, Han JH, Lee SY, Kim W, Myung SC. HNF1B polymorphism associated with development of prostate cancer in Korean patients. Urology. 2011 Oct;78(4):969.e1–6. doi: 10.1016/j.urology.2011.06.045.

[43] Nikolić ZZ, Branković AS, Savić-Pavićević DL, Preković SM, Vukotić VD, Cerović SJ, Filipović NN, Tomović SM, Romac SP, Brajušković GN. Assessment of association between common variants at 17q12 and prostate cancer risk-evidence from Serbian population and meta-analysis. Clin Transl Sci. 2014; 7(4):307–13. doi:10.1111/cts.12130.

[44] Chang BL, Spangler E, Gallagher S, Haiman CA, Henderson B, Isaacs W, Benford ML, Kidd LR, Cooney K, Strom S, Ingles SA, Stern MC, Corral R, Joshi AD, Xu J, Giri VN, Rybicki B, Neslund-Dudas C, Kibel AS, Thompson IM, Leach RJ, Ostrander EA, Stanford JL, Witte J, Casey G, Eeles R, Hsing AW, Chanock S, Hu JJ, John EM, Park J, Stefflova K, Zeigler-Johnson C, Rebbeck TR. Validation of genome-wide prostate cancer associations in men of African descent. Cancer Epidemiol Biomarkers Prev. 2011; 20(1): 23–32. doi: 10.1158/1055-9965.EPI-10-0698.

[45] Haiman CA, Chen GK, Blot WJ, Strom SS, Berndt SI, Kittles RA, Rybicki BA, Isaacs WB, Ingles SA, Stanford JL, Diver WR, Witte JS, Hsing AW, Nemesure B, Rebbeck TR, Cooney KA, Xu J, Kibel AS, Hu JJ, John EM, Gueye SM, Watya S, Signorello LB, Hayes

RB, Wang Z, Yeboah E, Tettey Y, Cai Q, Kolb S, Ostrander EA, Zeigler-Johnson C, Yamamura Y, Neslund-Dudas C, Haslag-Minoff J, Wu W, Thomas V, Allen GO, Murphy A, Chang BL, Zheng SL, Leske MC, Wu SY, Ray AM, Hennis AJ, Thun MJ, Carpten J, Casey G, Carter EN, Duarte ER, Xia LY, Sheng X, Wan P, Pooler LC, Cheng I, Monroe KR, Schumacher F, Le Marchand L, Kolonel LN, Chanock SJ, Van Den Berg D, Stram DO, Henderson BE. Genome-wide association study of prostate cancer in men of African ancestry identifies a susceptibility locus at 17q21. Nat Genet. 2011; 43(6):5703. doi: 10.1038/ng.839.

[46] Hooker S, Hernandez W, Chen H, Robbins C, Torres JB, Ahaghotu C, Carpten J, Kittles RA. Replication of prostate cancer risk loci on 8q24, 11q13, 17q12, 19q33, and Xp11 in African Americans. Prostate. 2010; 70(3):270-5. doi:10.1002/pros.21061.

[47] Chornokur G, Amankwah EK, Davis SN, Phelan CM, Park JY, Pow-Sang J, Kumar NB. Variation in HNF1B and obesity may influence prostate cancer risk in African American men: a pilot study. Prostate Cancer. 2013; 2013:384594. doi:10.1155/2013/384594.

[48] Zhang X, Cowper-Sal lari R, Bailey SD, Moore JH, Lupien M. Integrative functional genomics identifies an enhancer looping to the SOX9 gene disrupted by the 17q24.3 prostate cancer risk locus. Genome Res. 2012; 22(8):1437-46. doi:10.1101/gr.135665.111.

[49] Camp NJ, Farnham JM, Wong J, Christensen GB, Thomas A, Cannon-Albright LA. Replication of the 10q11 and Xp11 prostate cancer risk variants: results from a Utah pedigree-based study. Cancer Epidemiol Biomarkers Prev. 2009; 18(4):1290-4. doi: 10.1158/1055-9965.EPI-08-0327.

[50] Takata R, Akamatsu S, Kubo M, Takahashi A, Hosono N, Kawaguchi T, Tsunoda T, Inazawa J, Kamatani N, Ogawa O, Fujioka T, Nakamura Y, Nakagawa H. Genome-wide association study identifies five new susceptibility loci for prostate cancer in the Japanese population. Nat Genet. 2010; 42(9):751-4. doi: 10.1038/ng.635.

[51] Wang Y, Ray AM, Johnson EK, Zuhlke KA, Cooney KA, Lange EM. Evidence for an association between prostate cancer and chromosome 8q24 and 10q11 genetic variants in African American men: the Flint Men's Health Study. Prostate. 2011; 71(3):225–31. doi: 10.1002/pros.21234.

[52] Jin G, Lu L, Cooney KA, Ray AM, Zuhlke KA, Lange EM, Cannon-Albright LA, Camp NJ, Teerlink CC, Fitzgerald LM, Stanford JL, Wiley KE, Isaacs SD, Walsh PC, Foulkes WD, Giles GG, Hopper JL, Severi G, Eeles R, Easton D, Kote-Jarai Z, Guy M, Rinckleb A, Maier C, Vogel W, Cancel-Tassin G, Egrot C, Cussenot O, Thibodeau SN, McDonnell SK, Schaid DJ, Wiklund F, Grönberg H, Emanuelsson M, Whittemore AS, Oakley-Girvan I, Hsieh CL, Wahlfors T, Tammela T, Schleutker J, Catalona WJ, Zheng SL, Ostrander EA, Isaacs WB, Xu J; International Consortium for Prostate Cancer Genetics. Validation of prostate cancer risk-related loci identified from genome-wide association studies using family-based association analysis: evidence from the International Consortium for Prostate Cancer Genetics (ICPCG). Hum Genet. 2012; 131(7):1095–103. doi: 10.1007/s00439-011-1136-0.

[53] Teerlink CC, Thibodeau SN, McDonnell SK, Schaid DJ, Rinckleb A, Maier C, Vogel W, Cancel-Tassin G, Egrot C, Cussenot O, Foulkes WD, Giles GG, Hopper JL, Severi G, Eeles R, Easton D, Kote-Jarai Z, Guy M, Cooney KA, Ray AM, Zuhlke KA, Lange EM, Fitzgerald LM, Stanford JL, Ostrander EA, Wiley KE, Isaacs SD, Walsh PC, Isaacs WB, Wahlfors T, Tammela T, Schleutker J, Wiklund F, Grönberg H, Emanuelsson M, Carpten J, Bailey-Wilson J, Whittemore AS, Oakley-Girvan I, Hsieh CL, Catalona WJ, Zheng SL, Jin G, Lu L, Xu J; International Consortium for Prostate Cancer Genetics, Camp NJ, Cannon-Albright LA. Association analysis of 9,560 prostate cancer cases from the International Consortium of Prostate Cancer Genetics confirms the role of reported prostate cancer associated SNPs for familial disease. Hum Genet. 2014; 133(3):347–56. doi:10.1007/s00439-013-1384-2.

[54] Fernandez P, Salie M, du Toit D, van der Merwe A. Analysis of prostate cancer susceptibility variants in South African men: replicating associations on chromosomes 8q24 and 10q11. Prostate Cancer. 2015; 2015:465184. doi:10.1155/2015/465184.

[55] Jinga V, Csiki IE, Manolescu A, Iordache P, Mates IN, Radavoi D, Rascu S, Badescu D, Badea P, Mates D. Replication study of 34 common SNPs associated with prostate cancer in the Romanian population. J Cell Mol Med. 2016. doi:10.1111/jcmm.12729.

[56] Yeager M, Deng Z, Boland J, Matthews C, Bacior J, Lonsberry V, Hutchinson A, Burdett LA, Qi L, Jacobs KB, Gonzalez-Bosquet J, Berndt SI, Hayes RB, Hoover RN, Thomas G, Hunter DJ, Dean M, Chanock SJ. Comprehensive resequence analysis of a 97 kb region of chromosome 10q11.2 containing the MSMB gene associated with prostate cancer. Hum Genet. 2009; 126(6):743-50. doi:10.1007/s00439-009-0723-9.

[57] Lou H, Yeager M, Li H, Bosquet JG, Hayes RB, Orr N, Yu K, Hutchinson A, Jacobs KB, Kraft P, Wacholder S, Chatterjee N, Feigelson HS, Thun MJ, Diver WR, Albanes D, Virtamo J, Weinstein S, Ma J, Gaziano JM, Stampfer M, Schumacher FR, Giovannucci E, Cancel-Tassin G, Cussenot O, Valeri A, Andriole GL, Crawford ED, Anderson SK, Tucker M, Hoover RN, Fraumeni JF Jr, Thomas G, Hunter DJ, Dean M, Chanock SJ. Fine mapping and functional analysis of a common variant in MSMB on chromosome 10q11.2 associated with prostate cancer susceptibility. Proc Natl Acad Sci U S A. 2009; 106(19):7933-8. doi: 10.1073/pnas.0902104106.

[58] Pomerantz MM, Shrestha Y, Flavin RJ, Regan MM, Penney KL, Mucci LA, Stampfer MJ, Hunter DJ, Chanock SJ, Schafer EJ, Chan JA, Tabernero J, Baselga J, Richardson AL, Loda M, Oh WK, Kantoff PW, Hahn WC, Freedman ML. Analysis of the 10q11 cancer risk locus implicates MSMB and NCOA4 in human prostate tumorigenesis. PLoS Genet. 2010; 6(11):e1001204. doi:10.1371/journal.pgen.1001204.

[59] Parikh H, Wang Z, Pettigrew KA, Jia J, Daugherty S, Yeager M, Jacobs KB, Hutchinson A, Burdett L, Cullen M, Qi L, Boland J, Collins I, Albert TJ, Vatten LJ, Hveem K, Njølstad I, Cancel-Tassin G, Cussenot O, Valeri A, Virtamo J, Thun MJ, Feigelson HS, Diver WR, Chatterjee N, Thomas G, Albanes D, Chanock SJ, Hunter DJ, Hoover R, Hayes RB, Berndt SI, Sampson J, Amundadottir L. Fine mapping the KLK3 locus on chromosome

19q13.33 associated with prostate cancer susceptibility and PSA levels. Hum Genet. 2011; 129(6):675–85. doi:10.1007/s00439-011-0953-5.

[60] Xu J, Mo Z, Ye D, Wang M, Liu F, Jin G, Xu C, Wang X, Shao Q, Chen Z, Tao Z, Qi J, Zhou F, Wang Z, Fu Y, He D, Wei Q, Guo J, Wu D, Gao X, Yuan J, Wang G, Xu Y, Wang G, Yao H, Dong P, Jiao Y, Shen M, Yang J, Ou-Yang J, Jiang H, Zhu Y, Ren S, Zhang Z, Yin C, Gao X, Dai B, Hu Z, Yang Y, Wu Q, Chen H, Peng P, Zheng Y, Zheng X, Xiang Y, Long J, Gong J, Na R, Lin X, Yu H, Wang Z, Tao S, Feng J, Sun J, Liu W, Hsing A, Rao J, Ding Q, Wiklund F, Gronberg H, Shu XO, Zheng W, Shen H, Jin L, Shi R, Lu D, Zhang X, Sun J, Zheng SL, Sun Y. Genome-wide association study in Chinese men identifies two new prostate cancer risk loci at 9q31.2 and 19q13.4. Nat Genet. 2012; 44(11):1231–5. doi: 10.1038/ng.2424.

[61] Hsing AW, Chokkalingam AP. Prostate cancer epidemiology. Front Biosci. 2006; 11:1388-413.

[62] Dianat SS, Margreiter M, Eckersberger E, Finkelstein J, Kuehas F, Herwig R, Ayati M, Lepor H, Djavan B. Gene polymorphisms and prostate cancer: the evidence. BJU Int. 2009; 104(11):1560-72. doi: 10.1111/j.1464-410X.2009.08973.x.

[63] Sissung TM, Price DK, Del Re M, Ley AM, Giovannetti E, Figg WD, Danesi R. Genetic variation: effect on prostate cancer. Biochim Biophys Acta. 2014; 1846(2):446-56. doi: 10.1016/j.bbcan.2014.08.007.

[64] Chang CQ, Yesupriya A, Rowell JL, Pimentel CB, Clyne M, Gwinn M, Khoury MJ, Wulf A, Schully SD. A systematic review of cancer GWAS and candidate gene meta-analyses reveals limited overlap but similar effect sizes. Eur J Hum Genet. 2014; 22(3):402-8. doi: 10.1038/ejhg.2013.161.

[65] Slaby O, Bienertova-Vasku J, Svoboda M, Vyzula R. Genetic polymorphisms and microRNAs: new direction in molecular epidemiology of solid cancer. J Cell Mol Med. 2012; 16(1):8-21. doi: 10.1111/j.1582-4934.2011.01359.x.

[66] Lindström S, Ma J, Altshuler D, Giovannucci E, Riboli E, Albanes D, Allen NE, Berndt SI, Boeing H, Bueno-de-Mesquita HB, Chanock SJ, Dunning AM, Feigelson HS, Gaziano JM, Haiman CA, Hayes RB, Henderson BE, Hunter DJ, Kaaks R, Kolonel LN, Le Marchand L, Martínez C, Overvad K, Siddiq A, Stampfer M, Stattin P, Stram DO, Thun MJ, Trichopoulos D, Tumino R, Virtamo J, Weinstein SJ, Yeager M, Kraft P, Freedman ML. A large study of androgen receptor germline variants and their relation to sex hormone levels and prostate cancer risk. Results from the National Cancer Institute Breast and Prostate Cancer Cohort Consortium. J Clin Endocrinol Metab. 2010; 95(9):E121-7. doi: 10.1210/jc.2009-1911.

[67] Chamberlain NL, Driver ED, Miesfeld RL. The length and location of CAG trinucleotide repeats in the androgen receptor N-terminal domain affect transactivation function. Nucleic Acids Res. 1994; 22:3181-6. 10.1093/nar/22.15.3181.

[68] Price DK, Chau CH, Till C, Goodman PJ, Baum CE, Ockers SB, English BC, Minasian L, Parnes HL, Hsing AW, Reichardt JK, Hoque A, Tangen CM, Kristal AR, Thompson IM, Figg WD. Androgen receptor CAG repeat length and association with prostate cancer risk: results from the prostate cancer prevention trial. J Urol. 2010; 184(6): 2297-302. doi: 10.1016/j.juro.2010.08.005.

[69] Gu M, Dong X, Zhang X, Niu W. The CAG repeat polymorphism of androgen receptor gene and prostate cancer: a meta-analysis. Mol Biol Rep. 2012; 39(3):2615-24. doi: 10.1007/s11033-011-1014-9.

[70] Sun JH, Lee SA. Association between CAG repeat polymorphisms and the risk of prostate cancer: a meta-analysis by race, study design and the number of (CAG)n repeat polymorphisms. Int J Mol Med. 2013; 32(5):1195-203. doi:10.3892/ijmm.2013.1474.

[71] Hsing AW, Gao YT, Wu G, Wang X, Deng J, Chen YL, Sesterhenn IA, Mostofi FK, Benichou J, Chang C. Polymorphic CAG and GGN repeat lengths in the androgen receptor gene and prostate cancer risk: a population-based case-control study in China. Cancer Res. 2000; 60(18):5111-6.

[72] Brockschmidt FF, Nöthen MM, Hillmer AM. The two most common alleles of the coding GGN repeat in the androgen receptor gene cause differences in protein function. J Mol Endocrinol. 2007; 39(1):1-8.

[73] Zeegers MP, Kiemeney LA, Nieder AM, Ostrer H. How strong is the association between CAG and GGN repeat length polymorphisms in the androgen receptor gene and prostate cancer risk? Cancer Epidemiol Biomarkers Prev. 2004; 13(11 Pt 1):1765-71.

[74] Vijayalakshmi K, Thangaraj K, Rajender S, Vettriselvi V, Venkatesan P, Shroff S, Vishwanathan KN, Paul SF. GGN repeat length and GGN/CAG haplotype variations in the androgen receptor gene and prostate cancer risk in south Indian men. J Hum Genet. 2006; 51(11):998-1005.

[75] Mittal RD, Mishra DK, Thangaraj K, Singh R, Mandhani A. Is there an inter-relationship between prostate specific antigen, kallikrein-2 and androgen receptor gene polymorphisms with risk of prostate cancer in north Indian population? Steroids. 2007; 72(4): 335-41.

[76] Mittal RD, Mishra D, Mandhani AK. Role of an androgen receptor gene polymorphism in development of hormone refractory prostate cancer in Indian population. Asian Pac J Cancer Prev. 2007; 8(2):275-8.

[77] Lange EM, Sarma AV, Ray A, Wang Y, Ho LA, Anderson SA, Cunningham JM, Cooney KA. The androgen receptor CAG and GGN repeat polymorphisms and prostate cancer susceptibility in African-American men: results from the Flint Men's Health Study. J Hum Genet. 2008; 53(3):220-6. doi: 10.1007/s10038-007-0240-4.

[78] Rodríguez-González G, Cabrera S, Ramírez-Moreno R, Bilbao C, Díaz-Chico JC, Serra L, Chesa N, Cabrera JJ, Díaz-Chico BN. Short alleles of both GGN and CAG repeats at the exon-1 of the androgen receptor gene are associated to increased PSA staining and

a higher Gleason score in human prostatic cancer. J Steroid Biochem Mol Biol. 2009; 113(1–2):85-91. doi: 10.1016/j.jsbmb.2008.11.010.

[79] Akinloye O, Gromoll J, Simoni M. Variation in CAG and GGN repeat lengths and CAG/GGN haplotype in androgen receptor gene polymorphism and prostate carcinoma in Nigerians. Br J Biomed Sci. 2011; 68(3):138-42.

[80] Li J, Mercer E, Gou X, Lu YJ. Ethnical disparities of prostate cancer predisposition: genetic polymorphisms in androgen-related genes. Am J Cancer Res. 2013; 3(2):127-51.

[81] Cai Q, Wang Z, Zhang W, Guo X, Shang Z, Jiang N, Tian J, Niu Y. Association between glutathione S-transferases M1 and T1 gene polymorphisms and prostate cancer risk: a systematic review and meta-analysis. Tumour Biol. 2014; 35(1):247–56. doi: 10.1007/s13277-013-1030-6.

[82] Fang DH1, Fan CH, Ji Q, Qi BX, Li J, Wang L. Differential effects of paraoxonase 1 (PON1) polymorphisms on cancer risk: evidence from 25 published studies. MolBiol Rep. 2012; 39(6):6801–9.

[83] Zhang M, Xiong H, Fang L, Lu W, Wu X, Huang ZS, Wang YQ, Cai ZM, Wu S. Paraoxonase 1 (PON1) Q192R gene polymorphism and cancer risk: a meta-analysis based on 30 publications. Asian Pac J Cancer Prev. 2015; 16(10):4457-63.

[84] Ding G, Xu W, Liu H, Zhang M, Huang Q, Liao Z. CYP1A1 MspI polymorphism is associated with prostate cancer susceptibility: evidence from a meta-analysis. Mol Biol Rep. 2013; 40(5):3483-91.

[85] Wu B, Liu K, Huang H, Yuan J, Yuan W, Wang S, Chen T, Zhao H, Yin C.MspI and Ile462Val polymorphisms in CYP1A1 and overall cancer risk: a meta-analysis. PLoS One. 2013; 8(12):e85166.

[86] Ou C, Zhao Y, Liu JH, Zhu B, Li PZ, Zhao HL. Relationship Between Aldosterone Synthase CYP1A1 MspI Gene Polymorphism and Prostate Cancer Risk. Technol Cancer Res Treat. 2016 Jan 13. pii: 1533034615625519. [Epub ahead of print]

[87] Zhang H, Li L, Xu Y. CYP1B1 polymorphisms and susceptibility to prostate cancer: a meta-analysis. PLoS One. 2013; 8(7):e68634. doi:10.1371/journal.pone.0068634.

[88] He XF, Liu ZZ, Xie JJ, Wang W, Du YP, Chen Y, Wei W. Association between the CYP3A4 and CYP3A5 polymorphisms and cancer risk: a meta-analysis and meta-regression. Tumour Biol. 2014; 35(10):9859-77. doi:10.1007/s13277-014-2241-1.

[89] Feng YZ, Liu YL, He XF, Wei W, Shen XL, Xie DL.Association between the XRCC1 Arg194Trp polymorphism and risk of cancer: evidence from 201 case-control studies. Tumour Biol. 2014; 35(11):10677-97.

[90] Chen Y, Li T, Li J, Mo Z.X-ray repair cross-complementing group 1 (XRCC1) Arg399Gln polymorphism significantly associated with prostate cancer. Int J Biol Markers. 2015; 30(1):e12-21.

[91] Xuan G, Hui Y, Fang H. The association of XRCC3 Thr241Met genetic variant with risk of prostate cancer: a meta-analysis. Afr Health Sci. 2015; 15(1):117-22. doi: 10.4314/ahs.v15i1.16.

[92] Barry KH, Koutros S, Andreotti G, Sandler DP, Burdette LA, Yeager M, Beane Freeman LE, Lubin JH, Ma X, Zheng T, Alavanja MC, Berndt SI. Genetic variation in nucleotide excision repair pathway genes, pesticide exposure and prostate cancer risk. Carcinogenesis. 2012; 33(2):331-7. doi: 10.1093/carcin/bgr258.

[93] Henríquez-Hernández LA, Valenciano A, Foro-Arnalot P, Álvarez-Cubero MJ, Cozar JM, Suárez-Novo JF, Castells-Esteve M, Fernández-Gonzalo P, De-Paula-Carranza B, Ferrer M, Guedea F, Sancho-Pardo G, Craven-Bartle J, Ortiz-Gordillo MJ, Cabrera-Roldán P, Herrera-Ramos E, Rodríguez-Gallego C, Rodríguez-Melcón JI, Lara PC. Single nucleotide polymorphisms in DNA repair genes as risk factors associated to prostate cancer progression. BMC Med Genet. 2014;15:143.

[94] Meyer A, Coinac I, Bogdanova N, Dubrowinskaja N, Turmanov N, Haubold S, Schürmann P, Imkamp F, von Klot C, Merseburger AS, Machtens S, Bremer M, Hillemanns P, Kuczyk MA, Karstens JH, Serth J, Dörk T. Apoptosis gene polymorphisms and risk of prostate cancer: a hospital-based study of German patients treated with brachytherapy. Urol Oncol. 2013; 31(1):74-81. doi:10.1016/j.urolonc.2010.09.011.

[95] Ma Q, Qi C, Tie C, Guo Z. Genetic polymorphisms of xeroderma pigmentosum group D gene Asp312Asn and Lys751Gln and susceptibility to prostate cancer: a systematic review and meta-analysis. Gene. 2013; 530(2):309-14. doi:10.1016/j.gene.2013.08.053.

[96] Chen Y, Zhong H, Gao JG, Tang JE, Wang R. A systematic review and meta-analysis of three gene variants association with risk of prostate cancer: an update. Urol J. 2015; 12(3):2138-47.

[97] Kibel AS, Jin CH, Klim A, Luly J, A Roehl K, Wu WS, Suarez BK. Association between polymorphisms in cell cycle genes and advanced prostate carcinoma. Prostate. 2008; 68(11):1179-86. doi: 10.1002/pros.20784.

[98] Wei F, Xu J, Tang L, Shao J, Wang Y, Chen L, Guan X. p27(Kip1) V109G polymorphism and cancer risk: a systematic review and meta-analysis. Cancer Biother Radiopharm. 2012; 27(10):665-71. doi: 10.1089/cbr.2012.1229.

[99] Zheng M, Wan L, He X, Qi X, Liu F, Zhang DH. Effect of the CCND1 A870G polymorphism on prostate cancer risk: a meta-analysis of 3,820 cases and 3,825 controls. World J Surg Oncol. 2015;13:55.

[100] Hirata H, Hinoda Y, Kikuno N, Suehiro Y, Shahryari V, Ahmad AE, Tabatabai ZL, Igawa M, Dahiya R. Bcl2 -938C/A polymorphism carries increased risk of biochemical recurrence after radical prostatectomy. J Urol. 2009; 181(4):1907-12. doi: 10.1016/j.juro.2008.11.093.

[101] Bachmann HS, Heukamp LC, Schmitz KJ, Hilburn CF, Kahl P, Buettner R, Nückel H, Eisenhardt A, Rübben H, Schmid KW, Siffert W, Eggert A, Schramm A, Schulte JH.

Regulatory BCL2 promoter polymorphism (-938C>A) is associated with adverse outcome in patients with prostate carcinoma. Int J Cancer. 2011; 129(10):2390–9. doi: 10.1002/ijc.25904.

[102] Lu Y, Liu Y, Zeng J, He Y, Peng Q, Deng Y, Wang J, Xie L, Li T, Qin X, Li S. Association of p53 codon 72 polymorphism with prostate cancer: an update meta-analysis. Tumour Biol. 2014; 35(5):3997–4005. doi:10.1007/s13277-014-1657-y.

[103] Hodgson ME, Poole C, Olshan AF, North KE, Zeng D, Millikan RC.Smoking and selected DNA repair gene polymorphisms in controls: systematic review and meta-analysis. Cancer Epidemiol Biomarkers Prev. 2010;19(12): 3055–86.

[104] Langsenlehner T, Renner W, Gerger A, Hofmann G, Thurner EM, Kapp KS, Langsenlehner U. Association between single nucleotide polymorphisms in the gene for XRCC1 and radiation-induced late toxicity in prostate cancer patients. Radiother Oncol. 2011; 98(3):387–93.

[105] Song YZ, Han FJ, Liu M, Xia CC, Shi WY, Dong LH. Association between single nucleotide polymorphisms in XRCC3 and radiation-induced adverse effects on normal tissue: a meta-analysis. PLoS One. 2015; 10(6):e0130388.

[106] Kote-Jarai Z, Easton DF, StanfordJL, Ostrander EA, Schleutker J, Ingles SA, Schaid D, Thibodeau S, Dörk T, Neal D, Donovan J, Hamdy F, Cox A, Maier C, Vogel W, Guy M, Muir K, Lophatananon A, Kedda MA, Spurdle A, Steginga S, John EM, Giles G, Hopper J, Chappuis PO, Hutter P, Foulkes WD, Hamel N, Salinas CA, Koopmeiners JS, Karyadi DM, Johanneson B, Wahlfors T, Tammela TL, Stern MC, Corral R, McDonnell SK, Schürmann P, Meyer A, Kuefer R, Leongamornlert DA, Tymrakiewicz M, Liu JF, O'Mara T, Gardiner RA, Aitken J, Joshi AD, Severi G, English DR, Southey M, Edwards SM, Al Olama AA, PRACTICAL Consortium, Eeles RA. Multiple novel prostate cancer predisposition loci confirmed by an international study: the PRACTICAL Consortium. Cancer Epidemiol Biomarkers Prev. 2008; 17(8):2052–61.

[107] Chen T, Yi SH, Liu XY, Liu ZG. Meta-analysis of associations between the MDM2-T309G polymorphism and prostate cancer risk. Asian Pac J Cancer Prev. 2012; 13(9): 4327–30.

[108] Yang J, Gao W, Song NH, Wang W, Zhang JX, Lu P, Hua LX, Gu M. The risks, degree of malignancy and clinical progression of prostate cancer associated with the MDM2 T309G polymorphism: a meta-analysis. Asian J Androl. 2012; 14(5):726–31. doi: 10.1038/aja.2012.65.

[109] Stoehr R, Hitzenbichler F, Kneitz B, Hammerschmied CG, Burger M, Tannapfel A, Hartmann A. Mdm2-SNP309 polymorphism in prostate cancer: no evidence

for association with increased risk or histopathological tumour characteristics. Br J Cancer. 2008; 99(1):78–82. doi: 10.1038/sj.bjc.6604441.

[110] Yu CC, Lin VC, Huang CY, Liu CC, Wang JS, Wu TT, Pu YS, Huang CH, Huang CN, Huang SP, Bao BY. Prognostic significance of cyclin D1 polymorphisms on prostate-specific antigen recurrence after radical prostatectomy. Ann Surg Oncol. 2013; 20 Suppl 3:S492–9.

[111] Kidd LR, Coulibaly A, Templeton TM, Chen W, Long LO, Mason T, Bonilla C, Akereyeni F, Freeman V, Isaacs W, Ahaghotu C, Kittles RA. Germline BCL-2 sequence variants and inherited predisposition to prostate cancer. Prostate Cancer Prostatic Dis. 2006; 9(3):284–92.

[112] Yin M, Wei S, Wei Q. Vitamin D Receptor genetic polymorphisms and prostate cancer risk: a meta-analysis of 36 published studies. Int J Clin Exp Med. 2009; 2(2):159–75.

[113] Zhang Q, Shan Y. Genetic polymorphisms of vitamin D receptor and the risk of prostate cancer: a meta-analysis. J BUON. 2013; 18(4):961–9.

[114] Huang J, Yang J, Wang H, Xiong T, Zhang H, Ma Y, Wang X, Huang J, Du L. The association between the poly(A) polymorphism in the VDR gene and cancer risk: a meta-analysis. Tumour Biol. 2013 Jun;34(3):1833–8. doi:10.1007/s13277-013-0724-0.

[115] Guo Z, Wen J, Kan Q, Huang S, Liu X, Sun N, Li Z. Lack of association between vitamin D receptor gene FokI and BsmI polymorphisms and prostate cancer risk: an updated meta-analysis involving 21,756 subjects. Tumour Biol. 2013; 34(5):3189–200. doi: 10.1007/s13277-013-0889-6.

[116] Pao JB, Yang YP, Huang CN, Huang SP, Hour TC, Chang TY, Lan YH, Lu TL, Lee HZ, Juang SH, Huang CY, Bao BY. Vitamin D receptor gene variants and clinical outcomes after androgen-deprivation therapy for prostate cancer. World J Urol. 2013; 31(2):281–7. doi: 10.1007/s00345-011-0813-x.

[117] Tindall EA, Hayes VM, Petersen DC. Inflammatory genetic markers of prostate cancer risk. Cancers (Basel). 2010; 2(2):1198–220. doi:10.3390/cancers2021198.

[118] Cai Q, Tang Y, Zhang M, Shang Z, Li G, Tian J, Jiang N, Quan C, Niu Y. TGFβ1 Leu10Pro polymorphism contributes to the development of prostate cancer: evidence from a meta-analysis. Tumour Biol. 2014; 35(1):667–73. doi: 10.1007/s13277-013-1092-5.

[119] Wei BB, Xi B, Wang R, Bai JM, Chang JK, Zhang YY, Yoneda R, Su JT, Hua LX. TGFbeta1 T29C polymorphism and cancer risk: a meta-analysis based on 40 case-control studies. Cancer Genet Cytogenet. 2010; 196(1):68–75. doi:10.1016/j.cancergencyto.2009.09.016.

[120] Ewart-Toland A, Chan JM, Yuan J, Balmain A, Ma J. A gain of function TGFB1 polymorphism may be associated with late stage prostate cancer. Cancer Epidemiol Biomarkers Prev. 2004; 13(5):759–64.

[121] Faria PC, Saba K, Neves AF, Cordeiro ER, Marangoni K, Freitas DG, Goulart LR. Transforming growth factor-beta 1 gene polymorphisms and expression in the blood of prostate cancer patients. Cancer Invest. 2007; 25(8):726–32.

[122] Brand TC, Bermejo C, Canby-Hagino E, Troyer DA, Baillargeon J, Thompson IM, Leach RJ, Naylor SL. Association of polymorphisms in TGFB1 and prostate cancer prognosis. J Urol. 2008; 179(2):754–8.

[123] Teixeira AL, Ribeiro R, Morais A, Lobo F, Fraga A, Pina F, Calais-da-Silva FM, Calais-da-Silva FE, Medeiros R. Combined analysis of EGF+61G>A and TGFB1+869T>C functional polymorphisms in the time to androgen independence and prostate cancer susceptibility. Pharmacogenomics J. 2009; 9(5):341–6. doi:10.1038/tpj.2009.20.

[124] Hong TT, Zhang RX, Wu XH, Hua D. Polymorphism of vascular endothelial growth factor -1154G>A (rs1570360) with cancer risk: a meta-analysis of 16 case-control studies. Mol Biol Rep. 2012; 39(5):5283–9. doi: 10.1007/s11033-011-1326-9.

[125] Chen GQ, Luo JB, Wang GZ, Ding JE. Assessment of the associations between three VEGF polymorphisms and risk of prostate cancer. Tumour Biol. 2014; 35(3):1875–9. doi: 10.1007/s13277-013-1250-9.

[126] Chen Y, Li T, Yu X, Xu J, Li J, Luo D, Mo Z, Hu Y. The RTK/ERK pathway is associated with prostate cancer risk on the SNP level: a pooled analysis of 41 sets of data from case-control studies. Gene. 2014; 534(2):286–97. doi:10.1016/j.gene.2013.10.042.

[127] Shao N, Xu B, Mi YY, Hua LX. IL-10 polymorphisms and prostate cancer risk: a meta-analysis. Prostate Cancer Prostatic Dis. 2011; 14(2):129–35. doi:10.1038/pcan.2011.6.

[128] Yu Z, Liu Q, Huang C, Wu M, Li G. The interleukin 10 -819C/T polymorphism and cancer risk: a HuGE review and meta-analysis of 73 studies including 15,942 cases and 22,336 controls. OMICS. 2013; 17(4):200–14. doi: 10.1089/omi.2012.0089.

[129] Xu Y, Zhu S. Associations between vascular endothelial growth factor polymorphisms and prostate cancer risk: a meta-analysis. Tumour Biol. 2014; 35(2):1307–11. doi: 10.1007/s13277-013-1173-5.

[130] Sfar S, Saad H, Mosbah F, Chouchane L. Combined effects of the angiogenic genes polymorphisms on prostate cancer susceptibility and aggressiveness. Mol Biol Rep. 2009; 36(1):37–45.

[131] Jain L, Vargo CA, Danesi R, Sissung TM, Price DK, Venzon D, Venitz J, Figg WD. The role of vascular endothelial growth factor SNPs as predictive and prognostic markers for major solid tumors. Mol Cancer Ther. 2009; 8(9):2496–508. doi: 10.1158/1535-7163.MCT-09-0302.

[132] Orlandi P, Fontana A, Fioravanti A, Di Desidero T, Galli L, Derosa L, Canu B, Marconcini R, Biasco E, Solini A, Francia G, Danesi R, Falcone A, Bocci G. VEGF-A polymorphisms predict progression-free survival among advanced castration-resistant prostate cancer patients treated with metronomic cyclophosphamide. Br J Cancer. 2013; 109(4): 957–64. doi:10.1038/bjc.2013.398.

[133] Roberts E, Cossigny DA, Quan GM. The role of vascular endothelial growth factor in metastatic prostate cancer to the skeleton. Prostate Cancer. 2013; 2013:418340. doi: 10.1155/2013/418340.

[134] Ye Y, Wang M, Hu S, Shi Y, Zhang X, Zhou Y, Zhao C, Wang G, Wen J, Zong H. Hypoxia-inducible factor-1α C1772T polymorphism and cancer risk: a meta-analysis including 18,334 subjects. Cancer Invest. 2014; 32(4):126–35. doi: 10.3109/07357907.2014.883527.

[135] Xu B, Tong N, Chen SQ, Hua LX, Wang ZJ, Zhang ZD, Chen M. FGFR4 Gly388Arg polymorphism contributes to prostate cancer development and progression: a meta-analysis of 2618 cases and 2305 controls. BMC Cancer. 2011; 11:84. doi: 10.1186/1471-2407-11-84.

[136] Nikolić ZZ, Pavićević DLj, Romac SP, Brajušković GN. Genetic variants within endothelial nitric oxide synthase gene and prostate cancer: a meta-analysis. Clin Transl Sci. 2015; 8(1):23–31. doi: 10.1111/cts.12203.

[137] Forstermann U, Boissel JP, Kleinert H. Expressional control of the 'constitutive' isoforms of nitric oxide synthase (NOS I and NOS III) FASEB. J. 1998; 12:773–90.

[138] Burke AJ, Sullivan FJ, Giles FJ, Glynn SA. The yin and yang of nitric oxide in cancer progression. Carcinogenesis. 2013; 34(3):503–12. doi:10.1093/carcin/bgt034.

[139] Jacobs EJ, Hsing AW, Bain EB, Stevens VL, Wang Y, Chen J, Chanock SJ, Zheng SL, Xu J, Thun MJ, Calle EE, Rodriguez C. Polymorphisms in angiogenesis-related genes and prostate cancer. Cancer Epidemiol Biomarkers Prev. 2008; 17(4):972–7.

[140] Medeiros R, Morais A, Vasconcelos A, Costa S, Pinto D, Oliveira J, Lopes C. Endothelial nitric oxide synthase gene polymorphisms and genetic susceptibility to prostate cancer. Eur J Cancer Prev. 2002; 11(4):343–50.

[141] Medeiros RM, Morais A, Vasconcelos A, Costa S, Pinto D, Oliveira J, Ferreira P, Lopes C. Outcome in prostate cancer: association with endothelial nitric oxide synthase Glu-Asp298 polymorphism at exon 7. Clin Cancer Res. 2002;8(11): 3433–7.

[142] Marangoni K, Neves AF, Cardoso AM, Santos WK, Faria PC, Goulart LR. The endothelial nitric oxide synthase Glu-298-Asp polymorphism and its mRNA expression in the peripheral blood of patients with prostate cancer and benign prostatic hyperplasia. Cancer Detect Prev. 2006;30(1): 7–13.

[143] Marangoni K, Araújo TG, Neves AF, Goulart LR. The -786T>C promoter polymorphism of the NOS3 gene is associated with prostate cancer progression. BMC Cancer. 2008; 8:273.

[144] Lee KM, Kang D, Park SK, Berndt SI, Reding D, Chatterjee N, Chanock S, Huang WY, Hayes RB. Nitric oxide synthase gene polymorphisms and prostate cancer risk. Carcinogenesis. 2009; 30(4):621–5.

[145] Ziaei SA, Samzadeh M, Jamaldini SH, Afshari M, Haghdoost AA, Hasanzad M. Endothelial nitric oxide synthase Glu298Asp polymorphism as a risk factor for prostate cancer. Int J Biol Markers. 2013;28(1): 43–8.

[146] Safarinejad MR, Safarinejad S, Shafiei N, Safarinejad S. Effects of the T-786C, G894T, and Intron 4 VNTR (4a/b) polymorphisms of the endothelial nitric oxide synthase gene on the risk of prostate cancer. Urol Oncol. 2013;31(7): 1132–40.

[147] Branković A, Brajušković G, Nikolić Z, Vukotić V, Cerović S, Savić-Pavićević D, Romac S. Endothelial nitric oxide synthase gene polymorphisms and prostate cancer risk in Serbian population. Int J Exp Pathol. 2013; 94(6):355–61.

[148] Medeiros R, Morais A, Vasconcelos A, Costa S, Carrilho S, Oliveira J, Lopes C. Endothelial nitric oxide synthase gene polymorphisms and the shedding of circulating tumour cells in the blood of prostate cancer patients. Cancer Lett. 2003; 189(1):85–90.

[149] Sanli O, Kucukgergin C, Gokpinar M, Tefik T, Nane I, Seckin S. Despite the lack of association between different genotypes and the presence of prostate cancer, endothelial nitric oxide synthase a/b (eNOS4a/b) polymorphism may be associated with advanced clinical stage and bone metastasis. Urol Oncol. 2011; 29(2):183–8.

[150] Senthil D, Raveendran M, Shen YH, Utama B, Dudley D, Wang J, Wang XL. Genotype-dependent expression of endothelial nitric oxide synthase (eNOS) and its regulatory proteins in cultured endothelial cells. DNA Cell Biol. 2005; 24(4):218–24.

[151] Miyamoto Y, Saito Y, Nakayama M, Shimasaki Y, Yoshimura T, Yoshimura M, Harada M, Kajiyama N, Kishimoto I, Kuwahara K, Hino J, Ogawa E, Hamanaka I, Kamitani S, Takahashi N, Kawakami R, Kangawa K, Yasue H, Nakao K. Replication protein A1 reduces transcription of the endothelial nitric oxide synthase gene containing a -786T-->C mutation associated with coronary spastic angina. Hum Mol Genet. 2000; 9(18): 2629–37.

[152] Dos Reis ST, Pontes J Jr, Villanova FE, Borra PM, Antunes AA, Dall'oglio MF, Srougi M, Leite KR. Genetic polymorphisms of matrix metalloproteinases: susceptibility and prognostic implications for prostate cancer. J Urol. 2009; 181(5):2320–5. doi: 10.1016/j.juro.2009.01.012.

[153] dos Reis ST, Villanova FE, Andrade PM, Pontes J Jr, de Sousa-Canavez JM, Sañudo A, Antunes AA, Dall'oglio MF, Srougi M, Moreira Leite KR. Matrix metalloproteinase-2

polymorphism is associated with prognosis in prostate cancer. Urol Oncol. 2010; 28(6): 624–7. doi: 10.1016/j.urolonc.2008.10.012.

[154] Srivastava P, Lone TA, Kapoor R, Mittal RD. Association of promoter polymorphisms in MMP2 and TIMP2 with prostate cancer susceptibility in North India. Arch Med Res. 2012; 43(2):117–24. doi: 10.1016/j.arcmed.2012.02.006.

[155] Yaykaşli KO, Kayikçi MA, Yamak N, Soğuktaş H, Düzenli S, Arslan AO, Metın A, Kaya E, Hatıpoğlu ÖF. Polymorphisms in MMP-2 and TIMP-2 in Turkish patients with prostate cancer. Turk J Med Sci. 2014; 44(5):839–43.

[156] Adabi Z, Mohsen Ziaei SA, Imani M, Samzadeh M, Narouie B, Jamaldini SH, Afshari M, Safavi M, Roshandel MR, Hasanzad M. Genetic Polymorphism of MMP2 Gene and Susceptibility to Prostate Cancer. Arch Med Res. 2015; 46(7):546–50. doi:10.1016/j.arcmed.2015.08.004.

[157] Price SJ, Greaves DR, Watkins H. Identification of novel, functional genetic variants in the human matrix metalloproteinase-2 gene: role of Sp1 in allele-specific transcriptional regulation. J Biol Chem. 2001; 276(10):7549–58.

[158] Chang Z, Zhou H, Liu Y. Promoter methylation and polymorphism of E-cadherin gene may confer a risk to prostate cancer: a meta-analysis based on 22 studies. Tumour Biol. 2014; 35(10):10503–13. doi: 10.1007/s13277-014-2323-0.

[159] Li HC, Albert JM, Shinohara ET, Cai Q, Freyer A, Cai H, Cao C, Wang Z, Kataoka N, Teng M, Zheng W, Lu B. E-cadherin promoter polymorphisms are not associated with the aggressiveness of prostate cancer in Caucasian patients. Urol Oncol. 2006; 24(6): 496–502.

[160] Li LC, Chui RM, Sasaki M, Nakajima K, Perinchery G, Au HC, Nojima D, Carroll P, Dahiya R. A single nucleotide polymorphism in the E-cadherin gene promoter alters transcriptional activities. Cancer Res. 2000; 60(4):873–6.

[161] Kammerer S, Roth RB, Reneland R, Marnellos G, Hoyal CR, Markward NJ, Ebner F, Kiechle M, Schwarz-Boeger U, Griffiths LR, Ulbrich C, Chrobok K, Forster G, Praetorius GM, Meyer P, Rehbock J, Cantor CR, Nelson MR, Braun A. Large-scale association study identifies ICAM gene region as breast and prostate cancer susceptibility locus. Cancer Res. 2004; 64(24):8906–10

[162] Chen H, Hernandez W, Shriver MD, Ahaghotu CA, Kittles RA. ICAM gene cluster SNPs and prostate cancer risk in African Americans. Hum Genet. 2006; 120(1):69–76.

[163] Walsh AL, Tuzova AV, Bolton EM, Lynch TH, Perry AS. Long noncoding RNAs and prostate carcinogenesis: the missing "linc?" Trends Mol Med. 2014; 20(8):428–36. doi: 10.1016/j.molmed.2014.03.005.

[164] Fatima R, Akhade VS, Pal D, Rao SM. Long noncoding RNAs in development and cancer: potential biomarkers and therapeutic targets. Mol Cell Ther. 2015; 3:5. doi: 10.1186/s40591-015-0042-6.

[165] Jin G, Jielin S, Isaacs SD, Wiley KE, Kim S-T, Chu LW, et al. Human polymorphisms at long non-coding RNAs (lncRNAs) and association with prostate cancer risk. Carcinogenesis 2011; 32: 1655–9.

[166] Xue Y, Wang M, Kang M, Wang Q, Wu B, Chu H, Zhong D, Qin C, Yin C, Zhang Z, Wu D. Association between lncrna PCGEM1 polymorphisms and prostate cancer risk. Prostate Cancer Prostatic Dis. 2013; 16(2):139–44, S1. doi:10.1038/pcan.2013.6.

[167] Zhou W, Tao Z, Wang Z, Hu W, Shen M, Zhou L, Wen Z, Yu Z, Wu X, Huang K, Hu Y, Lin X. Long noncoding RNA PCA3 gene promoter region is related to the risk of prostate cancer on Chinese males. Exp Mol Pathol. 2014; 97(3):550–3. doi:10.1016/j.yexmp.2014.11.005.

[168] Cook MB, Wang Z, Yeboah ED, Tettey Y, Biritwum RB, Adjei AA, Tay E, Truelove A, Niwa S, Chung CC, Chokkalingam AP, Chu LW, Yeager M, Hutchinson A, Yu K, Rand KA, Haiman CA; African Ancestry Prostate Cancer GWAS Consortium, Hoover RN, Hsing AW, Chanock SJ. A genome-wide association study of prostate cancer in West African men. Hum Genet. 2014; 133(5):509–21. doi: 10.1007/s00439-013-1387-z.

[169] Chung S, Nakagawa H, Uemura M, Piao L, Ashikawa K, Hosono N, Takata R, Akamatsu S, Kawaguchi T, Morizono T, Tsunoda T, Daigo Y, Matsuda K, Kamatani N, Nakamura Y, Kubo M. Association of a novel long non-coding RNA in 8q24 with prostate cancer susceptibility. Cancer Sci. 2011; 102(1):245–52. doi:10.1111/j.1349-7006.2010.01737.x.

[170] Mishra PJ, Bertino JR. MicroRNA polymorphisms: the future of pharmacogenomics, molecular epidemiology and individualized medicine. Pharmacogenomics. 2009; 10(3): 399–416.

[171] Sun G, Yan J, Noltner K, Feng J, Li H, Sarkis DA, et al. SNPs in human miRNA genes affect biogenesis and function. RNA 2009; 15:1640–51.

[172] Ryan BM, Robles AI, Harris CC. Genetic variation in microRNA networks: the implications for cancer research. Nature Reviews Cancer 2010; 10:389–402.

[173] Xu B, Feng NH, Li PC, Tao J, Wu D, Zhang ZD, Tong N, Wang JF, Song NH, Zhang W, Hua LX, Wu HF. A functional polymorphism in Pre-miR-146a gene is associated with prostate cancer risk and mature miR-146a expression in vivo. Prostate. 2010; 70(5):467–72.

[174] George GP, Gangwar R, Mandal RK, Sankhwar SN, Mittal RD. Genetic variation in microRNA genes and prostate cancer risk in North Indian population. Mol Biol Rep. 2011; 38(3):1609-15.

[175] Nikolić ZZ, Savić Pavićević DLj, Vukotić VD, Tomović SM, Cerović SJ, Filipović N, Romac SP, Brajušković GN. Association between genetic variant in hsa-miR-146a gene and prostate cancer progression: evidence from Serbian population. Cancer Causes Control. 2014; 25(11):1571-5.

[176] Parlayan C, Ikeda S, Sato N, Sawabe M, Muramatsu M, Arai T. Association analysis of single nucleotide polymorphisms in miR-146a and miR-196a2 on the prevalence of cancer in elderly Japanese: a case-control study. Asian Pac J Cancer Prev. 2014; 15:2101-2107.

[177] Chu H, Zhong D, Tang J, Li J, Xue Y, Tong N, Qin C, Yin C, Zhang Z, Wang M. A functional variant in miR-143 promoter contributes to prostate cancer risk. Arch Toxicol. 2016; 90(2):403-14. doi: 10.1007/s00204-014-1396-2.

[178] Nikolić Z, Savić Pavićević D, Vučić N, Cidilko S, Filipović N, Cerović S, Vukotić V, Romac S, Brajušković G. Assessment of association between genetic variants in microRNA genes hsa-miR-499, hsa-miR-196a2 and hsa-miR-27a and prostate cancer risk in Serbian population. Exp Mol Pathol. 2015; 99(1):145-50. doi: 10.1016/j.yexmp. 2015.06.009.

[179] König IR. Validation in genetic association studies. Brief Bioinform. 2011; 12(3):253–8. doi: 10.1093/bib/bbq074.

[180] Chanock SJ, Manolio T, Boehnke M, Boerwinkle E, Hunter DJ, Thomas G, Hirschhorn JN, Abecasis G, Altshuler D, Bailey-Wilson JE, Brooks LD, Cardon LR, Daly M, Donnelly P, Fraumeni JF Jr, Freimer NB, Gerhard DS, Gunter C, Guttmacher AE, Guyer MS, Harris EL, Hoh J, Hoover R, Kong CA, Merikangas KR, Morton CC, Palmer LJ, Phimister EG, Rice JP, Roberts J, Rotimi C, Tucker MA, Vogan KJ, Wacholder S, Wijsman EM, Winn DM, Collins FS. NCI-NHGRI Working Group on Replication in Association Studies. Replicating genotype-phenotype associations. Nature. 2007; 447(7145):655–60.

[181] Garg AX, Hackam D, Tonelli M. Systematic review and meta-analysis: when one study is just not enough. Clin J Am Soc Nephrol. 2008; 3(1):253-60. doi:10.2215/CJN.01430307.

[182] Weed DL. Interpreting epidemiological evidence: how meta-analysis and causal inference methods are related. Int J Epidemiol. 2000; 29(3):387-90.

Chapter 11

Key Genes in Prostate Cancer Progression: Role of MDM2, PTEN, and TMPRSS2-ERG Fusions

Appu Rathinavelu and Arkene Levy

Additional information is available at the end of the chapter

http://dx.doi.org/10.5772/64337

Abstract

In recent years, multiple genes or their protein products have been linked to initiation and progression of prostate cancer. Such genes include TMPRSS2, ERG, PTEN, and MDM2. This chapter discusses the pathological roles as well as the potential diagnostic and therapeutic applications of these genes that are highly expressed in prostate cancer when compared to other cancer types. The presence of these genes and related defects are linked to growth, progression, metastasis, invasiveness and resistance in prostate cancers. While knowledge related to TMPRSS2, ERG, and PTEN have been accumulating in the last two decades, the prometastatic role of MDM2 has been emerging in the last few years and revealing important functions related to prostate cancer progression.

Keywords: prostate cancer, TMPRSS2-ERG, PTEN, MDM2

1. Introduction

Prostate cancer (PCa) is a long latency tumor that occurs in males that are typically aged 50 years and older. Globally, more than 1.1 million cases of prostate cancer were recorded in 2012, accounting for around 8% of all new cancer cases and 15% in men [1]. In 2015, an estimated 220,800 men will be diagnosed with PCa in the United States and an estimated 27,540 men will die due to the disease making this malignancy the second leading cause of cancer-related death in men [2]. In addition, African-American (AA) men have the highest incidence and mortality from PCa when compared to other races [2]. The pathophysiology of prostate cancer is not fully elucidated, but it is well established that this dreadful disease is primarily initiated by cellular proliferation within pre-existing ducts and glands, which is referred to as Prostatic intraepithelial neoplasia (PIN). The PIN eventually progresses to invasive prostate cancer [3]. Clinical manifestations of the disease are variable and based on the transport by blood or the lymphatic system to metastatic sites and the effects of localized tumor growth. Localized prostate cancer is typically curable with targeted local therapy such as radical prostatectomy or radiation therapy. In metastatic prostate cancer, one of the successful strategies of treatment is surgical or chemical castration leading to androgen deprivation therapy (ADT) [4]. Unfortunately, approximately 33% of patients develop resistance to these treatments with the eventual increases in the number of androgens, prostate specific antigen (PSA), and circulating tumor cells (CTCs), leading to the more progressive and metastatic castration resistant prostate cancer (CRPC) [5]. The poor prognosis associated with metastatic prostate cancers is attributable in part to the highly heterogeneous nature of the cancer cells, which provides a significant hurdle for treatment of the disease [6]. Multiple genomic alterations underlie the clinical heterogeneity of prostate cancer and such aberrations include, point mutations, microsatellite variations, and chromosomal alterations such as translocations, insertions, duplications, fusions, and deletions [6, 7]. Therefore, there is a heightened interest in understanding the role of these genetic changes in prostate cancer development and progression.

2. Key genes in prostate cancer progression

In the past decade, several genes associated with prostate cancer have been identified. Four such genes: the ETS-related gene (ERG), The Transmembrane Protease Serine 2 (TMPRSS2), Mouse double minute 2 homolog (MDM2), and Phosphatase and tensin homolog (PTEN) have gained recognition for their high specificity of expression in prostatic carcinomas.

2.1. Prostate cancer and PTEN

PTEN is a protein coding gene that encodes for phosphatidylinositol-3,4,5-trisphosphate 3-phosphatase. It contains a tensin-like domain in addition to a catalytic domain similar to that of the dual specificity protein tyrosine phosphatases. PTEN is one of the most commonly mutated tumor suppressor genes in human prostate cancer. Interestingly, many aspects of PTEN expression and function, including transcriptional and post-transcriptional regulation, post-translational modifications, and protein-protein interactions have been shown to be altered in human prostate cancer. PTEN is a non-redundant phosphatase that directly interferes with the phosphatidylinositol 3-kinase (PI3K)/AKT signaling pathway and thereby controls several processes that are important in the homeostasis of cell survival and a multitude of cellular functions, which includes growth, proliferation, metabolism, migration, and cellular architecture [8]. PTEN removes the phosphate from the D3 position of phosphatidylinositol-3,4,5-triphosphate (PIP3), a product of PI3K, thus, can lead to inhibition of downstream AKT activation in normal conditions. However, when PTEN is mutated there is sustained activation of AKT that can lead to cell proliferation, angiogenesis and other related events. AKT exists in three isoforms, namely AKT1, AKT2, and AKT3, which are typically activated by the phosphorylation at two specific sites: Thr308 by PDK1 [9] and Ser473 by the mammalian target of rapamycin complex 2 (mTORC2) [10]. Activated AKT can drive cell survival, proliferation, growth, angiogenesis, and metabolism by phosphorylating downstream signaling proteins, which include inhibitory phosphorylation of GSK3, FOXO, BAD, p21, p27, and PGC I and activating phosphorylation of mTORC I mammalian target of rapamycin complex I (mTORC I), IKK-β, MDM2, ENTPD5, SREBP1C, AS160, and SKP2, which eventually leads to cell cycle progression and proliferation [10, 11]. Inhibition of GSK3β has been shown to specifically prevent the degradation of cyclin D1 and β-catenin, which can further support G1 to S phase transition in different types of cancers including prostate cancers [11, 12]. Activation of AKT also helps to evade apoptosis directly by phosphorylation of the pro-apoptotic protein BAD [13]. Hence, re-expression of wild-type *PTEN* in *PTEN* null prostate cancer cell lines can lead to the initiation of apoptosis and regression of tumors [14]. In addition, AKT directly activates the mTOR pathway by phosphorylating TSC2, which dismantles the TSC1/TSC2 complex that keeps the Rheb in an inhibited state. Once released from the TSC1/TSC2 inhibition, the Rheb can stimulate the phosphotransferase activity of mTORC1 and phosphorylate the S6 kinase (S6K) and 4E-binding protein (4EBP1), which in turn initiates cap-dependent protein translation [15, 16]. Therefore, as a consequence of PTEN loss in prostate cancers, PI3K/AKT/mTOR pathway activation can strongly lead to enhanced translation of mRNAs involved in cell growth and proliferation.

The *PTEN* gene is comprised of nine exons and totally codes for 403 amino acids [17]. The substrate binding site of PTEN is in the C2 domain, which can bind to the phospholipid membranes. The C2 domain also contains a signature motif HCXXGXXR that is typically found in the protein tyrosine phosphateses (PTPs) and in the dual specific protein phosphatases (DPPs). In addition, there is a short phosphatidylinositol-4,5-bisphosphate (PIP2) binding domain (PDB) on the N terminus, a motif on the C-terminal tail that interacts with PDZ-BD domain-containing proteins, and regulates protein stability and two PEST domains containing proline (P), glutamic acid (E), serine (S), and threonine (T) amino acids, which acts as a signal peptide that is also involved in the stability and degradation of PTEN [18]. When PIP2 binds to the PDB domain of PTEN it produces a conformational change in the protein leading to allosteric activation of substrate binding site for attracting the substrates for de-phosphorylation [19]. In addition to the allosteric activation, the positive charge of the substrate binding pocket of PTEN's is also essential for accommodating larger substrates such as phosphoinositides. The phosphatase domain of PTEN is a evolutionarily conserved domain that harbors nearly 40% of its cancer-associated mutations, and the most common mutations are C124S mutation, which abolishes both lipid binding and protein phosphatase activity, and the G129E mutation that destroys the lipid phosphatase activity [20–22]. However, some of the important PTEN tumorigenic mutations occur on the C2 domain also, confirm the importance of the structural integrity of the C terminus in maintaining PTEN activity and protein stability [23, 24] (**Figure 1**). In prostate cancer, PTEN loss most commonly results from a somatic mutation generated through copy number loss rather than point mutation [25, 26], however, recent exome sequencing has identified several recurrent mutations also in the PTEN gene [27, 28].

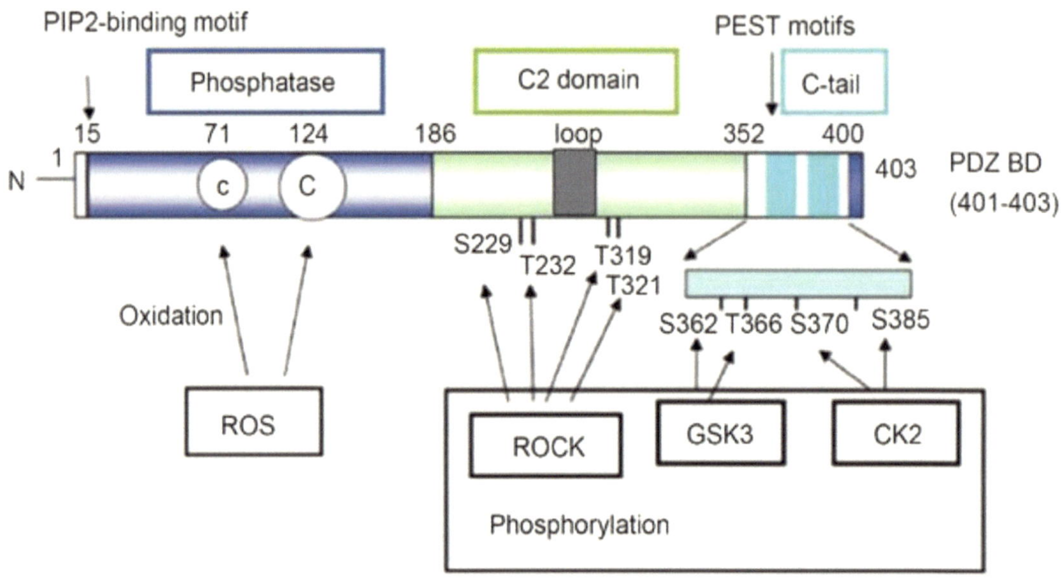

Figure 1. Different domains of PTEN and the phosphorylation sites. (Obtained from: Cell Res. 2008; 18: 807–816.)

2.1.1. PTEN loss combined with alterations in inflammatory pathway regulators

Various lines of evidence suggest that chronic inflammation is a closely associated event in the tumorigenic mechanisms of prostate cancer [29, 30] and to the several mutations that are causing this disease. A cytokine that is most commonly associated with tumor growth, proliferation, and angiogenesis in many cancers and also the most frequently found inflammatory mediator in prostate cancer is IL-6 [31]. When expressed at high levels, in addition to imposing the inflammatory functions, a strong correlation between the circulating levels of IL-6 and advancement in the stages of prostate cancer, therapeutic resistance, and as a result an overall poor prognosis has been well established until now [32]. Although one of the most important consequences of IL-6 expression is the stimulation of the JAK/STAT3 pathway [33], phosphorylation of STAT3 at Scr727 and activation of its function by the PI3K-AKT pathway cannot be ruled out completely because of the impact PTEN mutations can produce on this pathway [34]. Such activation of STAT3 can also lead to metastatic behavior of prostate cancer cells in both *in vitro* and *in vivo* conditions, through stimulation of angiogenesis and suppression of antitumor immune responses [35]. Many inflammatory cytokines and chemokines promote tumor progression by converging on and stimulating the IKK2/NF-κB signaling axis [36]. In addition to the above-mentioned mechanisms, constitutive activation of NF-κB has been correlated well with disease progression in prostate cancer [37], and therefore inhibition of NF-κB activity in prostate cancers can suppress angiogenesis and subsequent tumor invasion and metastasis by downregulating downstream targets such as VEGF and MMP9 [38]. In this context, it was determined using a mouse model that a constitutively active version of IKK2 alone is insufficient for promoting prostate tumorigenesis; however, in combination

http://dx.doi.org/10.5772/64337

with even heterozygous loss of *PTEN*, IKK2 activation can lead to an increase in tumor size, accompanied by increased inflammation [39]. Thus, earlier studies clearly demonstrate that the inflammatory cytokines secreted from the stromal microenvironment of the prostate cells can cooperate with PTEN loss to drive epithelial prostate tumor towards an invasive disease. Interestingly, recent studies have clearly indicated a greater role for the MDM2 oncogene in the progression of prostate cancer by impacting PI3K/AKT and NF-κB pathways [40, 41].

2.2. MDM2 and prostate cancer

Alterations in the *TP53* gene is one of the most commonly detected gene defects in a wide range of cancers; however, alterations of this gene is believed to be of low frequency in prostate cancer [42], and their clinical significance is also not fully investigated. On the contrary, the *MDM2* gene seems to be amplified in a significant fraction of prostate cancers, and overexpression of MDM2 protein without amplification is also observed as an alternate mechanism of p53 inactivation in these cancers [43, 44]. It has been widely reported that *p21/WAF1* gene expression could very well serve as an indicator of p53 activity because *p21/WAF1* is under the transcriptional control of p53 and therefore can be severely impacted when MDM2 is overexpressed. However, the *MDM2* gene itself is under the transcriptional control of p53, which creates an auto-regulatory feedback loop in many cancer types (**Figure 2**) [45]. An interesting fact that was revealed through mutation analysis of various cancer samples is that, in prostate cancers, alterations in the *TP53* gene seem to be uncommon, and therefore the clinical significance of *TP53* gene mutation has not been fully investigated for prostate cancers. Another important limitation of studies related to *TP53* gene defect in prostate cancer is that, in many cases their focus was confined to the analysis of p53 gene alterations without exploring other

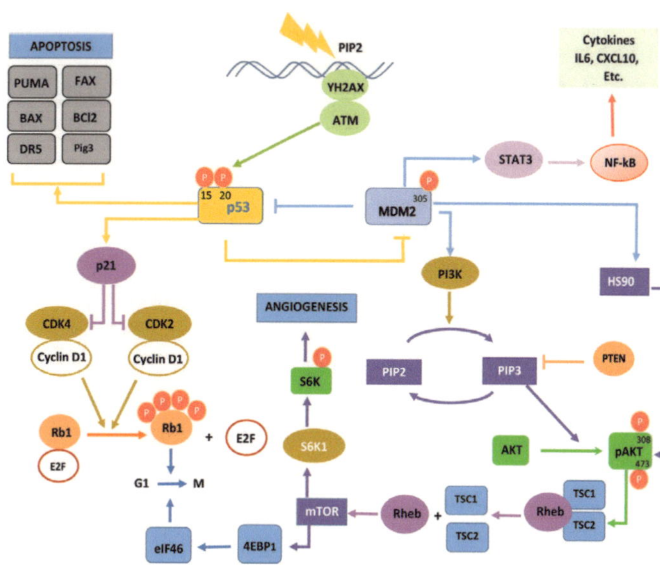

Figure 2. The pro-angiogenesis, apoptosis, cytokine release, and cell cycle pathways that are impacted by MDM2 expression.

possible mechanisms that might regulate its functions. For example, though the *MDM2* gene is amplified in a variety of tumors, MDM2 overexpression without amplification seems to be a common mechanism of p53 inactivation in certain cancers. As it was mentioned earlier in this section, it has been well established that *p21/WAF I* gene expression can serve as a good indicator of p53 activity, because *p21/WAFI* expression is under the transcriptional control of p53, and consequently indicate any related abnormality. However, several studies have analyzed the patterns of p53 expression and identified a correlation with MDM2 and p21 in prostate cancer patients. Results have confirmed a close association between levels of these markers and clinico-pathological parameters of poor outcome, including time to relapse and proliferative index. In addition, overexpression of MDM2 has been found to be associated with lack of response to chemoradiotherapy in oesophageal cancer and has been shown to exhibit androgen independence in prostate cancer cell lines [46, 47]. Thus, MDM2 overexpression was significantly associated with advanced stage prostate cancer (PCa) [48], a finding confirmed by several investigators [49, 50] validating the importance of MDM2 expression in prostate cancers. Recent studies have also shown that MDM2 expression enhances the angiogenic potential and proliferative capacity of PCa cells [51] and negatively impacts the effects of radiation and chemotherapy [52]. Thus, it is predictable that expression of MDM2 may play an important role, at least in part, in stimulating the aggressive nature of PCa in African-American (AA) patients. Recently, a single nucleotide polymorphism (SNP) referred as SNP309 was found at position 309 in the P2 promoter region of *MDM2* gene. This T > G polymorphism (rs22789744) which is located in the intronic portion of the promoter was shown to increase the binding affinity of the transcriptional activator Sp1, and increase the expression of MDM2 protein levels [53]. During the transcriptional activation of MDM2 gene, both the androgen receptor (AR) and estrogen receptors (ER) have been shown to form complexes with Sp1 and act as co-regulators and cause increase in protein expression [54, 55]. In addition, studies in ER-positive tumors such as breast and ovarian cancer have shown strong correlation between younger age of disease onset and the presence of *MDM2* SNP309 G allele [56, 57]. Interestingly, in the ovarian cancer patients, the age of onset in women with high level expression of ER and the presence of SNP309 G allele was 8 years earlier than those without the SNP309 G allele. Similarly, in a cohort of breast cancer patients with the G/G SNP309 genotype the age of onset was 7 years earlier than the patients with the T/T genotype. Furthermore, *MDM2* SNP309 G allele displayed early-onset of soft-tissue sarcoma, diffuse large B-cell lymphoma, colorectal cancer, and non-small cell lung cancer in premenopausal women with active estrogen signaling than the cohorts without the SNP309 polymorphism [58–61]. Hence, it is believed that SNP309 G allele found at the *MDM2* promoter region in AA patients may be responsible for the aggressive phenotype and early onset of their prostate cancers (48). Indeed, this appears to be one of the first studies of *MDM2* SNP309 showing the implication of this particular polymorphism to the racial differences in the clinic-pathologic presentation of the prostate cancer. Additionally, the above mentioned study is the first report that is closely correlating SNP309 genotype to MDM2 protein expression in a group of prostate cancer patients and showing its close correlation with tumor progression. Thus, several aspects of MDM2 expression and the gene polymorphisms seem to specifically impact the nature and progression of prostate cancers.

2.2.1. MDM2 and cytokine expression

In addition to being the trigger for developing cancers, MDM2 expression seems to be responsible for several events that promote cancer aggressiveness [48]. Increased expression of VEGF in cancer cells, which are positive for MDM2, is a well-established phenomenon that occurs through elevation of HIF-1alpha even during the absence of hypoxia in the tumor microenvironment [51]. In addition, many reports in the literature confirm that MDM2 overexpression could lead to activation of STAT3 and NF-κB pathways and cause elevation of cytokines that in-turn can stimulate cancer progression. One of the unique biological functions of MDM2 is its ability to induce sterile tissue inflammation, which is a major element of non-infectious tissue injury that occurs following exposure to toxins or reperfusion following ischemia. For example, an acute post-ischemic kidney injury that started as a sterile inflammatory response was reversed using the MDM2 blockade with nutlin-3 [62]. This effect was found to be totally independent of p53 that was observed in a p53-deficient mice. Also, MDM2 blockade effectively suppressed the post-ischemic induction of pro-inflammatory cytokines and chemokines as well as the infiltration of leukocytes to the site of injury. Following these observations, the mechanism underlying MDM2-mediated inflammation was identified under *in vitro* conditions showing that MDM2 could act as a co-factor for NF-NF-κB binding to its gene promoter binding sites [62]. This was actually confirmed by the electromobility shift assay in p53-deficient mouse embryonic fibroblasts using lipopolysaccharide (LPS) stimulation [62]. This observation is similar to several other reports which confirm that MDM2 blockade with nutlin-3 could effectively suppresses LPS-induced lung inflammation through interference of NF-NF-κB DNA binding in nutrophils; however this effect of nutlin-3 was dependent on the presence of intact p53 [62]. Similar to the activation of NF-κB pathway, MDM2 might release other cytokines like Interleukins (IL's) and support growth and progression of cancer.

2.3. TMPRSS2 and ERG fusions in prostate cancer

TMPRSS2 is an androgen regulated prostate-specific protein that is encoded in humans by the TMPRSS2 gene [63]. It is a 492 amino acid type II transmembrane serine protease (70 KDa) that is expressed at the cell surface in order to regulate cell-cell and cell-matrix interactions [64]. The serine protease gene family, play crucial roles in different physiological and pathological processes such as digestion, blood coagulation, remodeling of tissues, invasion of tumor cells, inflammatory responses, and apoptosis. The TMPRSS2 protein contains a Serine protease domain (aa 255-492) with three catalytic residues of histidine, aspartate, and serine, respectively, a Scavenger receptor cysteine-rich domain (SRDR, aa 149-242), an LDL receptor class A (LDLRA, aa 113-148) domain and a predicted transmembrane domain (aa 84-106) [65].

ERG is a member of the erythroblastosis virus E26 (ETS) oncogene family. There are over 20 ETS transcription factor family members, but ERG is the ETS transcription factor primarily involved in prostate cancer gene fusions [66]. The ERG protein interacts with ETS members as well as other transcription factors through its protein-protein interacting domain to regulate transcriptional activity of several downstream target genes that are crucial for DNA damage, cell invasion and proliferation, epithelial to mesenchymal transformation (EMT) as well as cellular differentiation and epigenetic control [66–68].

TMPRSS2 is expressed in normal and neoplastic prostate tissue and is strongly induced by androgens in androgen-sensitive prostate cell lines [65]. A major milestone in PCa research was the identification of recurrent fusions between TMPRSS2 and ERG [63]. TMPRSS2-ERG is fused in PCa through deletion of genomic DNA via a homogeneous deletion site between ERG and TMPRSS2 on chromosome 21q22.2 or through translocation or both [69–71]. These rearrangements (**Figure 1**) result in the formation of a TMPRSS2-ERG fusion transcript and the overexpression of ERG [63]. The TMPRSS2 and ERG genes are both located on the same chromosome (21q) and the distance between the TMPRSS2 and ERG oncogene is relatively short at 3 mega bases (MB) (**Figure 3**). This short distance has been suggested to account for the higher frequency of TMPRSS2: ERG fusions in prostate cancer [69, 73].

TMPRSS2-ERG fusion occurs early in prostate carcinogenesis at the transition between benign and prostatic intraepithelial neoplasia (PIN). Approximately 50% of PCas from prostate-specific antigen (PSA) screened surgical cohorts are TMPRSS2-ERG fusion-positive, and >90% of PCas over-expressing ERG harbor TMPRSS2-ERG fusions [74]. Over eight isoforms of the TMPRSS2-ERG fusion transcript have been identified with varying levels of expression in different PCa samples [75]. The most frequently found TMPRSS2-ERG fusion in PCa is the deletion between the 5 UTR end of TMPRSS2 exon 1 and 5 end of ERG exon 4 [76].

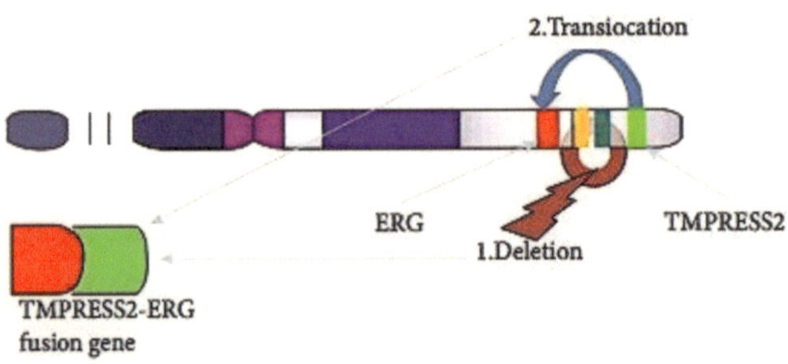

Figure 3. Mechanism of TMPRSS2-ERG fusion (chromosome 21). (1) Large deletion of intervening genetic region between ERG and TMPRSS2 genes (most common). (2) Translocation of TMPRSS2 and ERG genes. Reproduced with permission from the copyright holder: Hossain [72].

2.3.1. *Consequences of TMPRSS2-ERG fusion in prostate cancer*

TMPRSS2 is an androgen-responsive gene and AR regulated expression of the TMPRSS2-ERG fusion gene plays an early role in prostate cancer development and progression as its presence is required for prostate cancer initiation in ETS positive tumors [74]. The fusion results in the modulation of transcriptional patterns and cellular pathways causing the development of prostatic intraepithelial neoplasia (PIN) [77]. In particular, gene expression profiling has linked a deregulation of WNT and TGF-β/BMP signaling in fusion-positive prostate tumors [78]. It has also been shown in transgenic mice that overexpression of ERG as a result of TMPRSS2: ERG fusion leads to the formation of murine PIN (mPIN) by 5–6 months of age [74, 79]. Several studies have also confirmed that the overexpression of ERG leads to prostate cell migration and invasion that correlates with increased tumor metastasis and negative patient outcome [79, 80]. The most prominent role of ERG that has been consistently shown is its ability to increase cell migration and invasion via abrogating prostate epithelial differentiation and inducing epithelial to mesenchymal transition and motility-associated genes such as MMPs [81].

PCa specimens containing the TMPRSS2-ERG rearrangement are also significantly enriched for the loss of tumor suppressor gene phosphatase and tensin homologue PTEN [77], and it is already well established that aberrant PTEN activity is associated with poor prognosis in PCa [82]. Further studies have confirmed that TMPRSS2-ERG rearrangement cooperates with PTEN loss to promote prostate cancer progression from high-grade prostatic intraepithelial neoplasia (PIN) to invasive adenocarcinoma [77, 83].

2.3.2. *TMPRSS2-ERG fusions and ethnicity*

There are several studies evaluating the relationship between ethnicity and TMPRSS2-ERG expression in PCa. TMPRSS2-ERG gene fusion correlated with ethnicity in a multivariate analysis involving Caucasians [71], African-Americans, and Japanese men with PCa [71]. TMPRSS2-ERG gene fusion was present in 50% (21/42) of Caucasians, 31.3% (20/64) of African-Americans, and 15.9% (7/44) of Japanese patients. A subsequent study found that TMPRSS2-ERG gene fusions were identified in 48/112 tumors (42.9%) from a group of Caucasian men, while 28/105 tumors (26.7%; $p = 0.015$) from African-American men were positive for the gene fusion [84]. Interestingly, Mosquera and colleagues recognized that the TMPRSS2-ERG fusion through deletion, which has been associated with worse prognosis, is more common in PCa of African-American patients [73].

2.3.3. *Prognostic value of the TMPRSS2-ERG fusion gene*

The prognostic potential of TMPRSS2-ERG gene fusion is promising as it can be detected in urine, blood, and tissue using quantitative polymerase chain reaction [85, 86], Fluorescence in situ hybridization (FISH) [87], DNA sequencing, and Genechip [88]. This has significant applications toward understanding its role in PCa pathogenesis and developing novel diagnostics and targeted therapeutics. TMPRSS2 and TMPRSS2-ERG expression is decreased in response to ADT in primary PCa [89]. Interestingly, the ERG levels in TMPRSS2-ERG fusion-positive castration resistant prostate cancer CRPC are comparable with the levels in fusion gene-positive primary PC, and this confirms that TMPRSS2-ERG expression is reactivated by AR in CRPC [70]. These findings prove that restored AR receptor signaling contributes to the progression to CRPC in part through the TMPRSS2-ERG axis and highlights a therapeutic platform that can be explored in the management of CRPC. More recently, the TMPRSS2-ERG fusion has been linked to taxane resistance in preclinical models of castration-resistant prostate cancer, and TMPRSS2-ERG expression detection in the peripheral blood of metastatic castration-resistant prostate cancer patients correlates with docetaxel resistance [90]. Therefore, its presence predicts resistance to docetaxel, and it may be useful to select treatment and to avoid possible toxicities in refractory patients.

Acknowledgements

The author Appu Rathinavelu, Ph.D., would like to thank the Fulbright Scholar Program of the United States Department of State Bureau of Educational and Cultural Affairs and the USIEF (United States International Educational Foundation) for the Nehru—Fulbright Scholar Award during the completion of this book chapter. The author would also like to Thank Nova Southeastern University and the Royal Dames of Ft. Lauderdale Inc, Florida, USA for their support.

Author details

Appu Rathinavelu[1*] and Arkene Levy[2]

*Address all correspondence to: appu@nova.edu

1 Rumbaugh Goodwin Institute for Cancer Research, College of Pharmacy, Nova Southeastern University, Fort Lauderdale, Florida, USA

2 Pharmacology Section, Department of Basic Medical Sciences, University of the West Indies, Mona Campus, Jamaica

References

[1] Ferlay J, Dikshit R, Eser S, Mathers C, Rebelo M, Parkin D, et al. Cancer incidence and mortality worldwide: Sources, methods and major patterns in Globocan 2012. Int J Cancer. 2015; 136(5): E359–E386. doi:10.1002/ijc.29210

[2] Siegel R, Miller K, Jemal A. Cancer Statistics 2015. CA Cancer J Clin. 2015; 65: 5–29. doi: 10.3322/caac.21254

[3] Bostwick DG. High-grade prostatic intraepithelial neoplasia: The most likely precursor of prostate cancer. Cancer. 1995; 75: 1823–1836. doi:10.1002/1097-0142(19950401)75: 7+<1823::aid-cncr2820751612>3.0.co;2-7

[4] Massard C, Fizazi K. Targeting continued androgen receptor signaling in prostate cancer. Clin Cancer Res. 2011; 17(12): 3876–3883. doi:10.1158/1078-0432.ccr-10-2815

[5] Yap T, Swanton C, De Bono1 J. Personalization of prostate cancer prevention and therapy are clinically qualified biomarkers in the horizon? EPMA J. 2012; 3(1): 3. doi: 10.1007/s13167-011-0138-2

[6] Boyd L, Mao X, Lu Y. The complexity of prostate cancer: Genomic alterations and heterogeneity. Nat Rev Urol. 2012; 9: 652–664. doi:10.1038/nrurol.2012.185

[7] Shen MM, Abate-Shen C. Molecular genetics of prostate cancer: New prospects for old challenges. Genes Dev. 2010; 24(18): 1967–2000. doi:10.1101/gad.1965810

[8] Tindall D, editor. Prostate Cancer: Biochemistry, Molecular Biology and Genetics. 1st ed. Springer-Verlag: New York; 2013. 518 p. doi:10.1007/978-1-4614-6828-8

[9] Manning BD, Cantley LC. AKT/PKB signaling: Navigating downstream. Cell. 2007; 129(7): 1261–1274. doi:10.1016/j.cell.2007.06.009

[10] Zoncu R, Efeyan A, Sabatini D. MTOR: From growth signal integration to cancer, diabetes and ageing. Nat Rev Mol Cell Biol. 2011; 12(1): 21–35. doi:10.1038/nrm3025

[11] De la Taille A, Rubin M, Chen M, Vacherot F, De Medina S, Burchardt M, Buttyan R, Chopin D. Beta-catenin-related anomalies in apoptosis-resistant and hormone refractory prostate cancer cells. Clin Cancer Res. 2003; 9: 1801–1807.

[12] Lee H, Kwak H, Hur J, Kim I, Yang J, Park M, Yu J, Jeong S. Beta-catenin regulates multiple steps of RNA metabolism as revealed by the RNA aptamer in colon cancer cells. Cancer Res. 2007; 67: 9315–9321. doi:10.1158/0008-5472.CAN-07-1128

[13] Grunwald V, DeGraffenried L, Russel D, Friedrichs W, Ray R, Hidalgo M. Inhibitors of mTOR reverse doxorubicin resistance conferred by PTEN status in prostate cancer cells. Cancer Res. 2002; 62: 6141–6145.

[14] Wu X, Senechal K, Neshat M, Whang Y, Sawyers C. The PTEN/MMAC1 tumor suppressor phosphatase functions as a negative regulator of the phosphoinositide 3-kinase/Akt pathway. Proc Natl Acad Sci USA. 1998; 95: 15587–15591. doi:10.1073/pnas.95.26.15587

[15] Guertin D, Sabatini D. Defining the role of mTOR in cancer. Cancer Cell. 2007; 12: 9–22. doi:10.1016/j.ccr.2007.05.008

[16] Ma X, Blenis J. Molecular mechanisms of mTOR-mediated translational control. Nat Rev Mol Cell Biol. 2009; 10: 307–318. doi:10.1038/nrm2672

[17] Denu J, Stuckey J, Saper M, Dixon J. Form and function in protein dephosphorylation. Cell. 1996; 87: 361–364. doi:10.1016/S0092-8674(00)81356-2

[18] Lee J, Yang H, Georgescu M, Di Cristofano A, Maehama T, Shi Y, Dixon J, Pandolfi P, Pavletich N. Crystal structure of the PTEN tumor suppressor: Implications for its phosphoinositide phosphatase activity and membrane association. Cell. 1999; 99: 323–334. doi:10.1016/S0092-8674(00)81663-3

[19] Redfern R, Redfern D, Furgason M, Munson M, Ross A, Gericke A. PTEN phosphatase selectively binds phosphoinositides and undergoes structural changes. Biochemistry. 2008; 47: 2162–2171. doi:10.1021/bi702114w

[20] Liaw D, Marsh D, Li J, Dahia P, Wang S, Zheng Z, Bose S, Call K, Tsou H, Peacocke M, Eng C, Parsons R. Germline mutations of the PTEN gene in Cowden disease, an inherited breast and thyroid cancer syndrome. Nat Genet. 1997; 16: 64–67. doi:10.1038/ng0597-64

[21] Tonks N, Cicirelli M, Diltz C, Krebs E, Fischer E. Effect of microinjection of a low-Mr human placenta protein tyrosine phosphatase on induction of meiotic cell division in Xenopus oocytes. Mol Cell Biol. 1990; 10: 458–463. doi:10.1128/mcb.10.2.458

[22] Maehama T, Dixon J. The tumor suppressor, PTEN/MMAC1, dephosphorylates the lipid second messenger, phosphatidylinositol 3,4,5-trisphosphate. J Biol Chem. 1998; 273: 13375–13378. doi:10.1074/jbc.273.22.13375

[23] Waite KA, Eng C. Protean PTEN: Form and function. Am J Hum Genet. 2002; 70: 829–844. doi:10.1086/340026

[24] Georgescu M, Kirsch K, Kaloudis P, Yang H, Pavletich N, Hanafusa H. Stabilization and productive positioning roles of the C2 domain of PTEN tumor suppressor. Cancer Res. 2000; 60: 7033–7038.

[25] Taylor B, Schultz N, Hieronymus H, Gopalan A, Xiao Y, Carver BS, Arora VK, Kaushik P, Cerami E, Reva B, Antipin Y, Mitsiades N, Landers T, Dolgalev I, Major J, Wilson M, Socci N, et al. Integrative genomic profiling of human prostate cancer. Cancer Cell. 2010; 18: 11–22. doi:10.1016/j.ccr.2010.05.026

[26] Grasso C, Wu Y, Robinson D, Cao X, Dhanasekaran S, Khan A, Quist M, Jing X, Lonigro J, Brenner J, Asangani I, Ateeq B, Chun S, Siddiqui J, Sam L, Anstett M, et al. The mutational landscape of lethal castration-resistant prostate cancer. Nature. 2012; 487: 239–243. doi:10.1038/nature11125

[27] Barbieri C, Baca S, Lawrence M, Demichelis F, Blattner M, Theurillat J, White T, Stojanov P, Van Allen E, Stransky N, Nickerson E, et al. Exome sequencing identifies recurrent SPOP, FOXA1 and MED12 mutations in prostate cancer. Nat Genet. 2012; 44: 685–689. doi:10.1038/ng.2279

[28] Phin S, Moore MW, Cotter PD. Genomic rearrangements of PTEN in prostate cancer. Front Oncol. 2013; 3: 240. doi:10.3389/fonc.2013.00240

[29] Haverkamp J, Charbonneau B, Ratliff T. Prostate inflammation and its potential impact on prostate cancer: A current review. J Cell Biochem. 2008; 103: 1344–1353. doi:10.1002/jcb.21536

[30] De Marzo A, Platz E, Sutcliffe S, Xu J, Gronberg H, Drake C, Nakai Y, Isaacs W, Nelson W. Inflammation in prostate carcinogenesis. Nat Rev Cancer. 2007; 7: 256–269. doi:10.1038/nrc2090

[31] Blum D, Koyama T, M'Koma A, Iturregui JM, Martinez-Ferrer M, Uwamariya C, Smith JA Jr, Clark PE, Bhowmick NA. Chemokine markers predict biochemical recurrence of prostate cancer following prostatectomy. Clin Cancer Res. 2008; 14: 7790–7797. doi: 10.1158/1078-0432.CCR-08-1716

[32] Tassidis H, Culig Z, Wingren A, Harkonen P. Role of the protein tyrosine phosphatase SHP-1 in Interleukin-6 regulation of prostate cancer cells. Prostate. 2010; 70: 1491–1500. doi:10.1002/pros.21184

[33] Shariat S, Andrews B, Kattan M, Kim J, Wheeler T, Slawin K. Plasma levels of interleukin-6 and its soluble receptor are associated with prostate cancer progression and metastasis.Urology. 2001; 58: 1008–1015. doi:10.1016/S0090-4295(01)01405-4

[34] Chung T, Yu J, Kong T, Spiotto M, Lin J. Interleukin-6 activates phosphatidylinositol-3 kinase, which inhibits apoptosis in human prostate cancer cell lines. Prostate. 2000; 42: 1–7. doi:10.1002/(sici)1097-0045(20000101)42:1<1::aid-pros1>3.0.co;2-y

[35] Wen Z, Zhong Z, Darnell J. Maximal activation of transcription by Stat1 and Stat3 requires both tyrosine and serine phosphorylation. Cell. 1995; 82: 241–250. doi: 10.1016/0092-8674(95)90311-9

[36] Abdulghani J, Gu L, Dagvadorg A, Lutz J, Leiby B, Bonuccelli G, Lisanti M, Zellweger T, Alanen K, Mirtti T, Visakorpi T, Bubendorf L, Nevalainen M. Stat3 promotes metastatic progression of prostate cancer. Am J Pathol. 2008; 172: 1717–1728. doi: 10.2353/ajpath.2008.071054

[37] Blando J, Carbajal S, Abel E, Beltran L, Conti C, Fischer S, DiGiovanni J. Cooperation between Stat3 and Akt signaling leads to prostate tumor development in transgenic mice. Neoplasia. 2011; 13: 254–265. doi:10.1593/neo.101388

[38] Schmid J, Birbach A. IkappaB kinase beta (IKKbeta/IKK2/IKBKB)–a key molecule in signaling to the transcription factor NF-kappaB. Cytokine Growth Factor Rev. 2008; 19: 157–165. doi:10.1016/j.cytogfr.2008.01.006

[39] Shukla S, MacLennan G, Fu P, Patel J, Marengo S, Resnick M, Gupta S. Nuclear factor-kappaB/p65 (Rel A) is constitutively activated in human prostate adenocarcinoma and correlates with disease progression. Neoplasia. 2004; 6: 390–400. doi:10.1593/neo.04112

[40] Kong D, Li Y, Wang Z, Banerjee S, Sarkar F. Inhibition of angiogenesis and invasion by 3,3'-diindolylmethane is mediated by the nuclear factor-kappaB downstream target genes MMP-9 and uPA that regulated bioavailability of vascular endothelial growth factor in prostate cancer. Cancer Res. 2007; 67: 3310–3319. doi: 10.1158/0008-5472.CAN-06-4277

[41] Birbach A, Eisenbarth D, Kozakowski N, Ladenhauf E, Schmidt-Supprian M, Schmid J. Persistent inflammation leads to proliferative neoplasia and loss of smooth muscle cells in a prostate tumor model. Neoplasia. 2011; 13: 692–703. doi:10.1593/neo.11524

[42] Osman I, Drobnjak M, Fazzari M, Ferrara J, Scher H, Cordon-Cardo C. Inactivation of the p53 pathway in prostate cancer: Impact on tumor progression. Clin Cancer Res. 1999; 5(8): 2082–2088.

[43] Narasimhan M, Rose R, Karthikeyan M, Rathinavelu A. Detection of HDM2 and VEGF co-expression in cancer cell lines: Novel effect of HDM2 antisense treatment on VEGF expression. Life Sci. 2007; 81: 1362–1372. doi:10.1016/j.lfs.2007.08.029

[44] Rose R, Narasimhan M, Rathinavelu A. Identification of HDM2 as a regulator of VEGF expression in cancer cells. Life Sci. 2008; 82: 1231–1241. doi:10.1016/j.lfs.2007.08.029

[45] Ard P, Chatterjee C, Kunjibettu S, Adside L, Gralinski L, McMahon S. Transcriptional regulation of the mdm2 oncogene by p53 requires TRRAP acetyltransferase complexes. Mol Cell Biol. 2002; 22(16): 5650–5661. doi:10.1128/MCB.22.16.5650-5661.2002

[46] Okamoto H, Fujishima F, Kamei T, et al. Murine double minute 2 predicts response of advanced esophageal squamous cell carcinoma to definitive chemoradiotherapy. BMC Cancer. 2015; 15: 208. doi:10.1186/s12885-015-1222-0

[47] Udayakumar T, Hachem P, Ahmed M, Agrawal S, Pollack A. Antisense MDM2 enhances E2F1-induced apoptosis and the combination sensitizes androgen dependent and independent prostate cancer cells to radiation. Mol Cancer Res. 2008; 6(11): 1742–1754. doi:10.1158/1541-7786.MCR-08-0102

[48] Wang G, Firoz E, Rose A. Blochin E, Christos P, Pollens D, Mazumdar M, Gerald W, Oddoux C, Lee P, Osman I. MDM2 expression and regulation in prostate cancer racial disparity. Int J Clin Exp Pathol. 2009; 2(4): 353–360.

[49] Khor L, Desilvio M, Al-Saleem T, Hammond M, Grignon D, Sause W, Pilepich M, Okunieff P, Sandler H, Pollack A. Radiation therapy oncology group MDM2 as a predictor of prostate carcinoma outcome: An analysis of Radiation Therapy Oncology Group Protocol 8610. Cancer. 2005; 104: 962–967. doi:10.1002/cncr.21261

[50] Leite K, Franco M, Srougi M, Nesrallah A, Bevilacqua R, Darini E, Carvalho C, Meirelles M, Santana I, Camara-Lopes L. Abnormal expression of MDM2 in prostate carcinoma. Mod Pathol. 2001; 5: 428–436. doi:10.1038/modpathol.3880330

[51] Muthumani P, Alagarsamy K, Dhandayuthapani S, Venkatesan T, Rathinavelu A. Pro-angiogenic effects of MDM2 through HIF-1α and NF-κB mediated mechanisms in LNCaP prostate cancer cells. Mol Biol Rep. 2014; 41(8): 5533–5541. doi:10.1007/s11033-014-3430-0

[52] Khor LY, Desilvio M, Al-Saleem T, Hammond M, Grignon D, Sause W, Pilepich M, Okunieff P, Sandler H, Pollack A. MDM2 as a predictor of prostate carcinoma outcome: An analysis of radiation therapy. Cancer. 2005; 104(5): 962–967. doi: 10.1002/cncr.21261

[53] Bond G, Hu W, Bond E, Robins H, Lutzker S, Arva N, Bargonetti J, Bartel F, Taubert H, Wuerl P, Onel K, Yip L, Hwang S, Strong L, Lozano G, Levine

A. A single nucleotide polymorphism in the MDM2 promoter attenuates the p53 tumor suppressor pathway and accelerates tumor formation in humans. Cell. 2004; 119: 591–602. doi:10.1016/j.cell.2004.11.022

[54] Yuan H, Gong A, Young CY. Involvement of transcription factor Sp1 in quercetin-mediated inhibitory effect on the androgen receptor in human prostate cancer cells. Carcinogenesis. 2005; 26: 793–801. doi:10.1093/carcin/bgi021

[55] Saville B, Wormke M, Wang F, Nguyen T, Enmark E, Kuiper G, Gustafsson J, Safe S. Ligand, cell and estrogen receptor subtype (alpha/beta)-dependent activation at GC-rich (Sp1) promoter elements. J Biol Chem. 2000; 275: 5379–5387. doi:10.1074/jbc.275.8.5379

[56] Bartel F, Jung J, Bohnke A, Gradhand E, Zeng K, Thomssen C, Hauptmann S. Both germ line and somatic genetics of the p53 pathway affect ovarian cancer incidence and survival. Clin Cancer Res. 2008; 14: 89–96. doi:10.1158/1078-0432.CCR-07-1192

[57] Bond G, Hirshfield K, Kirchhoff T, Alexe G, Dond E, Robbins H, Bartel F, Taubert H, Wuerl P, Hait W, Toppmeyer D, Offit K, Levine AJ. MDM2 SNP309 accelerates tumor formation in a gender-specific and hormone-dependent manner. Cancer Res. 2006; 66: 5104–5110. doi:10.1158/0008-5472.CAN-06-0180

[58] Bond G, Menin C, Bertorelle R, Alhopuro P, Aaltonen L, Levine A. MDM SNP309 accelerates colorectal tumour formation in women. J Med Genet. 2006; 43: 950–952. doi:10.1136/jmg.2006.043539

[59] Lind H, Zienolddiny S, Ekstrom P, Skaug V, Haugen A. Association of a functional polymorphism in the promoter of the MDM2 gene with risk of non small cell lung cancer. Int J Cancer. 2006; 119: 718–721. doi:10.1002/ijc.21872

[60] Alhopuro P, Ylisaukko-Oja S, Koskinen W, Bono P, Arola J, Jarvinen H, Mecklin J, Atula T, Kontio R, Makitie A, Suominen S, Leivo I, Vahteristo P, Aaltonen L, Aaltonen L. The MDM2 promoter polymorphism SNP309T-->G and the risk of uterine leiomyosarcoma, colorectal cancer, and squamous cell carcinoma of the head and neck. J Med Genet. 2005; 42: 694–698. doi:10.1136/jmg.2005.031260

[61] Yarden R, Friedman E, Metsuyanim S, Olender T, Ben-Asher E, Papa MZ. MDM2 SNP309 accelerates breast and ovarian carcinogenesis in BRCA1 and BRCA2 carriers of Jewish-Ashkenazi descent. Breast Cancer Res Treat. 2008; 111: 497–504. doi:10.1007/s10549-007-9797-z

[62] Thomasova D, Mulay SR, Bruns H, Anders H-J. p53-Independent roles of MDM2 in NF-kB signaling: Implications for cancer therapy, wound healing, and autoimmune diseases. Neoplasia. 2012; 14(12): 1097–1101. doi:10.1593/neo.121534

[63] Tomlins S, Rhodes D, Perner S, Dhanasekaran S, Mehra R, Sun X, et al. Recurrent fusion of TMPRSS2 and ETS transcription factor genes in prostate cancer. Science. 2005; 310: 644–648. doi:10.1126/science.1117679

[64] Bugge T, Antalis T, Wu Q. Type II transmembrane serine proteases. J Biol Chem. 2009; 284(35): 23177–23181. doi:10.1074/jbc.R109.021006

[65] Paoloni-Giacobino A, Chen H, Peitsch M, Rossier C, Antonarakis S. Cloning of the TMPRSS2 gene, which encodes a novel serine protease with transmembrane,LDLRA, and SRCR domains and maps to 21q22.3. Genomics. 1997; 44(3): 309–320. doi:10.1006/geno.1997.4845

[66] Sreenath T, Dobi A, Srivastava S. Oncogenic activation of ERG: A predominant mechanism in prostate cancer. J Carcinog. 2011; 10: 37. doi: 10.4103/1477-3163.91122

[67] Carrere S, Verger A, Flourens A, Stehelin D, Duterque-Coquillaud M. Erg proteins, transcription factors of the Ets family, form homo heterodimers and ternary complexes via two distinct domains. Oncogene. 1998; 16(25): 3261–3268. doi:10.1038/sj.onc.1201868

[68] Basuyaux J, Ferreira E, Stehelin D, Buttice G. The Ets transcription factors interact with each other and with the c-Fos/c-Jun complex via distinct protein domains in a DNA-dependent and -independent manner. J Biol Chem. 1997; 272(42): 26188–26195. doi: 10.1074/jbc.272.42.26188

[69] Perner S, Demichelis F, Beroukhim R, Schmidt F, Mosquera J, Setlur S, et al. TMPRSS2:ERG fusion-associated deletions provide insight into the heterogeneity of prostate cancer. Cancer Res. 2006; 66(17): 8337–8341. doi: 10.1158/0008-5472.CAN-06-1482

[70] Cai C, Wang H, Xu Y, Chen S, Balk S. TMPRSS2: ERG gene expression in castration-resistant prostate cancer. Cancer Res. 2009; 69: 6027–6032. doi: 10.1158/0008-5472.CAN-09-0395

[71] Magi-Galluzzi C, Tsusuki T, Elson P, Simmerman K, LaFargue C, Esgueva R, et al. TMPRSS2–ERG gene fusion prevalence and class are significantly different in prostate cancer of caucasian, African-American and Japanese patients. The Prostate. 2011; 71: 489–497. doi:10.1002/pros.21265

[72] Hossain D, Bostwick D. Significance of the TMPRSS2:ERG gene fusion in prostate cancer. BJU Int. 2013; 111(5): 834–835. doi:10.1111/bju.12120

[73] Mosquera J, Mehra R, Regan M, Perner S, Genega E, Bueti G, et al. Prevalence of TMPRSS2-ERG fusion prostate cancer among men undergoing prostate biopsy in the United States. Clin Cancer Res 2009; 15(14): 4706–4711. doi: 10.1158/1078-0432.CCR-08-2927

[74] Tomlins S, Laxman B, Varambally S, Cao X, Yu J. Role of the TMPRSS2–ERG gene fusion in prostate cancer. Neoplasia. 2008; 10: 177–188.

[75] Nguyen P, Violette P, Chan S, Tanguay S, Kassouf W, Aprikian A, et al. A panel of TMPRSS2:ERG fusion transcript markers for urine-based prostate cancer detection

with high specificity and sensitivity. Eur Urol. 2011; 59(3): 407–414. doi:10.1016/j.eururo.2010.11.026

[76] Tu J, Rohan S, Kao J, Kitabayashi N, Mathew S, Chen J. Gene fusions between TMPRSS2 and ETS family genes in prostate cancer: Frequency and transcript variant analysis by RT-PCR and FISH on paraffin embedded tissues. Mod Pathol. 2007; 20: 921–928. doi: 10.1038/modpathol.3800903

[77] Carver B, Tran J, Gopalan A, Chen Z, Shaikh S, Carracedo A, et al. Aberrant ERG expression cooperates with loss of PTEN to promote cancer progression in the prostate. Nat Genet. 2009; 41(5): 619–624. doi:10.1038/ng.370

[78] Brase J, Johannes M, Mannsperger H, Fälth M, Metzger J, Kacprzyk L, Andrasiuk T, Gade S, Meister M, Sirma H, Sauter G, Simon R, et al. TMPRSS2-ERG -specific transcriptional modulation is associated with prostate cancer biomarkers and TGF-β signaling. BMC Cancer. 2011; 11: 507. doi:10.1186/1471-2407-11-507

[79] Klezovitch O, Risk M, Coleman I, Lucas J, Null M, True L, et al. A causal role for ERG in neoplastic transformationof prostate epithelium. Proc Natl Acad Sci U S A. 2008; 105(6): 2105–2110. doi:10.1073/pnas.0711711105

[80] Demichelis F, Fall K, Perner S, Andrén O, Schmidt F, Setlur S, et al. TMPRSS2: ERG gene fusion associated with lethal prostate cancer in a watchful waiting cohort. Oncogene. 2007; 26: 4596–4599. doi:10.1038/sj.onc.1210237

[81] Kim J, Wu L, Zhao JC, Jin H-J, Yu J. TMPRSS2-ERG gene fusions induce prostate tumorigenesis through modulating microRNA miR-200c. Oncogene. 2014; 33(44): 5183–5192. doi:10.1038/onc.2013.461

[82] Squire J. TMPRSS2-ERG and PTEN loss in prostate cancer. Nat Genet. 2009; 41: 509–510. doi:10.1038/ng0509-509

[83] King J, Xu J, Wongvipat J, Hieronymus H, Carver B, Leung D, et al. Cooperativity of TMPRSS2-ERG with PI3-kinase pathway activation in prostate oncogenesis. Nat Genet. 2009; 41(5): 524–526. doi:10.1038/ng.371

[84] Khani F, Mosquera J, Park K, Srivastava A, Tewari A, Mark R, et al. Differences in TMPRSS2-ERG gene fusion and SPINK1 overexpression in prostate cancer in African-American and Caucasian Men. J Urol. 2012; 187(4): e132. doi:10.1016/j.juro.2012.02.385

[85] Laxman B, Tomlins S, Mehra R, Morris D, Wang L, Helgeson B, et al. Noninvasive detection of TMPRSS2:ERG fusion transcripts in the urine of men with prostate cancer. Neoplasia. 2006; 8(10): 885–888. doi:10.1593/neo.06625

[86] Tavukcu HH, Mangir N, Ozyurek M, Turkeri L. Preliminary results of noninvasive detection of TMPRSS2:ERG gene fusion in a cohort of patients with localized prostate cancer. Korean J Urol. 2013; 54(6): 359–363. doi:10.4111/kju.2013.54.6.359

[87] Qu X, Randhawa G, Friedman C, et al. A novel four-color fluorescence in situ hybridization assay for the detection of TMPRSS2 and ERG rearrangements in prostate cancer. Cancer Genet. 2013; 206: 1–11. doi:10.016/j.cancergen.2012.12.004

[88] Smit F, Salagierski M, Jannink S, Schalken J. High-resolution ERG-expression profiling on Genechip exon 1.0 ST arrays in primary and castration-resistant prostate cancer. BJU Int. 2013; 111: 836–842. doi:10.1111/bju.12119

[89] Mostaghel E, Page S, Lin D, Fazli L, Coleman I, True L, et al. Intraprostatic androgens and androgen-regulated gene expression persist after testosterone suppression: Therapeutic implications for castration-resistant prostate cancer. Cancer Res. 2007; 67: 5033–5041. doi:10.1158/0008-5472.can-06-3332

[90] Reig Ò, Marín-Aguilera M, Carrera G, Jiménez N, Paré L, García-Recio S, Gaba L, Pereira M, Fernández P, Prat A, Mellado B. TMPRSS2-ERG in blood and docetaxel resistance in metastatic castration-resistant prostate cancer. Eur Urol. 2016; S0302–2838 (16): 00212–00218. doi:10.1016/j.eururo.2016.02.034

Chapter 12

Maspin Expression and its Metastasis Suppressing Function in Prostate Cancer

Eswar Shankar, Mario Candamo,
Gregory T. MacLennan and Sanjay Gupta

Additional information is available at the end of the chapter

http://dx.doi.org/10.5772/64336

Abstract

*Ma*mmary *S*erine *P*rotease *In*hibitor (Maspin) is a unique member of the serpin family with tumor suppressive properties. Maspin is a secreted protein encoded by a class II tumor suppressor gene, expressed in normal prostate luminal and basal cells but reduced or absent in prostate cancer. Currently, there is a consensus that maspin expression in prostate cancer is an indicator of a better prognosis and is a predictive marker for therapeutic response in prostate cancer. Experimental evidence consistently indicates that maspin suppresses tumor growth, invasion, and metastasis and promotes apoptosis in cancer cells. In this chapter, we discuss regulation of maspin expression, binding partners of maspin, and pathways through which maspin exerts its tumor suppressive properties. In addition, we summarize the progress that investigators have made in clarifying the role of maspin in prostate cancer biology and in assessing its role as a diagnostic marker and therapeutic agent.

Keywords: tumor suppressor, prognostic marker, SERPINB5, prostate cancer, maspin

1. Introduction

*Ma*mmary *S*erine *P*rotease *In*hibitor or Maspin (SERPINB5 or PI5 *Homo sapiens*) is a 42 kDa, non-classical, non-inhibitory member of the ovalbumin clade of serine protease inhibitors (serpins), encoded by the SERPIN5 gene [1]. Chromosome 18 encodes maspin along with gene cluster of other serpins in humans comprising squamous cell carcinoma antigens (SCCAs) 1 and 2 and plasminogen activator inhibitor type 2 (PAI-2) [1, 2]. Maspin has been characterized as a class II tumor suppressor gene, first recognized in 1994, in normal mammary tissue and breast cancer cell lines through subtractive hybridization, comparing genes expressed in different stages of a biological or pathological process [2]. Maspin has been shown to be downregulated in many metastatic tumor cell lines, without evidence of an underlying mutation [3]. Maspin contains a reactive center loop (RCL), which is used to trap the target protease and inhibit its activity, a common characteristic of inhibitory serpins [1, 2]. Recent studies suggest that serpins are involved in cell adhesion and play a role in extracellular remodeling [2, 3]. However, maspin has been found to be more closely related to the non-inhibitory clade B serpins. As maspin's RCL is shorter than those of inhibitory serpins and unlike multiple other serpins, maspin does not undergo a stressed-relaxed conformational change to inhibit protease activity. Despite the reported activity as a serine protease inhibitor, several studies argue that the tumor suppressor activity of maspin is due to its ability to inhibit proteolysis. Some studies demonstrate the efficacy of maspin in the inhibition of activity of tissue-type plasminogen activator [4]. Furthermore, maspin has been shown to mediate the inhibition of urokinase-type plasminogen activator (uPA) on the surface of prostate cancer cells [5]. Although maspin might lack the ability to inhibit serine proteases, its biological function can be attributed to RCL, which can be derived from its crystal structure [6]. Recent studies of maspin have provided evidence for its ability to regulate cell adhesion, motility, apoptosis, and angiogenesis, which has been of utmost interest in medical field attempting to use maspin as a method of therapeutic intervention for prostate cancer and other forms of malignancies [3–7].

2. Expression of maspin in normal prostate and cancer

Maspin has been localized to the cell surface, nucleus, cytoplasm, and extracellular matrix of epithelial cells of different tissues [8]. In normal breast and prostate epithelial cells, maspin is highly expressed and found to be localized mostly in the cytoplasm but has also been detected in the nucleus, secretory vesicles, and occasionally at the cell surface [6–8]. Maspin expression is almost completely suppressed in the human prostate cancer LNCaP, DU145, and PC-3 cell lines [9]. At the tissue level, maspin's function seems to be directly correlated with its localization. In benign prostate epithelium, maspin expression is uniformly noted in basal cells at high levels. In contrast, maspin expression is predominantly absent in benign secretory cells and elevated in secretory cells at the transition site between benign prostatic hyperplasia and high-grade PIN lesions [9, 10]. Pierson et al. noted higher expression of maspin in HGPIN lesions, particularly within secretory cells [11]. Elevated maspin immunoreactivity in the secretory cells appeared at the transition area between benign prostate tissue and HGPIN, whereas less intense maspin staining was observed in neoplastic cells adjacent to HGPIN. No change in maspin expression was observed in the basal cells near HGPIN, compared to normal basal cells [12]. Moreover, an inverse relationship between maspin expression and tumor progression was noted in clinical specimens with gradual disappearance in primary prostate cancer. Due to the loss of basal layer during prostate cancer progression, strong immunohistochemical staining of maspin was lost in the basal cells [12, 13]. A progressive decrease in maspin expression was noted with increase in Gleason grade, with complete loss of maspin in high grade and metastatic tumors (**Figure 1**). Maspin expression was significantly higher in tumor specimens of patients treated with neoadjuvant androgen ablation therapy before radical prostatectomy [14]. Prostate cancer patients whose tumors expressed maspin had a significantly longer recurrence-free survival [6, 12].

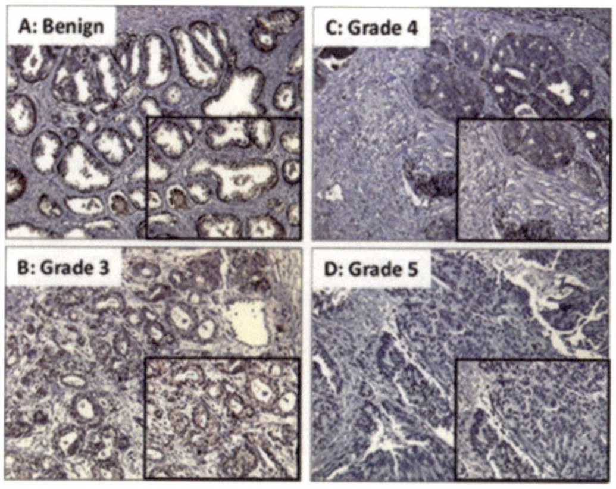

Figure 1. Expression of maspin in various representative human prostate specimens. Paraffin-embedded (4.0 μm) sections from benign *A*, and prostate cancer of various Gleason grades *B–D*, were used for maspin expression by immunohistochemistry. A strong nuclear and cytoplasmic staining was observed in benign tissue where the basal cell cytoplasm and nuclei were strongly and uniformly immunoreactive for maspin. Less intense cytoplasmic staining was noted in secretory cells. In low-grade cancer (Gleason grade 3), loss of nuclear maspin staining was observed and tumors progressively exhibited reduced maspin expression where the majority of high-grade tumors exhibit little or no cytoplasmic immunoreactivity. Magnified at ×20 and inset ×40.

3. Regulation of maspin expression

Maspin expression is regulated by a promoter with two response elements—Ets and a promiscuous hormone response element that binds glucocorticoid receptor and progesterone receptor [15]. Regulation of maspin by androgen receptor (AR) seems complex because the hormone response element of maspin's promoter appears to function as a negative regulator. Zou et al. have demonstrated that androgen-responsive LNCaP cells cultured in androgen-depleted medium exhibit induction of maspin promoter activity in a promoter luciferase reporter assay [16]. Furthermore, castration of nude mice induces maspin expression in LNCaP xenograft tumors. These data indicate that maspin may be transiently upregulated in early stages of prostate tumor development and remains sensitive to AR repression.

Another major regulatory mechanism for maspin is the involvement of p53 signaling pathway [16]. A consensus p53 site was identified in the maspin promoter, which induced its expression upon binding to p53. Maspin expression was increased in adenoviral-mediated expression of wild-type p53 in maspin-null prostate cancer cell lines. During cellular stress, p53-responsive pathways were induced in cells possessing wild-type p53, whereas mutant p53 failed to induce its expression. Purified p53 protein bound to regions within the promoter from −297 bp and p53 antibody supershifted maspin bands. In support of these data, a later study (using tissue microarray analysis) reported an inverse relationship between mutated p53 and maspin in human tumors [17]. The implication of maspin involvement in the p53 pathway demonstrated a potential hierarchy of tumor suppressor pathways. Studies suggest that maspin may act as an effector molecule downstream of the p53 stress-induced pathway. Interestingly, other proteins and signaling pathways related to maspin regulation were reported to be dependent on p53. Transforming growth factor β (TGFβ) was also found to increase maspin expression and required wild-type p53 activity [18]. This work demonstrated two p53 binding sites in the maspin promoter that were either in close proximity or overlapped with a Smad binding element, leading to recruitment of Smad2/3 and p53 to the maspin promoter following TGFβ signaling. In addition, Smad2/3 increased the binding of p53 to the maspin promoter demonstrating transcriptional co-regulation. Reports suggest that there are other factors that regulate maspin expression, independent of p53 function. Expression of the antioxidant manganese superoxide dismutase in prostate cells led to an increase in stability of maspin mRNA, and this effect persisted in the presence of wild-type or mutant p53 [19]. Furthermore, the activating transcription factor (ATF-2) was shown to induce maspin expression independently of p53 by binding to a CRE-like sequence downstream of the transcription start site [20]. In addition, other members of the p53 family, specifically the p63 isoform TAp63γ, induce expression of maspin by binding to the same consensus p53 promoter element and can substitute for activation in the absence of p53 [21]. Other transcription factors have also been noted to bind to maspin promoter and regulate its expression as shown in **Figure 2**.

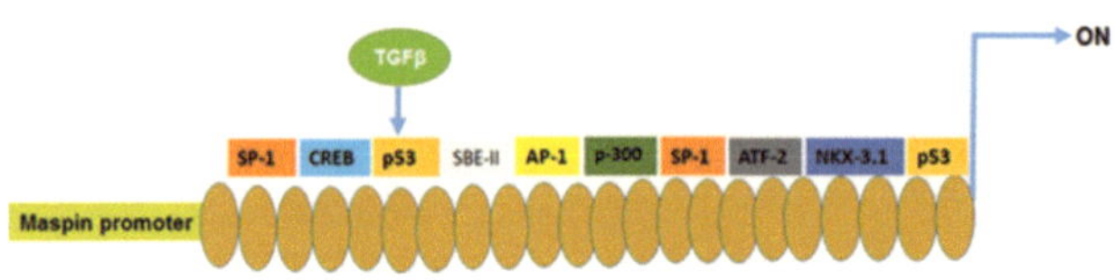

Figure 2. Regulation of maspin by various transcription factors. Maspin promoter has several transcription factor binding sites that regulate its expression and function. Most of maspin regulation by the transcription factors is unclear, but the regulation by p53 is widely studied and involves the TGF-β signaling.

Recent evidences suggest that maspin can be epigenetically regulated and that its expression in relationship with tissue specificity directly correlates with DNA methylation [2, 22]. Treatment of maspin-null cancer cell lines with 5-aza-2′-deoxycytidine resulted in the induction of maspin expression [22]. Furthermore, promoter methylation was found to serve as a mechanism for tissue and cell-specific expression of maspin [2, 22]. Epigenetic changes regulating maspin expression have been demonstrated to occur at the 5′ regulatory region of the maspin gene that involves methylation of cytosine, histone deacetylation, and the accessibility of chromatin. Two defining epigenetic events are DNA methylation and histone lysine methylation or deacetylation, which are categorized as chromatin modification events. In support of this, we and others have shown that treatment of prostate cancer cell lines with histone deacetylase (HDAC) inhibitors, namely sodium butyrate and trichostatin A, led to induction of maspin at mRNA and protein level [23]. Re-expression of maspin using demethylating agents and HDAC inhibitors in combination has been confirmed in additional studies. Furthermore, studies using prostate cancer cells and clinical specimens, we have further demonstrated that maspin expression was only induced by inhibition of class I histone deacetylases regardless of promoter methylation status, highlighting that chromatin condensation alone may determine its transcriptional activity [23].

Maspin is a non-glycosylated protein; however, phosphorylated forms have been identified and detected in various tumors [24]. Early studies demonstrate abundance of tyrosine phosphorylation in both endogenously expressed maspin in normal epithelial cells and after induction of maspin in transfected tumor cells [18]. Although the kinases responsible for this phosphorylation have yet to be identified, incubation of rMaspin with the TKD38 EGFR kinase domain led to tyrosine phosphorylation in a cell-free system. In addition, serine and threonine phosphorylation sites have been recently identified on maspin secreted from cornea cells using a mass spectrometry approach [25]. Whether this phenomenon is cell type specific requires further studies. In addition to phosphorylation studies, maspin also contains eight cysteine residues; however, intramolecular disulfide bonding had not previously been observed nor predicted from maspin crystallography. Under oxidative stress, maspin adopted an oxidized, disulfide-bonded structure, which was analyzed under non-reducing conditions in epithelial cells [26]. In this state, maspin was no longer able to bind glutathione *S*-transferase (GST), a binding partner for maspin, which suggested a potential difference in protein functionality.

4. Protein binding partners of maspin

Through the yeast two-hybrid assays, screening studies identified possible protein-protein interactions with maspin [27]. A short list of candidate intracellular partners of maspin include heat shock proteins (Hsp90 and Hsp70), glutathione *S*-transferase (GST), interferon regulatory factor 6 (IRF6), histone deacetylase 1 (HDAC1), early growth response protein 1 (Egr-1), and GC-binding factor 2 (GCF2). These studies provide new dimensions in understanding the role of maspin from that of a serine protease inhibitory serpin to that of a stress-responsive chaperone and role of maspin in tumor suppression.

Hsp90 is one of the most abundant stress-responsive chaperones that shuttle between the cytoplasm and nucleus to protect its client proteins from degradation [28]. Hsp90 binds and protects the native conformation of AR. AR attains activation and becomes functional as a consequence of agonists binding to its receptor, or when phosphorylated by Akt or due to mutation is ensued by its nuclear translocation. In the nucleus, AR employs co-activators that facilitate its binding to the promoter sequence of responsive genes to activate their expression [29]. Inhibition of Hsp90 destabilizes both wild type and mutant AR, presumably by releasing AR from the chaperone complex, to be subjected to degradation by the proteasome. Once in the nucleus, AR is acetylated, which may be mediated by its co-activators such as p300. Acetylated AR has been shown to specifically interact with and be deacetylated by HDAC1 [30]. Reports suggest that molecular interactions of maspin with HDAC1 and/or Hsp90 may underlie the positive correlation between nuclear maspin and better prognosis of cancer [31]. Inhibition of HDAC specifically upregulates genes that promote cell differentiation, cell cycle arrest, or cell death and downregulates genes that promote tumor survival and epithelial-mesenchymal transition, which correlate with higher levels of maspin, whereas both Hsp90 and HDAC have been implicated as key regulators of AR activity and stability. Lockett et al. have proposed a model where maspin may negatively regulate AR-dependent survival/ proliferation of both hormone-sensitive and hormone-refractory prostate epithelial cells [32]. This model proposes that genetic engineering approaches to induce maspin expression may prove to be effective in blocking Hsp90-mediated stability, and/or HDAC1-mediated transcriptional activation, of AR in prostate cancer cells.

The maspin/GST interaction was initially characterized [27]. Endogenous maspin has been shown to correlate with increased cellular GST activity, even though purified maspin does not affect the activity of GST *in vitro*. Furthermore, maspin transfected tumor cells exhibit markedly lower basal levels of ROS, compared to the control transfected cells. In contrast, siRNA knockdown of maspin in prostate cancer PC-3 cells increased the basal ROS level. Tahmatzopoulos et al. have shown that treatment of human prostate cancer DU145 cells with H_2O_2 (or PMA) but not with TRAIL further increases the maspin/GST interaction and significantly attenuated H_2O_2-induced ROS generation and VEGF expression [33]. This study further demonstrates that maspin transfected tumor cells produced less VEGF than the transfection control cells. Interestingly, a single point mutation at the RSL p1 position of maspin (MasR340A) greatly reduced the affinity for GST. Consistently, treatment with purified wild-type maspin, but not MasR340A, significantly increased cellular GST activity.

Studies by Bailey et al. reported specific interaction between maspin and interferon regulatory factor 6 (IRF6) [34, 35]. IRF6 is a member of the IRF family associated with epithelial-to-mesenchymal transition through increase in N-cadherin. The interaction between maspin and IRF6 appears to be regulated by IRF6 phosphorylation and may negatively regulate the IRF6 activity. Other maspin-binding proteins identified by yeast two-hybrid approach include transcription factors, such as early growth response protein 1 (Egr-1), GC-binding factor 2 (GCF2), and RNA-binding protein KHDRBS3 and FBX032, which are involved in ubiquitin protein ligase reactions [25]. Additional studies to understand how these proteins interact with maspin and their role during prostate cancer progression are needed.

5. Biological functions of maspin

Maspin downregulation correlates with increased tumor growth and metastasis [36]. Several published studies using cell lines and animal models underscore the critical role of maspin in tumor growth and invasion. Treatment with recombinant maspin protein was found to inhibit tumor invasion and motility of prostate cancer cells (LNCaP, DU145, and PC-3) in culture by binding specifically to the cell surface. This surface action was further supported by the ability of maspin to block urokinase-type plasminogen activator on cell surface of prostate cancer DU145 cells [5]. Cher et al. used a SCID human intraosseous tumor model that ectopically overexpresses maspin in prostate cancer DU145 cells to demonstrate maspin's ability to abrogate bone matrix remodeling, repress bone tumor growth, and prevent angiogenesis [37]. In another study, Hall et al. using maspin overexpressed PC-3 tumor cells injected to athymic nude mice demonstrated a decrease in bone metastasis but failed to suppress the ability of tumor cells spread/metastasize to distant sites providing new insight in the underlying inhibitory role of tumor cell homing into the bone [38]. Interestingly, in genetically engineered mouse model of prostate cancer, TRAMP the mechanism of maspin repression occurred through association of receptor activator of NF-kB (RANK) with ligand RANKL that facilitates IkB kinase α (IKKα) nuclear translocation, which in turn suppresses maspin transcription allowing progression of prostate cancer [39].

The anti-angiogenic effects of maspin were demonstrated by Zhang et al. using endothelial cells [40]. Increasing concentrations of rMaspin inhibited both the growth and migration of endothelial cells toward vascular endothelial growth factor (VEGF) and basic fibroblast growth factor (bFGF) *in vitro. In vivo* experiments using human prostate cancer LNCaP cells grown in immunodeficient xenograft model, tumor growth and neovascularization were reduced following rMaspin treatment [40]. A chimeric bone cancer model in which human cancer cells were injected into human bone that had been implanted into SCID/SCID mice demonstrated that DU145 human prostate cancer cells transfected with maspin exhibited less tumor neovascularization from murine endothelial cells compared to controls. This effect was associated with a decrease in tumor growth and bone destruction [36, 37]. Another study demonstrated that conditioned media (CM) from maspin-expressing human keratinocytes inhibited the ability of human endothelial cells to migrate toward angiogenic factors, namely VEGF, bFGF, and interleukin-8 (IL-8), in a dose-dependent manner [40]. Using maspin neutralizing antibody to the CM, the cells resumed their ability to migrate, providing evidence for a paracrine anti-angiogenic role of maspin.

Increased cell adhesion and cell-cell contact are negative factors for cell cycle progression. Increased cell adhesion to ECM is shown to cause certain cell types to arrest in G1 phase [41]. Studies suggest that maspin has ability to increase prostate epithelial cell adhesion to different matrix proteins and inhibit prostate tumor progression through increased cell adhesion to matrices. Recent study provides evidence that maspin controls cell adhesion through its interaction with integrin β1 [42]. Interestingly, loss of one copy of maspin gene in *Maspin*$^{+/-}$ heterozygous knockout mice leads to the development of prostate hyperplastic lesions, accompanied with a changed pattern of matrix deposition and a loss of epithelial cell polarity [41]. It was also demonstrated that maspin may be able to inhibit surface-bound urokinase plasminogen activator in prostate tumor cells. However, the aforementioned results were not easily observed *in vitro* or *in vivo*. *In vitro*, tumor suppression was not observed with the use of maspin, while *in vivo*, only 50% of tumors that expressed maspin showed a significant reduction [36, 37].

Maspin has been observed to be involved in the regulation of apoptosis. Pro-apoptotic effects from maspin have been demonstrated in prostate cancer cells. Studies by Mckenzie et al. underline maspin as a pertinent therapeutic target to overcome hypoxia in prostate cancer. Overexpression of maspin in DU145 cells leads to apoptosis by abrogating AKT activation induced by hypoxia. According to recent studies, it has been shown that maspin expression (endogenously) is able to sensitize prostate cancer LNCaP and DU145 cells to apoptosis [9]. Watanabe et al. used adeno-associated virus (AAV, serotype 2) vector encoding maspin as a means for introducing *in vivo* gene therapy subcutaneously formed human prostate cancer LNCaP or DU145 tumors in nude mice [43]. In this study, intratumoral AAV-mediated maspin expression significantly upregulated the number of apoptotic cells when compared with AAV-LacZ treatment. Moreover, significantly fewer CD31-positive micro-vessels were observed in AAV-maspin-treated tumors when compared with the control tumors, which correlated with persistent maspin expression. Studies on mechanics have demonstrated that maspin could possibly lead to apoptosis of tumor cells through the manipulation of mitochondrial permeability and the initiation of degradation through apoptosis [44]. Maspin has also been shown to induce prostate tumor cell dedifferentiation and to increase tumor cell sensitivity to drug-induced apoptosis. Suppression of maspin may partly be attributed to the involvement of AR in prostate tumorigenesis and cancer progression. Maspin's role as a tumor suppressor in prostate cancer cells irrespective of their AR status makes it an ideal candidate with therapeutic capabilities against hormone-refractory prostate cancer. Other biological functions of maspin are listed in **Figure 3**.

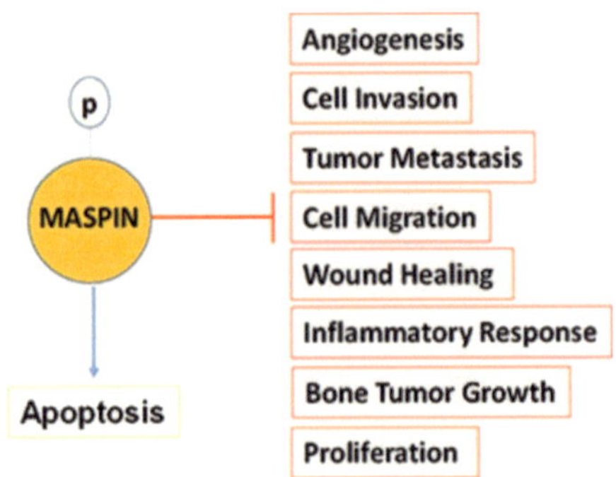

Figure 3. Biological functions of maspin. Post-translational modification of maspin and its nuclear localization suppresses angiogenesis, tumor metastasis, cell invasion, and migration and inhibits bone tumor growth and proliferation, while inducing apoptosis.

6. Therapeutic application of maspin

Recent studies have investigated the anticancer effects of maspin expression and the use of maspin as a therapeutic agent against cancer. Tumors with LNCaP cells expressing adenoviral maspin (AAV-GFP) resulted in a higher percentage of apoptotic cell death and a decrease in the number of CD31 positive vessels when compared with tumors with empty vector (GFP), thereby substantiating the role of maspin in gene therapy [44]. These results confirm maspin as a therapeutic agent/target in inhibiting prostate cancer progression. Furthermore, animal studies using targeted delivery of maspin by liposome/DNA and/or adenoviral constructs to tumor and/or tumor vasculature have supported a viable approach in cancer treatment [45].

Several reports suggest that exogenously added rMaspin, or maspin-derived peptide fragments, can act at the surface of numerous migratory cell types to suppress cell motility and movement by enhancing cellular adhesion to the extracellular matrix components laminin, fibronectin, and collagen [43, 45]. McGoven et al. have shown that purified recombinant maspin produced in baculovirus-infected *Spodoptera frugiperda* Sf9 insect cells [rMaspin] binds specifically to the surface of human prostate cancer DU145 cells, inhibits the DU145 cell surface-bound uPA, and forms a stable complex. Similar results with rMaspin were observed in *in vivo* studies transplanted with human prostate cells [5]. In fact, biological assays of invasion by prostate tumor cells through Matrigel membranes and of motility have shown that rMaspin inhibits invasion and migration of these cells [46].

Maspin expression in tumor cells can also be increased by the use of various phytochemicals. He et al. have demonstrated that gum mastic, a natural resin, can upregulate maspin expression in prostate cancer cells [47]. Gum mastic induced maspin mRNA and protein expression, as well as maspin promoter activity in LNCaP and DU145 cells by suppressing ARE binding activity and enhancing Sp1 binding activity, and the increased activity in the maspin promoter. Sheth et al. have demonstrated that resveratrol (trans-3,49,5-trihydroxystilbene), a polyphenolic antioxidant found in peanuts, grapes, and red wine inhibits cell proliferation, induces apoptosis of human prostate cancer cells mediated by increase in maspin levels through Akt/miR-21 pathway [48]. Natural compound curcumin, a hydrophobic polyphenol derived from turmeric (the rhizome of the herb *Curcuma longa*), has been shown to inhibit the AR gene activity in androgen-responsive human prostate cancer LNCaP cells suppressing AR transaction, thereby affecting AR-regulated genes including maspin [49]. As AR negatively regulates maspin expression, curcumin-mediated inhibition of AR may induce the expression of maspin through a mechanism, which is presently unclear. Nevertheless, increased expression of maspin occurs only in prostate cancer cells, which harbor wild-type p53. As p53 activates maspin promoter by binding directly to its p53 consensus-binding site [16], we studied the effect of apigenin, a natural plant flavonc in potentially restoring p53-mediated maspin levels. Exposure of LNCaP and 22Rv1 cells, harboring wild-type p53, with apigenin resulted in dose dependent increase in maspin expression and p53 activation through acetylation at the Lys305 residue by inhibiting class I HDACs. Apigenin withdrawal in LNCaP cells caused loss of maspin and p53 acetylation. Furthermore, proteasome inhibitor MG132 inhibited apigenin-mediated proteasomal degradation of class I HDACs in these cells. The increased apigenin-mediated p53 acetylation enhanced its binding on maspin promoter, which was associated with decrease in tumor cell invasion and migration. Apigenin treatment also caused accumulation of acetylated histone H3 in total cellular chromatin, increasing accessibility to bind with the promoter sequences of maspin, consistent with the effects elicited by HDAC inhibitor, trichostatin A. Similar observations were noted after feeding apigenin to 22Rv1 tumor xenograft implanted in nude mice [50]. Other natural compounds that have been reported to enhance prostate cancer suppression and inhibit invasion and migration through upregulation of maspin are tanshinone IIA and apple peel extract [51, 52].

A study by Jiang et al. revealed differential expression patterns of maspin mRNA and protein expression following treatment of cancer cells with essential fatty acids (EFAs) [53]. Addition of omega-6, EFAs arachidonic acid and α-linolenic acid had no effect on maspin expression, while treatment with γ-linolenic acid led to rapid increase in maspin mRNA [53]. Consumption of γ-linolenic acid has been linked to many beneficial effects in humans. Interestingly in the same study, another omega-6 EFA, linoleic acid, resulted in decreased maspin expression. This study highlighted specific effects of EFAs on maspin that may have significant implications in cancer biology as well as a role for maspin in lipid signaling and processing. Not surprisingly, *in vitro* promoter activity study showed that, in addition to p53 [16], a list of stress-related signals including DNA-damaging agents, cytotoxic drugs [16], peroxisome proliferator-activated receptor-gamma [54], nitric oxide [55], and manganese superoxide dismutase (MnSOD) [56] activates maspin expression. Consistently, several stress signals that induce maspin expression also induced more differentiated phenotypes [16, 54–56]. Furthermore, epigenetic treatment of prostate cancer cell lines with trichostatin A, a histone deacetylase (HDAC) inhibitor, led to induction of maspin mRNA [20, 50]. Re-expression of maspin using demethylating agents and HDAC inhibitors has been confirmed in additional studies [50, 57].

7. Conclusions and future directions

Much remains to be understood about the molecular mechanism(s) of action of maspin in the normal prostate and during cancer progression. Studies in our laboratory are ongoing to determine the post-translational modifications of maspin, which may help elucidate the role of maspin in signaling pathways relevant to cell adhesion and angiogenesis. The ability of maspin and its post-translationally modified forms to act as effective therapeutic agents in prostate cancer is also being pursued. Additional studies are required to unravel the multi-faceted interrogation of how maspin expression can alter the malignant phenotype of some cell types and not others. Nevertheless, recent findings and ongoing studies should encourage researchers to continue to explore the molecular mechanisms underlying maspin's biological effects in prostate cancer.

Clinical studies performed this far in prostate cancer demonstrate the significance of maspin expression as a useful prognostic and possibly predictive marker for patients undergoing definitive therapy. Focusing on the malignancies in which maspin exhibited a positive prognostic value, therapeutic approaches studied so far aimed to re-activate this dormant tumor suppressor gene by transcription factors that regulate its expression and/or to identify natural substances that can determine the activation and the expression of maspin or possibly deliver this molecule in tumor cell through gene therapy capable of upregulating maspin in an attempt to reduce invasiveness and the risk of metastasis. Maspin packaged as an adenoviral construct or a liposomal DNA has been utilized to reduce tumors and tumor vasculatures in *in vivo* studies corroborates as a feasible approach toward cancer therapy. Nevertheless, the approach using viral vectors or liposomal DNA complexes is accompanied with several safety and efficacy issues that modify their association upon interaction with serum components, which is a subject of rigorous studies, and further evaluation is required through clinical trials. The usefulness of rMaspin in targeted therapy is debatable because proteins undergo rapid clearance from the body through proteolysis, liver clearance and filtered through the kidneys. These issues can be resolved by the use of nanotechnology, which has provided a valuable option for targeted delivery of genes, drugs, and proteins.

Recently performed studies highlight reversible nature of epigenetic silencing of maspin in prostate cancer, which offers a unique opportunity for therapeutic intervention by several epigenetic modifiers. Considering the anti-angiogenic and pro-apoptotic properties of nuclear maspin shown by recent studies, re-activated nuclear maspin in association with anti-angiogenic or chemotherapeutic drugs may be effective in the treatment of advance-stage prostate cancer. Undoubtedly, the challenges are numerous, but the prospects for improved therapeutic approaches through maspin application for this debilitating disease could be immense.

Acknowledgements

The original work from author's laboratory outlined in this chapter was supported by the United States Public Health Service grants R01CA108512, R21CA193080, R03CA186179, Department of Defense grant W81XWH-15-1-0558, and Department of Veteran Affairs grant 1I01BX002494 to SG.

Conflict of interest

The authors have no competing interest.

Author details

Eswar Shankar[1], Mario Candamo[2], Gregory T. MacLennan[3] and Sanjay Gupta[1,4,5,6*]

*Address all correspondence to: sanjay.gupta@case.edu

1 Department of Urology, Case Western Reserve University, University Hospitals Case Medical Center, Cleveland, Ohio, United States

2 Department of Biology, School of Undergraduate Studies, Case Western Reserve University, Cleveland, Ohio, United States

3 Department of Pathology, Case Western Reserve University, University Hospitals Case Medical Center, Cleveland, Ohio,United States

4 Department of Nutrition, Case Western Reserve University, Cleveland, Ohio, United States

5 Division of General Medical Sciences, Case Comprehensive Cancer Center, Cleveland, Ohio, United States

6 Department of Urology, Louis Stokes Cleveland Veterans Affairs Medical Center, Cleveland, Ohio, United States

References

[1] Narayan M, Twining S. Focus on molecules: maspin. Exp Eye Res. 2010;90:2–3.

[2] Khalkhali-Ellis Z. Maspin: the new frontier. Clin Cancer Res. 2006;12:7279–83.

[3] Schaefer JS, Zhang M. Role of maspin in tumor metastasis and angiogenesis. Curr Mol Med. 2003;3:653–658.

[4] Sheng S, Truong B, Fredrickson D, Wu R, Pardee AB, Sager R. Tissue-type plasminogen activator is a target of the tumor suppressor gene maspin. Proc Natl Acad Sci U S A. 1998;95:499–504.

[5] McGowen R, Biliran H, Jr, Sager R, Sheng S. The surface of prostate carcinoma DU145 cells mediates the inhibition of urokinase-type plasminogen activator by maspin. Cancer Res. 2000;60:4771–4778.

[6] Berardi R, Morgese F, Onofri A, Mazzanti P, Pistelli M, Ballatore Z et al. Role of maspin in cancer. Clin Transl Med. 2013;2:8.

[7] McKenzie S, Sakamoto S, Kyprianou N. Maspin modulates prostate cancer cell apoptotic and angiogenic response to hypoxia via targeting AKT. Oncogene. 2008;27:7171–7179.

[8] Machowska M, Wachowicz K, Sopel M, Rzepecki R. Nuclear location of tumor suppressor protein maspin inhibits proliferation of breast cancer cells without affecting proliferation of normal epithelial cells. BMC Cancer. 2014;28:142.

[9] Bernardo MM, Meng Y, Lockett J, Dyson G, Dombkowski A, Kaplun A, et al. Maspin reprograms the gene expression profile of prostate carcinoma cells for differentiation. Genes Cancer. 2011;2:1009–1022.

[10] Shen M M, Abate-Shen C. Molecular genetics of prostate cancer: new prospects for old challenges. Genes Dev. 2010;24:1967–2000.

[11] Pierson, CR, McGowen R, Grignon D, Sakr W, Dey J, Sheng, S. Maspin is up-regulated in premalignant prostate epithelia. Prostate. 2002;53:255–262. doi: 10.1002/pros.10107

[12] Machtens S, Serth J, Bokemeyer C, Bathke W, Minssen A, Kollmannsberger C, Hartmann J, Knüchel R, Kondo M, Jonas U, Kuczyk M. Expression of the p53 and Maspin protein in primary prostate cancer: correlation with clinical features. Int J Cancer. 2001;95:337–342.

[13] Man YG, Zhao C, Chen X. A subset of prostate basal cells lacks the expression of corresponding phenotypic markers. Pathol Res Pract. 2006;202:651–662.

[14] Zou Z, Zhang W, Young D, Gleave MG, Rennie P, Connell T, Connelly R, Moul J, Srivastava S, Sesterhenn I. Maspin expression profile in human prostate cancer (CaP)

and in vitro induction of Maspin expression by androgen ablation. Clin Cancer Res. 2002;8:1172–1177.

[15] Zhang M, Magit D, Sager R. Expression of maspin in prostate cells is regulated by a positive ets element and a negative hormonal responsive element site recognized by the androgen receptor. Proc Natl Acad Sci U S A. 1997;94:5673–5678.

[16] Zou Z, Gao C, Nagaich AK, Connell T, Saito S, Moul JW, et al. p53 regulates the expression of the tumor suppressor gene maspin. J Biol Chem. 2000;275:6051–6054.

[17] Webber BA, Lawson D, Cohen C. Maspin and mutant p53 expression in malignant melanoma and carcinoma: use of tissue microarray. Appl Immunohistochem Mol Morphol. 2008;16:19–23.

[18] Wang SE, Narasanna A, Whitell CW, Wu FY, Friedman DB, Arteaga CL. Convergence of p53 and transforming growth factor beta (TGFbeta) signaling on activating expression of the tumor suppressor gene maspin in mammary epithelial cells. J Biol Chem. 2007;282:5661–5669.

[19] Duan H, Zhang HJ, Yang JQ, Oberley LW, Futscher BW, Domann FE. MnSOD upregulates maspin tumor suppressor gene expression in human breast and prostate cancer cells. Antioxid Redox Signal. 2003;5:677–688.

[20] Maekawa T, Sano Y, Shinagawa T, Rahman Z, Sakuma T, Nomura S, Licht JD, Ishii S. ATF-2 controls transcription of Maspin and GADD45 alpha genes independently from p53 to suppress mammary tumors. Oncogene. 2008;27:1045–1054.

[21] Kirschner R.D., Sänger K., Müller G.A., Engeland K. Transcriptional activation of the tumor suppressor and differentiation gene S100A2 by a novel p63-binding site. Nucleic Acids Res. 2008;36:2969–2980.

[22] Hurtubise A, Momparler RL. Evaluation of antineoplastic action of 5-aza-2′-deoxycytidine (Dacogen) and docetaxel (Taxotere) on human breast, lung and prostate carcinoma cell lines. Anticancer Drugs. 2004;15:161–167.

[23] Abbas A, Gupta S. The role of histone deacetylases in prostate cancer. Epigenetics. 2008;3:300–309.

[24] Nawata S, Shi HY, Sugino N, Zhang M. Evidence of post-translational modification of the tumor suppressor maspin under oxidative stress. Int J Mol Med. 2010;27:249–254.

[25] Narayan M, Mirza SP, Twining SS. Identification of phosphorylation sites on extracellular corneal epithelial cell maspin. Proteomics. 2011;11:1382–1390.

[26] Grek C.L., Townsend D.M., Uys J.D., Manevich Y., Coker W.J., III, Pazoles C.J. S-glutathionylated serine proteinase inhibitors as plasma biomarkers in assessing response to redox-modulating drugs. Cancer Res. 2012;72:2383–2393.

[27] Yin S, Li X, Meng Y, Finley RL Jr, Sakr W, Yang H, Reddy N, Sheng S. Tumor-suppressive maspin regulates cell response to oxidative stress by direct interaction with glutathione S-transferase. J Biol Chem. 2005;280:34985–34996.

[28] Vered M, Allon I, Tunis TS, Buchner A, Dayan D. Expression of the homeostasis-related markers, maspin, heat shock proteins 70 & 90, glutathione S-transferase, aquaporin 5 and NF-kB in young and old labial and palatal salivary glands. Exp Gerontol. 2013;48:444–450.

[29] Tan ME, Li J, Xu HE, Melcher K, Yong E-L. Androgen receptor: structure, role in prostate cancer and drug discovery. Acta Pharmacol Sin. 2015;36:3–23. doi: 10.1038/aps.2014.18.

[30] Gaughan L, Logan IR, Cook S, Neal DE, Robson CN. Tip60 and histone deacetylase 1 regulate androgen receptor activity through changes to the acetylation status of the receptor. J Biol Chem. 2002;277:25904–25913. doi: 10.1074/jbc.M203423200.

[31] Li X, Kaplun A, Lonardo F, Heath E, Sarkar FH, Irish J, Sakr W, Sheng S. HDAC1 inhibition by maspin abrogates epigenetic silencing of glutathione S-transferase pi in prostate carcinoma cells. Mol Cancer Res. 2011;9:733–745. doi: 10.1158/1541-7786.MCR-10-0505.

[32] Lockett J, Yin S, Li X, Meng Y, Sheng S. Tumor suppressive maspin and epithelial homeostasis. J Cell Biochem. 2006;97:651–660. doi:10.1002/jcb.20721.

[33] Tahmatzopoulos A, Sheng S, Kyprianou N. Maspin sensitizes prostate cancer cells to doxazosin-induced apoptosis. Oncogene. 2005;24:5375–5383. doi:10.1038/sj.onc.1208684.

[34] Bailey CM, Khalkhali-Ellis Z, Kondo S, Margaryan NV, Seftor RE, Wheaton WW, Amir S, Pins MR, Schutte BC, Hendrix MJ. Mammary serine protease inhibitor (Maspin) binds directly to interferon regulatory factor 6: identification of a novel serpin partnership. J Biol Chem. 2005;280:34210–34217.

[35] Bailey CM, Abbott DE, Margaryan NV, Khalkhali-Ellis Z, Hendrix MJ. Interferon regulatory factor 6 promotes cell cycle arrest and is regulated by the proteasome in a cell cycle-dependent manner. Mol Cell Biol. 2008;28:2235–2243. doi:10.1128/MCB.01866-07

[36] Dzinic SH, Chen K, Thakur A, Kaplun A, Bonfil RD, Li X, Liu J, Bernardo MM, Saliganan A, Back JB, Yano H, Schalk DL, Tomaszewski EN, Beydoun AS, Dyson G, Mujagic A, Krass D, Dean I, Mi QS, Heath E, Sakr W, Lum LG, Sheng S. Maspin expression in prostate tumor elicits host anti-tumor immunity. Oncotarget. 2014;5:11225–11236.

[37] Cher ML, Biliran HR, Jr, Bhagat S, Meng Y, Che M, Lockett J, Abrams J, Fridman R, Zachareas M, Sheng S. Maspin expression inhibits osteolysis, tumor growth, and angiogenesis in a model of prostate cancer bone metastasis. Proc Natl Acad Sci U S A. 2003;100:7847–7852. http://dx.doi.org/10.1073/pnas.1331360100

[38] Hall DC, Johnson-Pais TL, Grubbs B, Bernal R, Leach RJ, Padalecki SS. Maspin reduces prostate cancer metastasis to bone. Urol Oncol. 2008;26:652–658. doi:10.1016/j.urolonc.2007.07.017.

[39] Luo JL, Tan W, Ricono JM, Korchynskyi O, Zhang M, Gonias SL, Cheresh DA, Karin M. Nuclear cytokine-activated IKKalpha controls prostate cancer metastasis by repressing maspin. Nature. 2007;446:690–694.

[40] Zhang M, Volpert O, Shi YH, Bouck N. Maspin is an angiogenesis inhibitor. Nat Med. 2000;6:196–199. doi:10.1038/72303.

[41] Shao LJ, Shi HY, Ayala G, Rowley D, Zhang M. Haploinsufficiency of the maspin tumor suppressor gene leads to hyperplastic lesions in prostate. Cancer Res. 2008;68:5143–5151.

[42] Qin L, Zhang M. Maspin regulates endothelial cell adhesion and migration through an integrin signaling pathway. J Biol Chem. 2010;285:32360–32369. doi:10.1074/jbc.M110.131045.

[43] Watanabe M, Nasu Y, Kashiwakura Y, Nasu Y, Kashiwakura Y, Kusumi N, et al. Adeno-associated virus 2-mediated intratumoral prostate cancer gene therapy: long-term maspin expression efficiently suppresses tumor growth. Hum Gene Ther. 2005;16:699–710. doi:10.1089/hum.2005.16.699.

[44] Latha K, Zhang W, Cella N, Shi HY, Zhang M. Maspin mediates increased tumor cell apoptosis upon induction of the mitochondrial permeability transition. Mol Cell Biol. 2005;25:1737–1748. doi:10.1128/MCB.25.5.1737-1748.2005.

[45] Shi HY, Liang R, Templeton NS, Zhang M. Inhibition of breast tumor progression by systemic delivery of the maspin gene in a syngeneic tumor model. Mol Ther. 2002;5:755–761.

[46] Sheng S, Carey J, Seftor EA, Dias L, Hendrix MJ, Sager R. Maspin acts at the cell membrane to inhibit invasion and motility of mammary and prostatic cancer cells. Proc Natl Acad Sci U S A. 1996;93:11669–11674.

[47] He ML, Chen WW, Zhang PJ, Jiang AL, Fan W, Yuan HQ, Liu WW, Zhang JY. Gum mastic increases maspin expression in prostate cancer cells. Acta Pharmacol Sin. 2007;28:567–572.

[48] Sheth S, Jajoo S, Kaur T, Mukherjea D, Sheehan K, Rybak LP, Ramkumar V. Resveratrol reduces prostate cancer growth and metastasis by inhibiting the Akt/MicroRNA-21 pathway. PLoS One. 2012;7:e51655. doi:10.1371/journal.pone.0051655.

[49] Shi P, Chen WW, Hu XY, Yu CX, Zhang PJ, Jiang AL, Zhang JY. Up-regulates the expression of maspin gene in prostate cancer cell line LNCaP. Yao Xue Xue Bao. 2006;41:1152–1156.

[50] Shukla S., Abbas A., Gupta S. Apigenin increases maspin expression and suppresses invasiveness in prostate cancer cells [abstract]. In: Proceedings of the 106th Annual

Meeting of the American Association for Cancer Research; 2015 Apr 18–22; Philadelphia, PA. Philadelphia (PA): AACR; Cancer Res 2015;75(15 Suppl):Abstract nr 4649. doi: 10.1158/1538-7445.AM2015-4649

[51] Liu W, Zhou J, Geng G, Shi Q, Sauriol F, Wu JH. Antiandrogenic, maspin induction, and antiprostate cancer activities of tanshinone IIA and its novel derivatives with modification in ring A. J Med Chem. 2012;55:971–975. doi:10.1021/jm2015292

[52] Reagan-Shaw S, Eggert D, Mukhtar H, Ahmad N. Antiproliferative effects of apple peel extract against cancer cells. Nutr Cancer. 2010;62:517–524. doi: 10.1080/01635580903441253.

[53] Jiang WG, Hiscox S, Horrobin DF, Bryce RP, Mansel RE. γ-Linolenic acid regulates expression of maspin and the motility of cancer cells. Biochem Biophys Res Commun. 1997;237:639–644

[54] Burgermeister E, Tencer L, Liscovitch M. Peroxisome proliferator-activated receptor-gamma upregulates caveolin-1 and caveolin-2 expression in human carcinoma cells. Oncogene. 2003;22:3888–3900.

[55] Lam YW, Yuan Y, Isaac J, Babu CV, Meller J, Ho SM. Comprehensive identification and modified-site mapping of S-nitrosylated targets in prostate epithelial cells. PLoS One. 2010;5:e9075. doi:10.1371/journal.pone.0009075.

[56] Li JJ, Oberley LW, Fan M, Colburn NH. Inhibition of AP-1 and NF-kB by manganese-containing superoxide dismutase in human breast cancer cells. Carcinogenesis. 1998;19:833–839.

[57] Beltran AS, Sun X, Lizardi PM, Blancafort P. Reprogramming epigenetic silencing: artificial transcription factors synergize with chromatin remodeling drugs to reactivate the tumor suppressor mammary serine protease inhibitor. Mol Cancer Ther. 2008;7:1080–1090.

Chapter 13

The Emerging Role of PARP Inhibitors in the Treatment of Prostate Cancer

Jue Wang, Brent B. Freeman and Paul Mathew

Additional information is available at the end of the chapter

http://dx.doi.org/10.5772/63283

Abstract

Poly (ADPribose) polymerase (PARP) is a critical DNA repair enzyme involved in DNA single-strand break repair through the base excision repair pathway. PARP inhibitors have been shown to sensitize tumors to DNA-damaging agents and selectively kill homologous recombination repair-defective cancers, such as those arising in BRCA1 and BRCA2 mutation carriers. In addition to its well-documented role in DNA damage repair (DDR), emerging evidence has indicated that PARP1 plays an important role in mediating the transcriptional activities of androgen receptor (AR) and ETS gene rearrangement in prostate cancer. Preclinical and clinical research suggested that the activity of PARP inhibitors is not limited to those with BRCA mutations. PARP inhibitors may have activity in cancers deficient in other DNA repair genes or signaling pathways that mitigate DNA repair.

Based on results of the TOPARP-A Phase 2 trial, the US Food and Drug Administration (FDA) has granted Breakthrough Therapy designation to olaparib (Lynparza) for monotherapy treatment of BRCA1/2 or ataxia telangiectasia mutated (ATM) gene mutated in patients with metastatic castration-resistant prostate cancer who received a prior taxane-based chemotherapy and at least one newer hormonal agent. Future research is needed to address the optimal timing, combination, and to identify predictive biomarker for PARP inhibition.

Keywords: prostate cancer, BRCA1, BRCA2, poly(ADP-ribose) polymerases, PARP inhibitors

1. Introduction

Prostate cancer is the most commonly diagnosed cancer in men and is the second leading cause of cancer-related deaths in men each year [1]. Androgen-deprivation therapy has been the gold standard of care for metastatic prostate cancer for decades. While this treatment strategy initially shows benefit, the disease inevitably progresses to metastatic castration-resistant prostate cancer (mCRPC) for which there is limited treatment options [2]. Although chemo-therapies, immunotherapy, and novel androgen signaling pathway inhibitors therapies [3–7] have shown some benefit, mCRPC remain incurable with overall survival well under 5 years. Further development of novel agents is needed for the treatment of prostate cancer.

2. Poly(ADPribose) polymerase and DNA repair

Prostate cancer, like most other cancers, is a genetic disease resulting from the accumulation of genetic alterations that enable cancer cells to survive, proliferate, and metastasis [8, 9]. Such enrichment of genomic instability could be attributed to diminished DNA repair in mCRPC [8–11]. To maintain genomic integrity, there exists conserved checkpoint signaling pathways to facilitate cell cycle delay, DNA repair, and/or apoptosis in response to DNA damage [11].

BRCA1 and BRCA2 are the best characterized DNA repair genes associated with cancer development [12]. Germline-mutated prostate cancer is particularly frequent in young patients (<65 years), with BRCA2 more prevalent than BRCA1 (1.4 and 0.44% of all prostate cancer, respectively). Germline mutation carriers have higher Gleason scores, lower overall survival (OS) and cancer-specific survival, higher advanced stages, and globally a worse prognosis compared with noncarrier patients [13]. BRCA proteins have a crucial role in the regulation of homologous recombination (HR) repair, an accurate DNA double-strand break (DSB) repair process. In the absence of BRCAs (and other HR proteins), DNA DSBs increase which induce the accumulation of DNA mutations and thereby promotes tumorigenesis. Although BRCA dysfunction promotes an oncogenic advantage, it also renders cancer cells reliant on alterna-tive DNA repair pathways, such as base excision repair (BER).

Poly(ADPribose) polymerase (PARP) are a family of enzymes that catalyze Nicotinamide adenine dinucleotide (NAD) NAD+-dependent ADP ribosylation of DNA. PARP1 has been implicated in several DNA repair mechanisms, including DNA single-strand breaks (SSB) which repair through the BER pathway. PARP1 recognizes DNA SSB and orchestrates the recruitment and assembly of a DNA repair complex [14, 15]. As a result, PARP inhibition induces the accumulation of unrepaired SSB, which are subsequently converted into DSBs at fork replication. Cells with deficient HR repair systems (i.e., for BRCA1/2 mutations) treated with PARP inhibitors are overcome by DNA DSBs, which lead to further chromosomal instability, cell cycle arrest, and apoptosis [16]. Therefore, PARP-1 is an important therapeutic target in cancer therapy including prostate cancer, especially in patients harboring the BRCA mutations.

3. PARP-1 and prostate cancer

Several lines of evidence point to a potential role of PARP-1 in prostate cancer progression. PARP-1 expression is markedly elevated in prostate cancer relative to that in benign prostatic hyperplasia (BPH) tissues, which may imply the involvement of PARP-1 and PAR in the development of prostate cancer [17]. Augmented immunodetection of PARP-1 was associated with prostate cancer progression and biochemical recurrence [18].

In addition to its well-documented role in BER, emerging evidence has indicated that PARP1 plays an important role in mediating the transcriptional activities of androgen receptor (AR) and ETS gene rearrangement [19]. PARP inhibition results in antitumor activity in TMPRSS2-ERG rearranged cancer models and suppresses AR target gene expression and tumor proliferation [20]. PARP-1 regulates Smad-dependent responses to Transforming growth factor beta (TGF-β) signaling and potential AR activity, directing both toward epithelial-mesenchymal transition (EMT) in prostate cancer progression [21]. PARP-1 has also been implicated at the chromatin level in AR-mediated cell proliferation in the early and late-stage prostate cancer models [22], with suppression of PARP-1 resulting in reduced cell proliferation. In androgen-independent PC3 cells, PARP inhibition significantly decreased cell viability, migration, invasion, chromatin loop dimensions, and histone acetylation. Thus PARP could play a key role in the compartmentalization of chromatin and in the development of the more aggressive phenotype [23].

4. BRCAness and prostate cancer

McCabe et al. [24] demonstrated that deficiencies of several proteins in the HR DNA repair pathway, such as the DNA damage sensors ataxia telangiectasia mutated (ATM) and ataxia telangiectasia (ATR and RAD3-related protein), lead to HR deficiency and subsequent PARP inhibition sensitivity. This concept known as 'BRCAness' has been used to describe the phenotype arising in sporadic cancers that have intact BRCA1/2 genes but share features with the BRCA1/2 mutation-related tumors, such as profound platinum sensitivity [25]. For example, based on its high proliferation rate, sensitivity to platinum-based therapy and the rapid development of chemotherapy resistance [26], small cell/anaplastic prostate cancer clearly fits into the clinical phenotype of BRCAness. Studies of these tumor samples at the DNA level will likely reveal genetic alterations in DNA repair genes. Theoretically, PARP inhibitors may enhance the chemotherapy-induced DNA damage in anaplastic/small cell prostate cancer.

While only a minority of prostate cancer patients carry germline mutations, emerging data suggest that HR defects are common in prostate cancer, potentially conferring a BRCAness phenotype [26–29]. Recent genetic studies have shown somatic mutations of the DNA HR repair system in more than 20% of the patients with CRPC. The genes identified are involved in different steps and mechanisms of HR machinery [29]. In an extensive genome analysis, Robinson et al. compared genetic sequencing data of castration sensitive and CRPC. BRCA2 was the most frequent mutations occurring in 12.7% of cases. Interestingly, the analysis of other DNA repair genes showed overall DNA repair gene aberrations in 22.7% of patients, with ATM and BRCA1 alterations occurring most frequently (in 19.3% of patients). In addition, 3.4% of patients have CDK12, FANCA, RAD51B, and RAD51C mutations [29]. These patients represent a distinct subtype with unique clinical characteristics that have important implications for management.

5. Active clinical trials investigating PARP inhibitors in prostate cancer

The evidence correlating increased PARP-1 activity with tumor progression has opened a new avenue for the utilization of PARP inhibitors, which may impair the DNA repair machine. The clinical experiences with PARP inhibitors initially focused on patients carrying mutations of the BRCA1 or BRCA2 genes, which have been linked to increased sensitivity to PARP-1 inhibitors. Additional evidence has shown that tumors with other mechanisms of impaired DNA repair might benefit from treatment with PARP inhibitors. In addition to the use of single-agent, the PARP inhibitors have been studied in combination with a number of different agents in prostate cancer (**Table 1**) and other cancers (**Table 2**). Other areas of active investigation include the development of biomarkers that may predict clinical benefit from PARP inhibition, as well as the identification of resistance mechanisms to PARP inhibitor therapy.

Agent(s) [Phase]	Cancer	Identifier
Olaparib + Arbiraterone [II]	Metastatic castration-resistant prostate cancer	NCT01972217
Veliparib + Arbiraterone [II]	Metastatic castration-resistant prostate cancer	NCT01576172
Enzalutamide + Niraparib [I]	Metastatic castration-resistant prostate cancer	NCT02500901
Olaparib + Radical prostatectomy [I]	Intermediate/high-risk prostate cancer	NCT02324998

Table 1. Ongoing clinical trials (Phase I/II) with PARP-1 inhibitors combination for prostate cancers (www.clinicaltrials.gov).

5.1. PARP inhibitors as single-agent therapy

In a Phase I clinical trial with olaparib, 60 patients with various refractory caners were enrolled and treated. Objective antitumor activity was reported only in BRCA mutation carriers, all of whom had ovarian, breast, or prostate cancer and had received multiple treatment regimens. Three patients with mCRPC were recruited, and one of them had a BRCA2 mutation [30]. The patient with BRCA2 mutation had >50% decrease in serum prostate-specific antigen (PSA) levels and a complete response of bone lesions.

Niraparib was tested in a Phase 1 dose-escalation study of 21 mCRPC patients. The investigators reported 43% of the patients with stable disease, and a median duration of response of 254 days. In total, 30% of the patients had a decrease of circulating tumor cells (CTC), and one of the 21 patients enrolled had >50% PSA reduction. Importantly, the authors did not observe the hypothesized correlation between ERG rearrangements or loss of PTEN expression and treatment response [31].

Agent(s) [Phase]	Cancer	Identifier
PET imaging of PARP activity in cancer [0]	Solid tumors	NCT02469129
Veliparib and SCH727965 (Dinaciclib) [I]	Advanced solid tumors	NCT01434316
Olaparib and AKT inhibitor AZD5363 [I]	Solid tumors	NCT02338622
Olaparib (AZD2281) alone and in combination with AZD1775, AZD5363, or AZD2014 [I]	Molecularly selected patients with solid tumors	NCT02576444
Anti-PD-1 monoclonal antibody BGB-A317 in combination with the PARP inhibitor BGB-290 [I]	Solid tumors	NCT02660034
Molecular profiling-based assignment of cancer therapy Everolimus/Afinitor (mTOR inhibitor), Trametinib DMSO (MEK inhibitor), Temozolomide and ABT-888 (PARP inhibitor), and Carboplatin and MK-1775 (Wee1 inhibitor) [I]	Solid tumors that are metastatic or cannot be removed by surgery and liver or kidney dysfunction	NCT01366144
Veliparib + Topotecan [I/II]	Solid tumor, ovarian, peritoneal cavity tumors	NCT01012817
Olaparib + AZD5363 [I]	Solid tumor	NCT02338622
Rucaparib [I/II]	Patients with gBRCA mutation solid tumor, breast cancer	NCT01482715
Fluzoparib [I]	Solid tumors	NCT02575651
E7449; E7449 + TMZ; E7449 + Carbo + Pacli [I/II]	Solid tumor, ovarian, breast, melanoma, B-cell malignancy	NCT01618136

Table 2. Ongoing clinical trials (Phase I/II/III) with PARP-1 inhibitors for other cancers (www.clinicaltrials.gov).

In a Phase II clinical trial evaluating the efficacy and safety of olaparib in a spectrum of BRCA1/2-associated cancers, the authors reported 50% response rate, 25% stable disease, and an overall median duration response of 327 days in eight previously heavily treated mCRPC patients with germline BRCA1/2 mutations. Median progression-free survival was 7.2 months with 62.5% of the patients still progression-free at 6 months. Moreover, the Overall Survival (OS) was 18.4 months, with 50% of the patients was still alive at 12 months [32].

The publication of the Phase II clinical trial, TOPARP-A, which tests the efficacy of olaparib in mCRPC patients [33] generated a lot of excitement in prostate cancer field. Fifty mCRPC patients previously treated with docetaxel, most of whom had also been previously treated with abiraterone (Zytiga®) or enzalutamide (Xtandi®), received oral olaparib 400 mg twice daily in 28 day-cycles until disease progression. All patients had received docetaxel; 98% had received abiraterone or enzalutamide; and 58% had received cabazitaxel. Patients underwent biopsies at baseline and during therapy for whole-exome sequencing and transcriptome studies. The primary endpoint was response rate, PSA response, or conversion of the baseline circulating tumor cell count. Sixteen of the 49 patients who could be evaluated had a response rate of 33%, with 12 patients receiving the study treatment for more than 6 months. Median overall survival was 10.1 months. Next-generation sequencing identified homozygous deletions, deleterious mutations, or both in DNA-repair genes--including BRCA1/2, ATM, Fanconi's anemia genes, and CHEK2—in 16 of the 49 patients who could be evaluated (33%). Of these 16 patients, 14 (88%) had a response to olaparib, including all 7 patients with BRCA2 loss (four with biallelic somatic loss and three with germline mutations) and 4 of 5 with ATM aberrations. Anemia and fatigue were the major treatment-related adverse effects. The mutational status of the ERG oncogene and that of the PTEN tumor suppressor gene was not associated with olaparib responses. TOPARP-B, the second stage of this trial, is ongoing and aiming to validate findings of TOPARP-A. Part B of TOPARP (TOPARP-B) is open to the recruitment and aims to recruit a total of 88 patients. Potential participants will have their tumor tissue analyzed and only those with biomarkers predictive of olaparib response will go on to enter TOPARP-B. Forty-four patients will receive 300 mg twice daily, and 44 will receive 400 mg of olaparib twice daily. Part C (TOPARP-C) will be the subsequent Phase II randomized, double-blind, placebo-controlled evaluation of olaparib and is currently in development.

5.2. PARP inhibitors in combination therapy

5.2.1. Combining the PARP inhibitor with cytotoxic chemotherapy

Preclinical research has provided a strong rationale for employing PARP inhibitors as chemosensitizers in combination with cytotoxic agents. The PARP inhibitor veliparib has been shown to enhance the antitumor activity of Temozolomide (TMZ) in prostate cancer xenografts [34]. This formed the rationale for testing the safety and efficacy of veliparib and TMZ in 26 patients with mCRPC pretreated with docetaxel [35]. Despite the promising preclinical activity, this combination showed modest activity over TMZ monotherapy. Two patients had a confirmed PSA response and four patients had stable disease (SD) for at least 4 months. The median progression-free survival (PFS) and OS were 2.1 and 9.1 months, respectively. One patient had the TMPRSS2:ERG gene fusion, and this patient achieved stable disease with a progression-free survival of 70 days and overall survival of 277 days. Grade III/IV thrombocytopenia was noted in 15% of patients.

5.2.2. Combining the PARP inhibitor with androgen deprivation therapy

The preclinical findings of PARP1 in mediating transcriptional regulation by AR and the ETS fusion protein [20–23] and the potential preclinical synergy of targeting of the PARP and AR pathways provide a strong rationale for the clinical evaluation of combining of these two classes of anticancer drugs.

The primary objective of a multicenter randomized Phase II trial (NCT01576172) is to evaluate whether adding veliparib to abiraterone acetate and prednisone would improve the PSA response rate of the standard abiraterone acetate and prednisone regimen in patients with

http://dx.doi.org/10.5772/63283

mCRPC. Secondary and exploratory objectives include PSA decline rate, objective response rate, progression-free survival and toxicity. The investigators will evaluate ETS fusion status in metastatic tumor tissue, and a logistic model will be used to determine the association of TMPRSS2-ERG fusion status with the PSA response in the veliparib plus abiraterone and prednisone arm. This study will provide validation on the value of ETS gene rearrangement as a predicative biomarker for PARP inhibitor-based therapy for mCRPC.

Another Phase I trial evaluating the combination of PARP inhibitor niraparib and enzalutamide (NCT02500901) was recently activated. The primary goal of this study is to assess whether patients with AR-regulated CRPC can be assessed for synergistic clinical benefit from dual AR blockade and PARP-1 inhibition, with the combination of enzalutamide and niraparib. Secondary and exploratory objectives include PSA kinetics, progression-free survival, and objective response. Correlative studies using quantitative and qualitative measures of CTCs to identify a predictive biomarker of response to the combination. These include dynamic studies of AR and AR splice variant nuclear localization and feasibility studies aim to assess homologous repair deficiency in CTCs.

5.2.3. Combining the PARP inhibitors with radiotherapy

Preclinical study with prostate cancer cell lines reported that combining the PARP inhibitor rucaparib with radiation enhanced the DNA damage and antitumor effects compared with radiation alone. The strongest synergistic activities were observed in LNCaP and VCaP cells, which contain the TMPRSS2-ERG fusion gene [36–38]. However, no association was noted between the loss of PTEN expression and ETS rearrangements, with radiologic assessment of the antitumor activity of niraparib in a Phase I trial [31]. At the present time, there are no active clinical trials investigating the combination of radiation therapy with PARP inhibition in mCRPC.

The combination of a PARP inhibitor with radiation would be an attractive strategy for newly diagnosed ETS fusion-positive, locally advanced, high-risk prostate cancer in adjuvant or neoadjuvant setting, or nonmetastatic CRPC at recurrent setting. However, the risk of overtreatment and long-term safety are the main concerns of testing this strategy.

Combining PARP inhibitors with radiation or radiopharmaceuticals such like Xofigo®(radium 223) could be another reasonable combination for patients with mCRPC to the bone. Currently, there is no active trial testing the combination.

5.2.4. Combining the PARP inhibitors with molecularly targeted drugs

In a Phase II clinical trial (NCT02576444), the investigators evaluated the safety of combining the AKT inhibitor AZD5363 with olaparib. The authors reported that the novel combination of olaparib and AZD5363 was safe and yielded responses in patients with a variety of cancer types, including breast, ovarian, and prostate cancers, regardless of BRCA1/2 mutation status. One patient with BRCA1/2-mutant advanced prostate cancer had a sustained response both by MRI and PSA Working Group 2 response criteria at 11 months. The most commonly observed side effects were nausea, vomiting, fatigue, diarrhea, and anemia.

Several other trails combining the PARP inhibitor with other molecularly targeted drugs are ongoing (**Tables 1** and **2**).

5.2.5. preoperative (neoadjuvant) studies of PARP1 inhibitors

The testing of novel agents in the preoperative (neoadjuvant) setting approach offers a potentially rapid and efficient strategy for drug development. Neoadjuvant studies allow the assessment of drug effects on the target (pharmacodynamic response) and the development of predictive biomarkers of response.

A Phase I study investigating the feasibility and tolerability of a short course of neoadjuvant treatment with olaparib given prior to radical prostatectomy in men with localized intermediate-/high-risk prostate cancer is ongoing (NCT02324998). The primary objective is to determine the pharmacodynamic biomarker effects of olaparib in this patient population. Participants will receive either single-agent olaparib, or olaparib in combination with degarelix (androgen deprivation), for one week prior to routine radical prostatectomy. The degree of PARP inhibition will be measured by the change in immunohistochemistry (IHC) levels of biomarkers such as PAR, gamma H2AX, pH2A (s129), Rad51 foci, FancD2 foci, and ATM/ATR/CHK1/2 in tumor samples taken at baseline and following treatment with olaparib (either alone or in combination with degarelix). Secondary outcome measures include the incidence and severity of adverse events caused by treatment for 7 days with olaparib (either alone or in combination with degarelix) prior to radical prostatectomy [41].

5.3. Safety of PARP inhibitors

The toxicity profile of PARP inhibitor monotherapy appears to be similar to cytotoxic chemotherapeutic agents [30–33, 39]. The most frequently reported adverse events in published studies are grade 1–2 nausea, vomiting, diarrhea, fatigue, headache, and anemia. Grade 3 or 4 toxicities are rare in early phase clinical trials in patients with prostate cancer being treated with a single-agent. The most common grade 3–4 toxicities were nausea, vomiting, and hematological toxicity, with anemia, lymphopenia, and thrombocytopenia being the most common dose-limiting toxicities in dose-finding studies [31, 32]. In a Phase II trial, in which patients with mCRPC were treated with olaparib tablets at a dose of 400 mg twice a day, anemia (20%) and fatigue (12%) were the most common grade 3 or 4 adverse events. These findings are consistent with previous studies of olaparib [33].

Conversely, dose-limiting toxicities observed in trials of PARP inhibitors in combination with cytotoxic agents include primarily hematologic toxicities. For example, olaparib in combination with cisplatin and gemcitabine is associated with myelosuppression even at relatively low doses in a Phase I study of patients with advanced solid tumors [40]. An intermittent schedule of PARP inhibition instead of continuous dosing was investigated [41].

At this time, the long-term safety data on the PAPR inhibitors is still lacking. Enhanced DNA damage with a PARP inhibitor and radiation may lead to genomic instability and more aggressive prostate cancer and secondary malignancy. Few cases of myelodysplastic syndrome and acute myeloid leukemia have been reported in PARP inhibitor trials; most of the

http://dx.doi.org/10.5772/63283

patients had been treated with DNA-damaging classic chemotherapeutic agents. Nonetheless, the potential increased risk of developing secondary cancer from DNA damage warrants close attention in future development of PARP inhibitors, especially in the neoadjuvant and adjuvant settings [42].

5.4. Biomarkers for PARP-directed therapy

The ultimate clinical need in the development of PARP-directed therapy is to identify biomarkers to enrich selection of patients who are most likely to respond to therapy [43]. As monotherapy, findings from clinical trials with olaparib showed that genetic biomarkers could be used to select the patients with mCRPC who will respond to PARP inhibitor therapy. The HR/PARP synthetic lethality model may be more widely applicable in prostate cancer with germline or somatic inactivating mutations in the HR DNA repair genes, CHK2, BRIPI/FANCJ, NBS1, BRCA1, and ATM, collectively estimated to occur in 20–25% of prostate cancer cases. Two of the most common genetic alterations in prostate cancer, TMPRSS2: ERG gene fusion ETS gene rearrangement, and loss of PTEN, have also been linked to increased sensitivity to PARP inhibitor in preclinical models [37, 38]. However, this association has not been confirmed in clinical study [31]. Regardless, these results underscore the complexity and challenge in developing a biomarker for PARP inhibitor activity. Although additional synthetic lethal strategies have been explored in preclinical, or early clinical trial setting [44–47], development of a clinically validated biomarker (companion diagnostic) will depend on the results of well-designed and conducted Phase III clinical trials.

It is clear that the individual clinical response to PARP inhibition is varied and that currently accepted markers of response (progression-free survival, RECIST, PARP inhibition in peripheral blood mononuclear cells, or hair follicles) are not ideal [48]. The availability of direct imaging tests capable of measuring PARP inhibition locally would thus be of enormous value in such settings [49]. A new radiolabeled compound (18°F) FluorThanatrace ([18 F] FTT), has been generated which can be used to measure PARP1 activity noninvasively and quantitatively using positron emission tomography (PET). Preclinical models show that the uptake of this compound is specific for PARP1 activity and correlates with biochemically determined PARP1 activity. Additional data also suggests that decreased (18 F) FTT uptake predicts tumor response to PARP inhibition with olaparib. A Phase 0 study investigating the feasibility of PET imaging of PARP activity in cancer (NCT02469129) recently opened for enrollment. This technology provides both a biomarker for patient selection as well as a means of monitoring PARP activity during treatment.

6. Conclusion

Approximately 30% of mCRPC exhibit defective DNA repair via HR, representing a distinct subtype with unique clinical characteristics that have important implications for management. PARP inhibitors are an exciting new class of agents that have already demonstrated promising preclinical and clinical activity in mCRPC. Recent Phase I and II studies have reported single-agent activities with favorable side effect profiles in sporadic and in BRCA-mutant prostate cancers. Based on results of the TOPARP-A Phase II trial, the US FDA has granted Breakthrough Therapy designation to olaparib (Lynparza) [50]., for monotherapy treatment of BRCA1/2 or ATM gene mutated mCRPC in patients who received a prior taxane-based chemotherapy and at least one newer androgen signaling inhibitor. Currently, there are seven different PARP inhibitors in clinical development for cancer. As we learn more about these agents through ongoing trials, it will be important to identify biomarkers that predict patients who may benefit the most from PARP inhibitor therapy. In addition, it will be important to determine the optimal timing, sequence and clinical setting (neoadjuvant, adjuvant, or maintenance), either as monotherapy or in combination.

Author details

Jue Wang*, Brent B. Freeman and Paul Mathew

*Address all correspondence to: jue.wang@dignityhealth.org

University of Arizona Cancer Center at Dignity Health St. Joseph's, Phoenix, AZ, USA

References

[1] Siegel R, Naishadham D, Jemal A. Cancer statistics, 2013. CA Cancer J Clin. 2013;63(1): 11–3010.

[2] Attard G, Sarker D, Reid A, Molife R, Parker C, de Bono JS. Improving the outcome of patients with castration-resistant prostate cancer through rational drug development. Br J Cancer. 2006;95(7):767–774.

[3] Tannock IF, de Wit R, Berry WR, et al. Docetaxel plus prednisone or mitoxantrone plus prednisone for advanced prostate cancer. N Engl J Med. 2004;351:1502–1512

[4] de Bono JS, Oudard S, Ozguroglu M, et al. Prednisone plus cabazitaxel or mitoxantrone for metastatic castration-resistant prostate cancer progressing after docetaxel treatment: a randomised open-label trial. Lancet. 2010;376:1147–1154

[5] de Bono JS, Logothetis CJ, Molina A, et al. Abiraterone and increased survival in metastatic prostate cancer. N Engl J Med. 2011;364:1995–2005

[6] Kantoff PW, Higano CS, Shore ND, et al. Sipuleucel-T immunotherapy for castration-resistant prostate cancer. N Engl J Med. 2010;363:411–422

[7] Fizazi K, Carducci M, Smith M, et al. Denosumab versus zoledronic acid for treatment of bone metastases in men with castration-resistant prostate cancer: a randomised, double-blind study. Lancet. 2011;377:813-822

[8] Taylor BS, Schultz N, Hieronymus H, Gopalan A, Xiao Y, et al. Integrative genomic profiling of human prostate cancer. Cancer Cell. 2010; 18: 11–22.

[9] Grasso CS, Wu YM, Robinson DR, Cao X, Dhanasekaran SM, et al. The mutational landscape of lethal castration-resistant prostate cancer. Nature 2012; 487: 239–243.

[10] Chen Y, Wang J, Fraig MM, Metcalf J, Turner WR, et al. Defects of DNA mismatch repair in human prostate cancer. Cancer Res. 2001; 61: 4112–4121.

[11] Fan R, Kumaravel TS, Jalali F, Marrano P, Squire JA, et al. Defective DNA strand break repair after DNA damage in prostate cancer cells: implications for genetic instability and prostate cancer progression. Cancer Res. 2004; 64: 8526–8533.

[12] Consortium TB. Cancer risks in BRCA2 mutation carriers. J Natl Cancer Inst. 1999;91:1310–1316.

[13] Castro E, Goh C, Olmos D et al. GermlineBRCA mutations are associated with higher risk of nodal involvement, distant metastasis, and poor survival outcomes in prostate cancer. J. Clin. Oncol. 2013, 31(14), 1748–1757.

[14] Do K, Chen AP. Molecular pathways: targeting PARP in cancer treatment. Clin Cancer Res. 2013;19(5):977–984.

[15] Durkacz BW, Omidiji O, Gray DA, Shall S. (ADP-ribose) n participates in DNA excision repair. Nature. 1980;283(5747):593–610.

[16] Menissier-de Murcia J, Molinete M, Gradwohl G, Simonin F, de Murcia G 1989. Zinc-binding domain of poly(ADP-ribose)polymerase participates in the recognition of single strand breaks on DNA. J Mol Biol. 1989; 210(1): 229–233.

[17] Salemi M, Galia A, Fraggetta F, La Corte C, Pepe P, La Vignera S, Improta G, Bosco P, Calogero AE. Poly (ADP-ribose) polymerase 1 protein expression in normal and neoplastic prostatic tissue. Eur J Histochem. 2013; 57(2):e13.

[18] Thomas E, Gannon PO, Koumakpayi IH, Latour M, Mes-Masson A, Saad.F. Implication of PARP-1 expression in prostate cancer progression. J Clin Oncol. 2011;29(suppl); abstr e15025

[19] Brenner JC, Ateeq B, Li Y, et al. Mechanistic rationale for inhibition of poly(ADP-ribose) polymerase in ETS gene fusion-positive prostate cancer. Cancer Cell 2011;19:664–678.

[20] Schiewer MJ, Goodwin JF, Han S, Brenner JC, Augello MA, Dean JL, Liu F, Planck JL, Ravindranathan P, Chinnaiyan AM, McCue P, Gomella LG, Raj GV, Dicker AP, Brody JR, Pascal JM, Centenera MM, Butler LM, Tilley WD, Feng FY, Knudsen KE. Dual roles of PARP-1 promote cancer growth and progression. Cancer Discov. 2012, 2(12):1134–1149.

[21] Pu H, Horbinski C, Hensley PJ, Matuszak EA, Atkinson T, Kyprianou N. PARP-1 regulates epithelial-mesenchymal transition (EMT) in prostate tumorigenesis. Carcinogenesis. 2014;35(11):2592–2601.

[22] Barboro P, Ferrari N, Capaia M, Petretto A, Salvi S, Boccardo S, Balbi C. Expression of nuclear matrix proteins binding matrix attachment regions in prostate cancer. PARP-1: New player in tumor progression. Int J Cancer. 2015;137(7):1574–1586.

[23] Salemi M, Condorelli RA, La Vignera S, Barone N, Ridolfo F, Giuffrida MC, Vicari E, Calogero AE. PARP-1 and CASP3 genes are up-regulated in LNCaP and PC-3 prostate cancer cell lines. Hum Cell. 2014;27(4):172–175.

[24] McCabe, Turner NC, Lord CJ, et al. Deficiency in the repair of DNA damage by homologous recombination and sensitivity to poly(ADP-ribose) polymerase inhibition. Cancer Res. 2006;66(16):8109–8115.

[25] Turner N, Tutt A, Ashworth A. Hallmarks of 'BRCAness' in sporadic cancers. Nat Rev Cancer. 2004;4(10):814–819.

[26] Aparicio AM, Harzstark AL, Corn PG, Wen S, Araujo JC, et al. Platinum-based chemotherapy for variant castrate-resistant prostate cancer. Clin Cancer Res. 2013;19: 3621–3630.

[27] Beltran H, Yelensky R, Frampton GM, Park K, Downing SR, MacDonald TY, Jarosz M, Lipson D, Tagawa ST, Nanus DM, Stephens PJ, Mosquera JM, Cronin MT, Rubin MA. Targeted next-generation sequencing of advanced prostate cancer identifies potential therapeutic targets and disease heterogeneity. Eur Urol. 2013;63(5):920–926.

[28] Farmer H, McCabe N, Lord CJ, Tutt AN, Johnson DA, Richardson TB, et al. Targeting the DNA repair defect in BRCA mutant cells as a therapeutic strategy. Nature. 2005; 434(7035):917–2110.

[29] Robinson D, Van Allen EM, Wu YM, et al. Integrative clinical genomics of advanced prostate cancer. Cell. 2015;161(5):1215–1228.

[30] Fong PC, Boss DS, Yap TA, Tutt A, Wu P, Mergui-Roelvink M, Mortimer P, Swaisland H, Lau A, O'Connor MJ, Ashworth A, Carmichael J, Kaye SB, Schellens JH, de Bono JS. Inhibition of poly(ADP-ribose) polymerase in tumors from BRCA mutation carriers. N Engl J Med. 2009;361(2):123–134.

[31] Sandhu SK, Schelman WR, Wilding G, Moreno V, Baird RD, Miranda S, Hylands L, Riisnaes R, Forster M, Omlin A, Kreischer N, Thway K, Gevensleben H, Sun L, Loughney J, Chatterjee M, Toniatti C, Carpenter CL, Iannone R, Kaye SB, de Bono JS, Wenham RM. The poly(ADP-ribose) polymerase inhibitor niraparib (MK4827) in BRCA mutation carriers and patients with sporadic cancer: a phase 1 dose-escalation trial. Lancet Oncol. 2013;14(9):882–892.

[32] Kaufman B, Shapira-Frommer R, Schmutzler RK et al. Olaparib monotherapy in patients with advanced cancer and a germline BRCA1/2 mutation. J. Clin. Oncol. 2015;33(3), 244–250.

[33] Mateo J, Carreira S, Sandhu S, Miranda S, Mossop H, Perez-Lopez R, NavaRodrigues D, Robinson D, Omlin A, Tunariu N, Boysen G, Porta N, Flohr P, Gillman A, Figueiredo

I, Paulding C, Seed G, Jain S, Ralph C, Protheroe A, Hussain S, Jones R, Elliott T, McGovern U, Bianchini D, Goodall J, Zafeiriou Z, Williamson CT, Ferraldeschi R, Riisnaes R, Ebbs B, Fowler G, Roda D, Yuan W, Wu YM, Cao X, Brough R, Pemberton H, A'Hern R, Swain A, Kunju LP, Eeles R, Attard G, Lord CJ, Ashworth A, Rubin MA, Knudsen KE, Feng FY, Chinnaiyan AM, Hall E, de Bono JS. DNA-repair defects and olaparib in metastatic prostate cancer. N Engl J Med. 2015;373(18):1697–1708.

[34] Palma JP, Wang YC, Rodriguez LE, Montgomery D, Ellis PA, Bukofzer G, et al. ABT-888 confers broad in vivo activity in combination with temozolomide in diverse tumors. Clin Cancer Res. 2009;15(23):7277–9010.

[35] Hussain M, Carducci MA, Slovin S, Cetnar J, Qian J, McKeegan EM, Refici-Buhr M, Chyla B, Shepherd SP, Giranda VL, Alumkal JJ. Targeting DNA repair with combination veliparib (ABT-888) and temozolomide in patients with metastatic castration-resistant prostate cancer. Invest New Drugs 2014; 32: 904–912.

[36] Chatterjee P, Choudhary GS, Sharma A, Singh K, Heston WD, Ciezki J, et al. PARP inhibition sensitizes to low dose-rate radiation TMPRSS2-ERG fusion gene-expressing and PTEN-deficient prostate cancer cells. PLoS One. 2013;8(4):e60408.

[37] Verhagen CV, de Haan R, Hageman F, Oostendorp TP, Carli AL, O'Connor MJ,Jonkers J, Verheij M, van den Brekel MW, Vens C. Extent of radiosensitization by the PARP inhibitor olaparib depends on its dose, the radiation dose and the integrity of the homologous recombination pathway of tumor cells. Radiother Oncol. 2015;116(3):358–365.

[38] Han S, Brenner JC, Sabolch A, Jackson W, Speers C, Wilder-Romans K, Knudsen KE, Lawrence TS, Chinnaiyan AM, Feng FY. Targeted radiosensitization of ETS fusion-positive prostate cancer through PARP1 inhibition. Neoplasia. 2013;15(10): 1207–1217.

[39] Rajan A, Carter CA, Kelly RJ, Gutierrez M, Kummar S, Szabo E, Yancey MA, Ji J,Mannargudi B, Woo S, Spencer S, Figg WD, Giaccone G. A phase I combination study of olaparib with cisplatin and gemcitabine in adults with solid tumors. Clin Cancer Res. 2012;18(8):2344–2351.

[40] Balmana J, Tung NM, Isakoff SJ, Grana B, Ryan PD, Saura C, et al. Phase I trial of olaparib in combination with cisplatin for the treatment of patients with advanced breast, ovarian and other solid tumors. Ann Oncol. 2014;25:1656–1663.

[41] Murray J, Thomas H, Berry P, Kyle S, Patterson M, Jones C, Los G, Hostomsky Z, Plummer ER, Boddy AV, Curtin NJ. Tumour cell retention of rucaparib, sustained PARP inhibition and efficacy of weekly as well as daily schedules. Br J Cancer. 2014 Apr 15;110(8):1977-84.

[42] Sonnenblick A, de Azambuja E, Azim HAJr, Piccart M. An update on PARP inhibitors – moving to the adjuvant setting. Nat Rev Clin Oncol. 2015;12(1):27–41.

[43] Tan DS, Thomas GV, Garrett MD, Banerji U, de Bono JS, Kaye SB, Workman P.Biomarker-driven early clinical trials in oncology: a paradigm shift in drug development. Cancer J. 2009;15(5):406–420.

[44] Duan W, Gao L, Zhao W, Leon M, Sadee W, Webb A, et al. Assessment of FANCD2 nuclear foci formation in paraffin-embedded tumors: a potential patient-enrichment strategy for treatment with DNA interstrand crosslinking agents. Transl Res. 2013;161(3):156–6410.

[45] Mukhopadhyay A, Elattar A, Cerbinskaite A, Wilkinson SJ, Drew Y, Kyle S, et al. Development of a functional assay for homologous recombination status in primary cultures of epithelial ovarian tumor and correlation with sensitivity to poly(ADP-ribose) polymerase inhibitors. Clin Cancer Res. 2010,16(8):2344–5110. DOI: 10.1158/1078–0432.

[46] Mukhopadhyay A, Plummer ER, Elattar A, Soohoo S, Uzir B, Quinn JE, et al. Clinicopathological features of homologous recombination-deficient epithelial ovarian cancers: sensitivity to PARP inhibitors, platinum, and survival. Cancer Res. 2012; 72(22):5675–8210.

[47] Ji J, Kinders RJ, Zhang Y, Rubinstein L, Kummar S, Parchment RE, et al. Modeling pharmacodynamic response to the poly(ADP-ribose) polymerase inhibitor ABT-888 in human peripheral blood mononuclear cells. PLoS One. 2011; 6(10):e26152. 10.1371/journal.pone.0026152.

[48] Reiner T, Lacy J, Keliher EJ, Yang KS, Ullal A, Kohler RH, Vinegoni C, Weissleder R. Imaging therapeutic PARP inhibition in vivo through bioorthogonally developed companion imaging agents. Neoplasia. 2012;14(3):169–177.

[49] Tunariu N, Kaye SB, deSouza NM. Functional imaging: what evidence is there for its utility in clinical trials of targeted therapies? British J Cancer. 2012;106(4):619–628.

[50] Lynparza™ (Olaparib) granted Breakthrough Therapy designation by US FDA for treatment of BRCA1/2 or ATM gene mutated metastatic Castration Resistant Prostate Cancer [news release]. AstraZeneca. January 28, 2016. https://www.astrazeneca.com/our-company/media-centre/press-releases/2016/Lynparza-Olaparib-granted-Breakthrough-Therapy-Designation-by-US-FDA-for-treatment-of-BRCA1-2-or-ATM-gene-mutated-metastatic-Castration-Resistant-Prostate-Cancer-28012016.html#main. Accessed February 1, 2016.

Chapter 14

Rehabilitation of Patients with Prostate Cancer

Meral Huri, Burcu Semin Akel and Sedef Şahin

Additional information is available at the end of the chapter

http://dx.doi.org/10.5772/63989

Abstract

Cancer rehabilitation involves helping an individual with cancer to regain maximum psychological, physical, cognitive, social, and vocational functioning with the limits up to disease and its treatments in an interdisciplinary team concept. Prostate cancer is one of the most frequent male malignancies in the world. Prostate cancer treatment options have the risk of some side effects including loss of muscle strength, fatigue, pain, urinary incontinence, erectile dysfunction, cognitive problems, decrease in bone density, weight loss, gynecomastia, and hot flushes with stress-related psychosocial problems. Relative to other cancers, the prognosis of men with prostate cancer is much better and the potential treatment-related side effects have important implications which can affect the health-related quality of life (QOL) of this population. Recent studies support the efficiency of multimodal treatment to recognize, prevent, and increase functional recovery with an interdisciplinary rehabilitation team which includes physical and occupational therapists. This chapter describes briefly cancer rehabilitation and rehabilitation approaches at every stage of patients with prostate cancer for minimizing the morbidity rate associated with prostate cancer treatment to increase occupational participation and improve QOL.

Keywords: prostate cancer, rehabilitation, physiotherapy, occupational therapy

1. Introduction

Cancer rehabilitation involves helping an individual with cancer to regain maximum psychological, physical, cognitive, social, and vocational functioning with the limits up to disease and its treatments in an interdisciplinary team concept [1]. Prostate cancer is one of the most frequent male malignancies in the world [2]. The development of serum prostate-specific antigen (PSA) and advanced cancer treatment modalities increased 10-year survival rates from ~60% to >70%. Prostate cancer can occur as a local disease or an advanced metastatic disease. Surgical removal of the prostate gland, hormonal therapy, radiation therapy, cryoablation, and expectant monitoring are some of the treatment options for patients with prostate cancer [3].

These treatment options are associated with the risk of some side effects including fatigue, pain, urinary incontinence, erectile dysfunction, cognitive problems, decrease in bone density, weight loss, gynecomastia, and hot flushes with stress-related psychosocial problems [4]. Relative to other cancers, the prognosis of men with prostate cancer is much better, and the potential treatment-related side effects have important implications which can affect the health-related quality of life (QOL) of the patients; besides, these treatment-related side effects are significant in this population [5].

Increased rates of survival and support required for functional, physical, and psychological status led to a considerable interest in rehabilitation needs and the approaches used to increase the QOL of the patients with prostate cancer [5]. Recent studies support the efficiency of multimodal treatment to recognize, prevent, and increase functional recovery with an interdisciplinary rehabilitation team which includes physical and occupational therapists. These professionals provide inpatient care, outpatient follow-up and education, and services in home care, palliative, and hospice care settings [6].

Physical therapists play a vital role in the rehabilitation of patients with prostate cancer by teaching and implementing weight-bearing and gentle exercise, resistive exercises, and vibration exercises which transmit energy to the body with special techniques that strengthen the posture, balance, and body fitness, maintain or improve bone density, and prevent falls [6, 7]. In addition, pelvic floor training helps alleviate symptoms of urinary incontinence and maintain normal pelvic floor muscle functions [8]. Physical therapy also focuses on restoring the cardiovascular system which helps improve blood flow; this has been shown to improve symptoms associated with cancer-related fatigue and erectile dysfunction. Physical therapists assess the patients and develop individualized intervention programs including exercise programs to increase the endurance, muscle strength, mobility, and balance of patients with prostate cancer [6–8].

Occupational therapists play a vital role in increasing the occupational participation of the patients with prostate cancer [5]. Occupational therapists use training in activities of daily living, assistive technology approaches, education of energy conservation techniques, management of treatment-related problems such as pain, fatigue, and nausea. Moreover, occupational therapists give occupational balance training for regaining value of engagement in meaningful activities with a holistic view of creative and therapeutic use of activity [5, 9]. Occupational therapists focus on adaptations and offer education assistance for sexual activity for patients where certain sexual positions are limited or impossible due to pain, fatigue, or positioning issues. This complication in prostate cancer treatments is one of the most important limitations of activities of daily living that men face [9]. Occupational therapists offer ways to help patients with prostate cancer to confirm, express, accept, and use problem-solving techniques to present the changes due to prostate cancer and its treatment. Effective stress management must include relaxation and social support in a supportive environment. Such interventions decrease treatment-related symptoms, reduce the physiological accompaniments of stress, and improve mood. Patients who participate in such rehabilitation interventions are shown to have improved mental health by feeling more controlled and experiencing reduced interpersonal conflicts and distress related to cancer-related intrusive thinking [5]. In addition, cognitive therapy and changing life style with cognitive behavioral therapy are the mostly used occupational therapy interventions for patients with prostate cancer [5]. Futher-more, remaining in or returning to work is increasingly important for patients with and survivors of prostate cancer. Occupational therapists support men to remain in or return to work by providing fast-track care, counseling, and monitoring the men in work environment [10].

This chapter describes briefly cancer rehabilitation and rehabilitation approaches for prostate cancer patients at every stage of the disease for minimizing the morbidity rates associated with prostate cancer treatment to increase occupational participation and improve QOL. The chapter also focuses on physical and occupational therapy approaches for patients with prostate cancer with psychosocial and vocational rehabilitation after prostate cancer treatment.

2. Cancer rehabilitation

Conventionally, function is the most important indicator of activity and is strongly associated with physical performance and interrelated areas such as range of motion, muscular strength, and endurance [11]. The more contemporary function is a perspective that encompasses individual's physical conditions, emotional and psychological states, and the environmental and social circumstances of the individual [12]. The World Health Organization's International Classification of Functioning, Disability and Health (ICF) describes a framework that focuses this multidimensional or biopsychosocial approach for a deeper understanding of function [11, 12]. Within the ICF framework, function is defined as the interactions between an individual, their health conditions, and the social and personal situations in which they thrive [13]. The complex interactions between these variables determine function and disability. In the context of prostate cancer, morbidity associated with the disease and its treatments can lead to functional problems or impairments in physiological, psychological, or behavioral attributes (body functions and structures), potentially leading to limitations in the ability to execute desired tasks (activity) and participation in social demands (participation) [14]. A variety of approaches and a framework for cancer rehabilitation are based on the ICF to diagnosis and treatment of function for prostate cancer survivors [15].

The overall aim in rehabilitation of all cancer types is to overcome all symptoms causing functional difficulties and increase QOL [16]. De Lisa mentioned the importance of maintaining QOL at a high level; therefore, rehabilitation should not only focus on improving function and prognosis [17]. In general, cancer rehabilitation goals are classified as restorative, supportive, palliative, and preventive according to progression and the nature of cancer. *Restorative care* aims at maximal recovery of residual function of the patients. *Supportive* efforts seek to increase ability in daily life and mobility using effective methods such as decrease in functional difficulties and compensate for permanent deficits. In this stage, rehabilitation also aims to prevent disuse for secondary problems such as contractures and loss of muscle strength. *Palliative treatment* aims to reduce or eliminate symptoms such as pain and dyspnea. In the terminal stage of the patient, physical, psychological, and social high QOL as well as wishes of the patient are important, and positioning, heat modalities, low-frequency therapy, breathing– relaxation exercises, or assistive devices can be used. The primary goal of *preventive rehabilitation* is to prevent impairments. Rehabilitation in this stage must include preoperative education, maintenance of strength, and range of motion after treatment. This rehabilitation process starts right after diagnosis [18]. This framework can guide a therapist in all types of cancer.

Body functions and body structures
Somatic
Direct operation sequences (wound healing, lymphocele, urinary retention, urinary)
Radiation effects (cystitis, proctitis, lymphedema)
Treatment-related hormone deficiency symptoms
Urinary incontinence
Post-therapeutic pain syndromes
Sequelae cytostatic chemotherapy (polyneuropathy), myelosuppression
Sexual dysfunction (erectile dysfunction)
Psychosocial
Problems of coping
Depression
Relapse fears
Sleep disorders
Partnership problems
Fatigue syndrome
Post-traumatic stress disorder
Activities
Reduction in exercise capacity
Restriction in the field of transportation (incontinence, bone pain, edema)
Social withdrawal
Participation
Problems in integrating into the social environment
Problems with the reintegration
Limitation of mobility and participation in cultural life (incontinence)

Table 1. Impairment of functional health in prostate cancer.

http://dx.doi.org/10.5772/63989

General rehabilitation goals	Evaluation instruments
Physical performance	WHO Activity Index, Karnofsky Performance Score, Harvard Step Test, Ergometry, Muscle Strength Measurement (Vigorimeter, Digimax Muscle Testing), Quality of Life Questionnaires (EORTC-QLQ-C30), Functional Assessment of Cancer Therapy (G: General, F: Fatigue, P: Prostate-FACT)
Function-related treatment goals	Direct Assessment of Functional Abilities (DAFA) Direct Assessment of Functional Status (DAFS)
Reducing post-surgical problems (scars discomfort, seroma)	Clinical observation
Reducing symptoms after radiotherapy (cystitis, proctitis)	Micturition, Chair Diary
Reducing hormone deficiency symptoms (vasomotor reactions, osteoporosis)	Visual Analog Scale (VAS) *Osteodensitometry must be checked
Reducing symptoms after cytostatic chemotherapy (polyneuropathy)	Common Toxicity Criteria of the National Cancer Institute (NCI-CTC), Sensitivity Measurement, Vibration Sense
Reduction of fatigue	Multidimensional fatigue Inventory (MFI), Functional Assessment of Cancer Therapy, Fatigue (FACT-F), Visual Analog Scale (VAS), EORTC-QLQ-C30, Fatigue Module
Reducing pain	Visual Analog Scale (VAS), Pain Diary
Reduction of lymphedema	Clinical observation, Rating scale
Bladder in post therapeutic Urge symptoms	Voiding diary *Must be checked with the urologist
Improvement in urinary incontinence	Miktions protocol, PAD test, Biofeedback, *Residual urine and results of uroflowmetry must be checked with the urologist.
Dealing with sexual dysfunction, improvement of erectile dysfunction	Diary, International Index of Erectile Function (IIEF)
Improvement of functional disorders of the musculoskeletal system	Range of motion
Improving self-sufficiency	Detailed activity analysis, Functional Independence Measure (FIM), Barthel Index (BI), Instrumental Activities of Daily Living Scale (IADL), Role Checklist (RL)
Reduction of long-term care	Functional Independence Measure (FIM), Barthel Index (BI)
Learning proper movement, sporting and leisure activities	OQ (Occupational Questionnaire), Interest Checklist and Activity Checklist (ICAC)
Improvement of cognitive performance	d2-test (attention stress test), Benton test (visual memory-BT), Multiple Choice Vocabulary Intelligence Test (MWT-B),

General rehabilitation goals	Evaluation instruments
	Loewenstein Occupational Therapy Cognitive Assessment (LOTCA)
Promoting disease management, improving self-awareness and self-acceptance, emotional stabilization	EORTC, SF-36, Functional Assessment of Cancer Therapy (G: General, F: Fatigue, P: Prostate-FACT),
Coping with stress and anxiety depressive states and relaxation	"Stress thermometer", Hospital Anxiety and Depression Scale (HADS-D), Beck Depression Inventory (BDI), Beck Anxiety Inventory (BAI), Visual Analog Scale (VAS)
Reduction of Progression	Fear of Progression Questionnaire
Assistance in transition and when dealing with stroke-related disabilities (incontinence, erectile dysfunction)	QLQ-C30, prostate module
Breakdown of family and partnership problems	Interview, Couples Climate Scales
Reduction of insomnia	SF, Diary
Construction of meaning and objective perspectives	Interview
Treatment goals in the social sphere and Preparation of reintegration, possibly initiating professional promotions	CIO Community Integration Questionnaire, ISSI (Interview Schedule For Social Interaction)
Obtaining self-sufficiency, financial management and participation in social life and counseling and assistance for reintegration, placement of self-help groups	Reintegration to Normal Living Index, Instrumental Activities of Daily Living Scale (IADL)
Learning to continence training and transfer in activities of daily living	Miktions protocol, Diary, Barthel Index (BI), Instrumental Activities of Daily Living Scale (IADL)
Reduction of risk behavior (smoking alcohol abuse, overwork)	Life Habits Assessment (LIFE-H), Questionnaires
Positive influence of eating habits within the meaning of health promotion	Diet Protocol, Body Mass Index (BMI), Bioelectrical Impedance Analysis (BIA)
Vocational rehabilitation	Worker Role Interview, Valpar Component Work Samples (VCWS), COPM

Table 2. Rehabilitation goals and the evaluation instruments mostly used for patients with prostate cancer.

In patients with prostate cancer, fatigue, urinary incontinence, sexual dysfunction, impaired physical performance, psychological distress, weight gain, and changes in male body image are stated as the long-term sequelae of disease. Therefore, while considering general rehabilitation framework, special attention has to be given and specific methods must be used while making a treatment plan for patients with prostate cancer.

http://dx.doi.org/10.5772/63989

The evaluation for rehabilitation program of patients with prostate cancer for determining the individual rehabilitation needs can be identified after completion of the primary treatment of prostate cancer to verify the success of rehabilitation intervention [19]. During the follow-up treatment in patients who are taken directly from the acute care settings, the results of the current status of malignancy and PSA levels must be recorded in addition to the results of special rehabilitation evaluation tests, instruments, or interviews on the day of admission to check the rehabilitation capacity of patients with prostate cancer. Patients must be evaluated by functional and goal-oriented evaluation instruments in the somatic, psychosocial, and vocational rehabilitation and participation in daily living activities and public life with contextual factor areas; thus, the therapist can obtain a top-down view of these patients [20]. **Table 1** shows the impairment areas of functional health in prostate cancer which must be analyzed by rehabilitation therapists.

Evaluation tests for assessing body structure and functions, activity, and participation conducted at the beginning and end of rehabilitation to assess the level of achieving success in terms of the rehabilitation goals. **Table 2** shows the rehabilitation goals and the evaluation instruments which are mostly used by the therapists for patients with prostate cancer.

Cancer rehabilitation must include different therapies from different specialists to improve muscle strength and cardiopulmonary endurance, preserve energy for daily living activities, decrease stress, and especially decrease the effects of prostate cancer and its treatments. Physical therapy and occupational therapy specialists may be involved in the care of prostate cancer patients from the beginning of treatment to the end of a patient's life. They provide evidence-based interventions during inpatient care, outpatient follow-up, education, and services in home care and hospice care settings.

3. Physical therapy

Herein, it is important to remember that rehabilitation programs are driven for men with prostate cancer. Therefore, physical therapists should also be aware of the factors threatening men's health. These factors are stated as obesity, overweight, and bad habits (smoking and drug or alcohol abuse). Epidemics in many diseases are directly related to smoking, poor diet, excess alcohol consumption, and sedentary lifestyles [21]. For a man with prostate cancer and life-threatening habits, the rehabilitation program must also include preparation of a healthy life plan for him as well as his partner. Smoking and other substance abuse should be avoided and such patients can be referred to psychotherapy or cognitive behavioral therapy to redesign their lifestyle. A coordinated plan of rehabilitation team aiming at a healthy diet and lifestyle can lead to good recovery after cancer diagnosis. The main role of physical therapy is to inhibit sedentary behavior and maintain adequate exercise for patients with prostate cancer.

3.1. Muscle strength and loss of bone mineral density

Prostate cancer and its treatments can cause inactivity and disuse syndrome which must be avoided, while fitness and active lifestyles should be encouraged [16]. It is important to preserve and restore function through exercise as exercise has several, evident positive effects on patients with cancer. Graded exercise has been suggested as a treatment strategy for cancer-related fatigue that has the strongest evidence [22]. Aerobic exercise has been found to have effects on not only fatigue but also psychological well-being, QOL, physical performance, and weight control [16, 22, 23]. Improvements in the sense of personal worth, self-esteem, self-image, and confidence have also been stated as good results of exercise. Therefore, exercise improves the positive mood of people and decreases negative moods such as depression and anxiety [16, 22–24]. Some studies also stated the reduced risk of disease recurrence [22–24].

It is stated that aerobic exercise is helpful if it is given in low to moderate intensity (50–70 heart rate%), starting from 15 minutes to 30 minutes duration 3–5 times a week in a progressive way. The current exercise guidelines indicate that cancer survivors should achieve 150-min aerobic exercise per week and resistance (strength) training twice weekly [24, 25]. Most importantly, exercise needs to become a habit. Patients can be encouraged to start exercise with a short duration (15 min a day, several times a week) and then shape the pattern. Electronic monitoring bracelets can be helpful while following this pattern [21]. The patient can also control himself via this bracelet.

Berglund offered a physical training program for men with prostate cancer for an hour lasting for 7 weeks. This training started with light physical training, breathing exercises, and relaxation, and then included exercises of the pelvic floor [26]. The participants stated the benefit of this exercise program. The physical therapist should prepare a patient-specific aerobic exercise plan. Strengthening and endurance exercises should be performed in addition to aerobic training to improve participation in the activities of daily living [16]. Pelvic floor exercises must be added to physical therapy program for prostate cancer patients. These exercises will be mentioned during the management of urinary incontinence.

3.2. Incontinence

Urinary incontinence is common in patients with prostate cancer who underwent surgery or radiation therapy. Stress incontinence characterized with loss of urine with a cough, sneeze, or laugh is the most common type of urine leakage after prostate surgery, while the need to frequently urinate with episodes of leakage is the most common type seen after radiation therapy [27]. The treatments are as follows:

a. *Pelvic floor exercises*: Pelvic floor muscle training was found to be evident in speeding the recovery of continence [27, 28]. Recovery of normal urinary control after surgery normally takes 1 or 2 years. Pelvic-floor reeducation should be used for treating incontinence effectively [16]. First, it is important to train men to control their ability to hold in their urine. For this purpose, men are instructed on the identification and function of the pelvic floor muscles. Training men prior to prostate surgery can help men use their muscles more actively following surgery [27]. Kegel exercises are taught to men to strengthen the pelvic floor muscles. These exercises consist of repeated, high-intensity contractions of the muscles. Similar to providing training, introducing the exercises before surgery is also very beneficial. If possible, the patient is advised to start exercises before the medical treatment. Pelvic floor exercises can be combined with biofeedback programs. In a study, the authors showed positive results on incontinence after a single session of biofeedback-assisted behavioral training. The use of biofeedback may improve a man's ability to isolate the pelvic floor muscle and differentiate between muscle contraction and relaxation [29, 30].

b. *Supportive care, behavioral therapy*: This treatment includes behavior modification to prevent urine leakage. Men are advised to drink fewer fluids, avoid caffeine, alcohol, or spicy foods, and limit drink before bedtime. Patients must be encouraged to urinate regularly and not wait until the last moment possible. Conservative behavioral treatments by changing patients' behavior or environment or by teaching new skills can make improvements in symptoms [31].

c. *Neuromuscular electrical stimulation*: Stimulation can be used to retrain and strengthen weak urinary muscles and improve bladder control. A probe is inserted into the anus and a current is passed through the probe at a level below the pain threshold, causing a contraction. The patient is instructed to squeeze the muscles when the current is on. After the contraction, the current is switched off [28, 30].

3.3. Fatigue management

Most cancer patients experience fatigue and loss of energy. This severe and activity-limiting symptom is also common among patients with prostate cancer. Fatigue is mostly related with cancer treatment [16, 31]; however, it may also be present after or before treatment due to cancer [32, 33]. From our experience, in the presence of fatigue, patients, their relatives, and even some professionals suggest to rest and slow down activities. During the day time, many patients sleep a lot and cannot sleep well at night. Prolonged rest and inactivity induces muscular catabolism and the time of being fatigue increases [16]. Therefore, cancer patients suffering from primary fatigue should not be advised to increase the amount of daily rest. As we have mentioned earlier, exercise has a positive effect on fatigue. Therefore, patients should not be advised to rest more but carry out aerobic exercise [34]. It is supported that an 8-week cardiovascular exercise program in patients with localized prostate cancer undergoing radiotherapy improved the overall QOL and helped prevent fatigue [31].

Occupational therapists follow other strategies in terms of physical, psychological, cognitive, and social dimensions of fatigue. Graded activity and diversional should be planned in the manner of giving exercise [33]. Other interventions to reduce the degree of fatigue are stress management, nutritional management, and energy conservation techniques [16]. During energy conservation, patients should be taught to spread out activities through the use of timetables, organize activities to the energy level required, ensure breaks during activities, and use adaptive devices [33]. Providing good rest/sleep patterns, teaching structured sleep is also an important role of a therapist [16]. The patient should be recommended to maintain a schedule of sleeping and waking times, avoid sleeping constantly during day time, open curtains in the morning, and avoid doing things that can affect night sleep [33]. Therapists should remember that fatigue is an important symptom of cancer and help their patients to manage this symptom.

3.4. Lymphedema management

Lymphedema can be observed in patients with prostate cancer as a result of radiation damage or following the removal of lymph nodes during surgery. It is characterized with the collection of fluids in the lower extremities, and compression therapy helps the fluid to move and reduce swelling which can help the patient move easily and comfortably [34, 35].

Both occupational and physical therapists may decide the kind of compression therapy and the effective manual techniques for patients with prostate cancer. Elevation, exercise, and using custom-fitted compression wear can help increase the lymph flow in the early stages of lymphedema. Compression wears are worn continuously throughout the day and removed at night. They are reapplied as soon as the patient awakens in the early morning. Additionally; to drain the lymph from the extremity pneumatic pump compression which provides sequential, active compression can be used in the home [34, 35]. For severe edema, compression bandaging after manual lymphatic drainage using light massage (complete decongestive therapy) can be effective. Manual massage can help collateral lymph vessels to milk the lymphedema. To determine the effectiveness of the treatment, the size of the extremity always must be monitored by the therapist [36–38].

3.5. Peripheral neuropathy

Peripheral neuropathy is one of the side effects of chemotherapy. It is characterized with tingling, burning, or shooting pain sensation of hands and feet depending on nerve damage. Patients with prostate cancer may also experience loss of sensation which can cause problems on somatosensory perception, finger movements and grasping problems, balance problems, tripping, and/or decreased reflexes. Physical and occupational therapy can help the patients with prostate cancer to improve coordination, balance and gait, fine motor skills, and dexterity. The primary aim of treating peripheral neuropathy is to decrease the risk of falling and injuries [39].

3.6. Scar tissue management

Radiation therapy can cause scar tissue which may increase pain and decrease the flexibility of the skin. Physical therapists can use manual therapy and tissue techniques for stretching and tissue and nerve mobilization to decrease pain and increase the tissue mobility of the patients with prostate cancer [39].

3.7. Early ambulation

If patients underwent surgery, early postoperative ambulation and improving physical functions is the main goal of physical therapy [22]. During chemotherapy, physical strength

http://dx.doi.org/10.5772/63989

tends to diminish; hence, rehabilitation aims to encourage ambulation consistent with the patient's condition even during chemotherapy and prevent disuse syndrome and maintain physical and muscle strength by performing early ambulation [24, 26].

4. Occupational therapy

Occupational therapy (OT) offers a client-centered approach to patients with prostate cancer. OT clinical reasoning assessments and interventions focus on functioning and participation by rehabilitating the abilities of the patients with prostate cancer. Therapists guide goal-directed activities that give meaning to the patient's life [40]. According to the ICF, the affected performance areas of prostate cancer on which OT focuses are shown in **Table 3**.

ICF			
Body structure/body function	**Impairment**	**Activity**	**Participation**
Prostate	Sensory	Basic ADL* Instrumental ADL*	Loss of sense of self as a sexual being
	Cognitive		Loss of ability to participate in activities (self-care, sport, and leisure)
	Psychological		Loss of occupational roles: work/ family
	Motor		Inability to be independently involved in daily occupations

*ADL = Activities of Daily Living.

Table 3. Affected performance areas and occupational therapy focus in patients with prostate cancer.

As shown in **Table 3**, OT mainly focuses on activity and participation limitations in the rehabilitation phase. Patients with prostate cancer generally require activity education, sensory training breathing and relaxation education, stress management education, sensory stimuli and praxis skills, cognitive therapy, erectile dysfunction and sexual rehabilitation, cognitive therapy, vocational rehabilitation, patient education and counseling, and also rehabilitation during palliative care and supportive care to engage in activities independently.

4.1. Daily living activities education

Reasons of limitation of activity are both dysmotility and muscle weakness. Activity limitation interventions are important for improving the activity performance of patients with cancer. The occupational therapist describes and measures activity performance necessitated to be carried out by patients with prostate cancer. After the activity for individual needs is identified, intervention strategies may be determined. The practitioner must determine the appropriate intervention approach for each patient. These strategies are divided into four parts: restoration, compensation, environmental modification, and education of patient [41].

4.1.1. Restoration

Patients have many different activities related to their roles. It is important to determine the most important activities for their life. The focus of the restorative approach is to develop patient skills and abilities or restore the activity performance of the patient with prostate cancer. A restorative approach is planned specifically to the situation of the patient. In this stage, grading of the activity level can be done. Grading can be done according to the following parameters:

- *Physical assistance*: If the patient with prostate cancer is in need of help, practitioner or caregiver can provide assistance. In this way, patients' skill to complete task may be increased. The presence of some symptoms such as fatigue or pain can cause the patient with prostate cancer to take physical support. This support does not mean that caregiver do all of the tasks instead of the patient.
- *Supervision and cuing*: This involves a number and types of cues. For example, if the patient forgets some tasks of activity due to cognitive impairment, patient can be supported by verbal, tactile, and written material cues to help the patient with cancer finalize the activity.
- *Activity demands*: The activity can be changed due to complexity of performance skills. Generally, for patients with prostate cancer, it will be better to select an activity with low-motor and high-cognitive demands by the reason of symptoms. In activity education, the motor and cognitive demands of the activity can be increased step by step.
- *Sequencing of activity*: Activity is divided in order of priority and sequence. The number of steps in tasks and the total number of steps can be purposed to increase. Thus, patient with prostate cancer can complete the activity easily without fatigue or pain.
- *Type of activity*: During activity education, activities can be graded from familiar to unfamiliar or from former to new. This method can help the patient with prostate cancer feel more comfortable during activity education.
- *Environment*: Activity environment can affect participation in the activities. For instance, patients with prostate cancer may have urinary incontinence. Therefore, patients may need to use toilet frequently. This situation can affect men in a negative way. To avoid negative symptoms such as stress or unhappiness, patients may limit themselves to only familiar environments to find a toilet. In intervention programs, the activity can be graded from a familiar to unfamiliar environment.

4.1.2. Compensation

The compensation approach focuses on using the patients' skills to achieve the highest possible stage of functioning in the activities. Therapists may teach the patients with prostate cancer new methods for modifying task performance to compensate for deficient areas of occupation, performance, and individual factors. If the patients still require help for participation in new activities, the occupational therapist should also give some advice regarding the use of adapted techniques or equipment. Patients with prostate cancer may need to use some assisted technology devices such as activity facilitator or computer-aided software to perform the activities. These instruments can help decrease symptoms (i.e., fatigue and pain) of cancer and increase participation in the activities of patients.

4.1.3. *Environmental modification*

Environmental modifications consist of compensation, modification, and adaptation strategy. The compensation approach directly influences patient functioning. However, environmental modification approach influences patients' functioning indirectly. Patients with prostate cancer will need help for home or work environment. Occupational therapists should give advice to redesign the home or work environment of the patient with prostate cancer where the patients can participate in activity easier than before. Modifications can include low-cost and easily accessible strategies to improve participation in domestic and community activities. Patients can also have problems in a social environment. They might not want to participate in social activities owing to general reluctance to do any activities. Besides, they may be exposed to stigma and pity from other people. For these reasons, occupational therapists must consider both physical and social aspects. Daily living activity education needs to be holistic and must integrate the activity, environment, and the patient with prostate cancer. Using occupation-based activity, education improves participation and supports wellness and QOL of patients with prostate cancer.

4.2. Sensory training

Treatment modalities such as surgery (e.g., radical prostatectomy), androgen deprivation therapy, radiation therapy, and chemotherapy affect the sensory–neural ways in body. After treatment, some deficiencies can occur in sensory skills. In particular, body composition may be affected if patients receive ADT. The generally observed side effects such as fatigue and pain might negatively affect patient body. Literature evidence demonstrates that sensory training is an important part of intervention program in patients with prostate cancer [42]. The purpose of sensory training is to develop body image by increasing body awareness. The body awareness includes these trainings and sensory stimuli, breathing, and relaxation techniques.

4.3. Breathing and relaxation education

Cancer and its treatment can be stressful for patients with prostate cancer and their partners and caregivers. Relaxation techniques and other body/mind practices can help calm the patient's mind, reduce stress, and sharpen the ability to focus to maintain inner peace. Some patients with prostate cancer use these techniques to help themselves relax while they wait for the results of treatments or tests. Breathing techniques include slow inhalation and exhalation to reduce tension in the shoulders, trunk, and abdomen. The process begins with focusing on normal breathing in a quiet and comfortable place when the patients feel stressful. Patients should perform deep inhalation and slow exhalation. During this phase, the abdominal muscles should be relaxed during inhalation; the abdominal muscles should be contracted during exhalation [41]. Relaxation techniques involve teaching the patient with prostate cancer to cope with stress which results in deficiency of body composition. During relaxation education, the patient with prostate cancer is instructed to contract and relax his major skeletal muscles systematically and then asked to repeat phases silently and finally asked to use purposeful images to achieve the goals [41]. OT practitioners have a core role in providing therapeutic activities that enable the patients with sensory problems to develop body imagination in occupational performance.

4.4. Stress management

Occupational therapists help patients with prostate cancer to acknowledge, express, accept, and use problem-solving techniques to address the changes that result from prostate cancer and its treatments. Effective stress management can include relaxation training, education, a supportive environment, social support, and participation in daily living activities. It is supported that these interventions can help decrease the treatment-related symptoms, the physiological accompaniments of stress, and improve mood of the patient with prostate cancer. Patients who participate in such rehabilitation programs are shown to control and experience reduced interpersonal conflicts and distress related to cancer-related intrusive thinking and have improved mental health [5].

4.5. Sensory stimuli

The patients involve in many activities which include various sensory stimuli. The basic activities involve tactile and proprioceptive inputs. Occupational therapists impart sensory training to patients with prostate cancer and also suggest somatosensoriel perception activities that involve tactile and proprioceptive inputs especially after chemotherapy or hormonal therapy. Patients use these senses during routines of activity in daily life. In addition, mirror activities and visual perception skills must be added to intervention programs to promote sensorial perception, harmony with the environment, and the body imagination of patients with prostate cancer [43–45].

4.6. Cognitive therapy

Cognitive therapy approach was generally used in patients with mental health problems. However, patients with prostate cancer may have some deficiencies in cognitive skills owing to cancer and its treatments [16]. OT intervention should focus on cognitive skills and activity function, and it includes orientation, memory, attention, motor planning, and executive functions of the patient with prostate cancer [44, 45].

Orientation is the ability to understand the self and the relationship between self and past–present environment time. After receiving the cancer treatments, patients might have orientation problems about place or time. In the intervention, verbal and external cues are used as reminders and therapy advances by changing numbers and types of cues [46]. *Memory* is described in terms of sensory memory, working or immediate memory, and long-term memory. If there are any problems on these types of memory, patients' tasks may be affected. Occupational therapists evaluate and improve memory abilities. They may also advice to use verbal, visual, and external cues for activity independently [46]. *Attention* is a multidimension that includes five components: sustained attention (concentration), selective attention, divided attention, alternating attention, and shifting of attention. Patients may have problems pertaining to not only each component of attention but also several components of attention [46]. The occupational therapist provides examples of basic and complex tasks for each component of attention. *Motor planning or praxis* is the ability of individuals to point at how to get their body to do what they want it to do. Motor planning involves the cognitive skills of intending to move, selecting a goal, planning the movement, and anticipating the end result. Impaired motor planning is disabling in cancer patients so that they may not be able to initiate or follow through on tasks [46]. The occupational therapist may give information about the functional properties of an activity. Besides, they might inform about conceptual errors related to creating the idea of the movement, involving object usage information, and sequencing of activity. When evaluating or treating patients with prostate cancer for motor planning abilities, it is important to identify the patients' activities. A series of cues (visual, verbal, or tactile) may be used if the patient experiences difficulty in performing an activity demand in the OT [46]. *Executive functions* consist of organization, problem-solving, and coping skills. It may significantly influence performance of activities of daily living. Occupational therapist using a dynamic interactional approach to the intervention of executive functions and organizational, problem- solving, and coping skills would focus on self-awareness and ability to perform new, unexpected or routine tasks [46]. In conclusion, cognitive impairments can be seen, caused either by cancer or its treatments in patients with prostate cancer. Hence, cognitive skills of prostate cancer patients should not be ignored.

4.7. Erectile dysfunction and sexual rehabilitation

Rehabilitation approach to erectile dysfunction is focused on pelvic floor muscle training and the muscle strength at the base of the penis. After the initial examination and determining an intervention plan, the physical therapist may guide the patient to perform specific pelvic floor muscle exercises and indirectly related muscles such as abdominal and gluteal muscles. These exercises help increase oxygen supply to the tissues. Vacuum therapy can also be used to generate negative pressure that increases the blood flow to the penis [47].

Sexual rehabilitation is one of the most important components of rehabilitation of patients with prostate cancer and significantly related to quality of life. Men with prostate cancer are more stressed about sexual dysfunction if they are younger. Both younger and older men are in need of physical, social, emotional, and psychological treatment assistance for this issue [28].

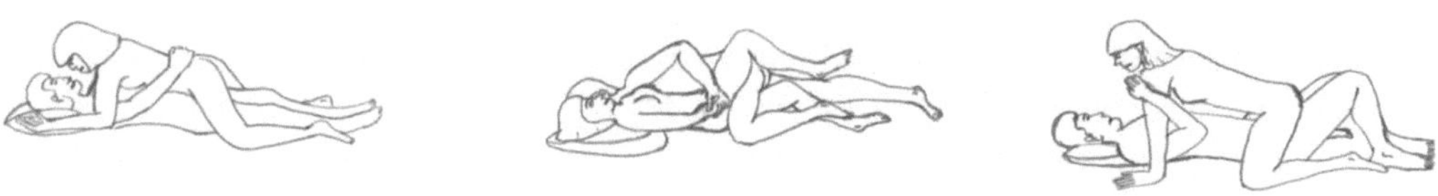

Figure 1. Safe and less fatigue sex positions for patients with prostate cancer.

Sexuality is an intimate issue and occupational therapy practitioners can examine both societal attitudes toward patients with prostate cancer and their own beliefs, values, and attitudes about sexuality. Patients can be emotionally vulnerable and recessive. The occupational therapists may provide information about the sexual rehabilitation. Rehabilitation should consists of an interdisciplinary team including nurses, physiotherapists, occupational therapists, social workers, sexologists, dieticians, massage therapists and psychologists. Die Perink et al. had conducted a rehabilitation program, with a 4-day course developed based on the experience with rehabilitation of more than 7000 cancer survivors, included physical activity, pelvic floor exercises, couples massage and relaxation, diet, and education of sexuality. They advise to practice sexual rehabilitation about sexual dysfunction [28]. Occupational therapists may give physically advice not only patients, but also partners regarding favorable sex positions (**Figure 1**). These positions can be more comfortable and safe for men. Thus, the occurrence of symptoms such as fatigue and pain will be reduced with occupational therapy intervention. Patients with prostate cancer will thus have normal sexual function. The patients and their partners should be informed about social support. It has many dimensions, including emotional, material assistance, and information. The occupational therapist should give lifestyle advice to patients for applying to their daily life. Thus, the patients and their partners will be improved.

4.8. Vocational Rehabilitation

Long survival with good quality of life make the patient with prostate cancer to think about returning to work after prostate cancer treatment and also 6 months after the radical prostatectomy surgery, men can return to their work. This may be a big positive step for men, and men might look forward to re-establishing his usual routine and it is understandable if they feel anxious or worried. But from a view of occupational therapy, having a return-to-work plan can help the patient to make the transition easier. Most of the mentally and physically healthy prostate cancer survivors do not require a job change, while others need some adjustments such as reduced working hours, modified duties, trying to do similar jobs, making self to do lists with time use with fatigue management, or the use of assistive technology. An occupational therapist can help the man determine if he is ready to go back to work, identify accommodations that will help him do his job, and help him get training or seek new employment if needed. In addition, improving self-management skills of prostate cancer survival helps him identify his needs and borders which can help him prepare for independent daily life and social reinteraction [48].

4.9. Patient education and counseling

Patient, partner, family, and caregiver education are an important part of occupational therapy because nearly all of the approaches (restoration, compensation, environmental modification, etc.) involve learning new strategies and combining these strategies into persons' lifestyles. Education contains information about prostate cancer; symptoms create and raise awareness about management skills. At the same time, an occupational therapist can use various materials such as demonstration, written format, pictures, and videotapes to help the patient and family participate in their activities. In addition to general education, it is supported that the main education resource of the patient with prostate cancer is internet but this way may not be

http://dx.doi.org/10.5772/63989

helpful for psychosocial healing of the patient with prostate cancer or the survivor. Hence, in recent studies, new education programs were designed such as "Between men," which offers group online therapy sessions and education. The aims of these programs were to give the patients all the available information about prostate cancer, treatment, side effects, and how to deal with the side effects. Program planned once a week for 7 weeks and it included patients' experiences and reactions, patients' communication difficulties especially sexual and emotional effects, prostate cancer disease and treatments, incontinence, sexuality, importance, and problem solving. Online education programs must be improved and generalized for patients and survivors with prostate cancer [5, 49].

5. Rehabilitation in palliative care and hospice care

In palliative and hospice care, both physical and occupational therapists support men with prostate cancer by minimizing the secondary symptoms related to cancer and its treatments. The role of the occupational therapist and physical therapist in palliative and hospice care is quite similar and important.

At the end of life, physical therapy offers functional training, therapeutic exercise, and soft tissue mobilization. The goals of physical therapy are to improve overall strength, range of motion, and endurance of the patient with prostate cancer. Physical therapists may use heat, cold, and TENS (transcutaneous electrical nerve stimulation) for pain relief and design exercises that improve endurance and positioning regimens that help the patient maintain functional range of motion [50, 51].

In this stage, occupational therapists identify the roles and activities which are meaningful to the patient with prostate cancer and try to present the barriers that limit their performance. Occupational therapists support the patient both for physical and psychosocial/behavioral health requirements and pay close attention to what is most important for the patient. They look at the available activity and environmental resources to increase patient participation. The main goal of occupational therapy is to improve the quality of life according to patients' values and maximize residual functional abilities [50].

6. Conclusion

Patients with prostate cancer can face problems about body structure and functions, activity, and participation which may limit their participation to life. Patients with prostate cancer require skilled rehabilitation and supportive care from the initial process of diagnosis through clinical reasoning and treatment to posttreatment periods. Qualified interdisciplinary rehabilitation interventions may help men regain their performance and independency and maintain the highest quality of life.

Author details

Meral Huri*, Burcu Semin Akel and Sedef Şahin

*Address all correspondence to: meralhuri@yahoo.com

Hacettepe University, Faculty of Health Sciences, Department of Occupational Therapy, Ankara, Turkey

References

[1] Cheville AL. Cancer rehabilitation. Semin Oncol. 2005; 32 (2): 219–224. DOI:10.1053/j.seminoncol.2004.11.009

[2] Jemal A, Bray F, Center MM, Ferlay J, Ward E, Forman D. Global cancer statistics. CA Cancer J Clin. 2011; 61: 69–90. DOI: 10.3322/caac.20107.

[3] Bray F, Lortet-Tieulent J, Ferlay J, Forman D, Auvinen A. Prostate cancer incidence and mortality trends in 37 European countries: an overview. Eur J Cancer. 2010; 46 (17): 3040–3052. DOI:10.1016/j.ejca.2010.09.013

[4] Heidenreich A, Bastian PJ, Bellmunt J, Bolla M, Joniau S, Kwast TV. EAU guidelines on prostate cancer. Part 1: screening, diagnosis, and treatment of clinically localised disease. Eur Urol. 2011; 59: 61–71. DOI: 10.1016/j.eururo.2013.09.046

[5] Huri M, Huri E, Kayihan H, Altuntas O. Effects of occupational therapy on quality of life of patients with metastatic prostate cancer: a randomized controlled study. Saudi Med J. 2015; 36 (38): 954–61. DOI: 10.15537/smj.2015.8.11461

[6] Keogh J W, Patel A, MacLeod RD, Masters J. Perceived barriers and facilitators to physical activity in men with prostate cancer: possible influence of androgen deprivation therapy. Eur J Cancer Care. 2014; 23 (2): 263–273. DOI: 10.1111/ecc.12141.

[7] Friedenreich C, Kopciuk K, Wang Q, McGregor S, Angyalfi S, Courneya K. Pre-and post-diagnosis physical activity and survival after prostate cancer. J Sci Med Sport. 2012; 15: 334–335.

[8] Baumann FT, Zopf EM, Bloch W. Clinical exercise interventions in prostate cancer patients—A systematic review of randomized controlled trials. Supp Care Cancer. 2012; 20 (2): 221–233. DOI 10.1007/s00520-011-1271-0

[9] Silver JK, Gilchrist LS. Cancer rehabilitation with a focus on evidence-based outpatient physical and occupational therapy interventions. Am J Phys Med Rehabil. 2011; 90 (5): 5–15.

[10] Knoll N, Wiedemann AU, Schultze M, Schrader M, Heckhausen J. Prostate cancer patients gradually advance goals for rehabilitation after radical prostatectomy:

applying a lines-of-defense model to rehabilitation. Psychol Aging. 2014; 29 (4): 787. DOI: 10.1037/a0038311.

[11] Chasen M, Jacobsen PB. Rehabilitation in cancer. In: Olver IN, editor. The MASCC Textbook of Cancer Supportive Care and Survivorship. New York: Springer; 2011. P. 389–396.

[12] Dalton SO, Johansen C. New paradigms in planning cancer rehabilitation and survivorship. Acta Oncol. 2013; 52 (2): 191–194. DOI:10.3109/0284186X.2012.748216

[13] Egan MY, McEwen S, Sikora L, Chasen M, Fitch M, Eldred S. Rehabilitation following cancer treatment. Disabil Rehabil. 2013; 35(26): 2245–2258. DOI: 10.3109/09638288.2013.774441

[14] Weis J, Giesler JM. Rehabilitation for cancer patients. In: Goerling U, editor. Psycho-Oncology. Berlin Heidelberg: Springer; 2014; 87–101.

[15] Holm LV, Hansen DG, Kragstrup J, Johansen C, dePont Christensen R, Vedsted P. Influence of comorbidity on cancer patients' rehabilitation needs, participation in rehabilitation activities and unmet needs: a population-based cohort study. Supp Care Cancer. 2014; 22(8): 2095–2105.

[16] Fialka-Moser V, Crevenna R, Korpan M, Quittan M. Cancer rehabilitation particularly with aspects on physical impairments. J Rehabil Med. 2003; 35: 153–162. DOI 10.1080/16501970310000511

[17] DeLisa JA. A history of cancer rehabilitation. Cancer. 2001; 92(4): 970–974. DOI: 10.1002/1097-0142

[18] Dietz JJ. Adaptive rehabilitation in cancer. Postgrad Med. 1980; 68: 145–153.

[19] Ture M, Barth J, Angst F, Aeschlimann A, Schnyder U, Zerkiebel N. Use of inpatient rehabilitation for cancer patients in Switzerland: who undergoes cancer rehabilitation? Swiss Med Wkly. 2014; 145: 14214. DOI:10.4414/smw.2015.14214

[20] Lehmann C, Beierlein V, Hagen-Aukamp C, Kerschgens C, Rhee M, Frühauf S. Psychosocial predictors of utilization of medical rehabilitation services among prostate cancer patients. Die Rehabil. 2012; 51 (3): 160–170. DOI: 10.4414/smw.2015.14214

[21] Pelman RS, Elterman DS. Lifestyle and disease, male health and risks. Rev Med Clin Condes. 2014; 25(1): 25–29. DOI:10.1016/S0716-8640(14)70006-9

[22] Shin KY, Guo Y, Konzen B, Fu J, Yadav R, Bruera E. Inpatient cancer rehabilitation: the experience of a national comprehensive cancer center. Am J Phys Med Rehabil. 2011; 90 (5): 63–S68. DOI: 10.1097/PHM.0b013e31820be1a4

[23] Bourke L, Homer KE, Thaha MA, Steed L, Rosario DJ, Robb KA. Interventions to improve exercise behaviour in sedentary people living with and beyond cancer: a systematic review. Br J Cancer. 2014; 110: 831–841. DOI: 10.1038/bjc.2013

[24] Bourke L, Sohanpal R, Nanton V, Crank H, Rosario DJ, Saxton JM. A qualitative study evaluating experiences of a lifestyle intervention in men with prostate cancer undergoing androgen suppression therapy. Trials. 2012; 13: 208. DOI: 10.1186/1745-6215-13-208

[25] Hunter EG, Baltisberger J. Functional outcomes by age for inpatient cancer rehabilitation: a retrospective chart review. J Appl Gerontol. 2013; 32(4): 443–456. DOI: 10.1177/0733464811432632

[26] Berglund G, Petersson LM, Eriksson KRN, Häggman M. "Between men": patient perceptions and priorities in a rehabilitation program for men with prostate cancer. Patient Educ Counsel. 2003; 49 (3):285–292. DOI:10.1016/S0738-3991(02)00186-6

[27] Newman DK, Guzzo T, Lee D, Jayadevappa R. An evidence-based strategy for the conservative management of the male patient with incontinence. Curr Opin Urol. 2014; 24: 553–559. DOI:10.1097/MOU.0000000000000115

[28] Dieperink KB, Mark K, Mikkelsen TB. Marital rehabilitation after prostate cancer – a matter of intimacy. Int J Urol Nurs. 2016; 10 (1): 21–29. DOI: 10.1111/ijun.12091

[29] Mina DS, Au D, Alibhai SMH, Jamnicky L, Faghani N, Hilton WJ. A pilot randomized trial of conventional versus advanced pelvic floor exercises to treat urinary incontinence after radical prostatectomy: a study protocol. BMC Urol. 2015; 15: 94. DOI 10.1186/s12894-015-0088-4

[30] Wang W, Huang QM, Liu FP, Mao Q. Effectiveness of preoperative pelvic floor muscle training for urinary incontinence after radical prostatectomy: a meta-analysis. BMC Urol. 2014; 14: 99. DOI: 10.1186/1471-2490-14-99

[31] Donna B, Greenberg MD, Jennifer L, Gray BA, Catherine M, Mannix RN. Treatment-related fatigue and serum interleukin-1 levels in patients during external beam irradiation for prostate cancer. J Pain Sympt Manage. 1993; 8 (4): 196–200. DOI: 10.1016/0885-3924(93)90127-H

[32] Monga U, Garber SL, Thornby J, Vallbona C, Kerrigan AJ, Monga TN. Exercise prevents fatigue and improves quality of life in prostate cancer patients undergoing radiotherapy. Arch Phys Med Rehabil. 2007; 88(11): 1416–22. DOI: 10.1016/j.apmr.2007.08.110

[33] Cooper J. Occupational therapy in oncology and palliative care. In: Lowrie D. Occupational Therapy and Cancer Related Fatigue. John Wiley Sons, 2006.

[34] Courneya KS, Keats MR, Turner AR. Physical exercise and quality of life in cancer patients following high dose chemotherapy and autologous bone marrow transplantation. Psychooncology. 2000; 9: 127–136. DOI:10.1002/(SICI)1099-1611

[35] Wollin DA, Makarov D. Extended pelvic lymph node dissection for prostate cancer: do more nodes mean better survival? Oncology. 2014; 8 (7): 601–601.

[36] Rasmusson E, Kjellén E, Blom R, Björk-Eriksson T, Nilsson P, Gunnlaugsson A. EP-1081: low rate of lymphedema after pelvic lymphadenectomy followed by pelvic

irradiation of node positive prostate cancer. Radiother Oncol. 2013; 106 (2): 410. DOI: 10.1016/S0167-8140(15)33387-9

[37] Shaitelman SF, Cromwell KD, Rasmussen JC, Stout NL, Armer JM, Lasinski BB. Recent progress in the treatment and prevention of cancer-related lymphedema. Cancer J Clin. 2015; 65 (1): 55–81. DOI: 10.3322/caac.21253

[38] Preston, NJ, Seers, K, Mortimer, PS. Physical therapies for reducing and controlling lymphoedema of the limbs. Cochrane Database Syst Rev, 2004; 4.

[39] Choi, M, Craft, B, Geraci, SA. Surveillance and monitoring of adult cancer survivors. Am J Med. 2011; 124 (7): 598-601.

[40] Burhardt A. Oncology. In: Pendleton HM, Schultz-Krohn W, editors. Pedretti's Occupational Therapy Practice Skills for Physical Dysfunction. 6th ed. USA: Elsevier; 2006; 1157–1168.

[41] Pergolotti M, Deal AM, Williams GR, Bryant AL, Reeve BB, Muss HB. A randomized controlled trial of outpatient CAncer REhabilitation for older adults: the CARE Program. Contemporary Clinical Trials. 2015; 44: 89–94. DOI:10.1016/j.cct.2015.07.021

[42] Keogh JWL, MacLeod RD. Body composition, physical fitness, functional performance, quality of life, and fatigue benefits of exercise for prostate cancer patients: a systematic review. J Pain Sympt Manage. 2012; 43 (1): 96–110. DOI: 10.1016/j.jpainsymman.2011.03.006

[43] Rhodes VA, McDaniel RW, Hanson B, Markway E, Johnson M. Sensory perception of patients on selected antineoplastic chemotherapy protocols. Cancer Nurs. 1994; 17 (1): 45–51.

[44] Dolhi C, Leibold ML, Schreiber J. Interventions to improve personal skills and abilities, sensorimotor techniques. In: Crepeau EB, Cohn ES, Schell BAB, editors. Willard and Spackman's Occupational Therapy. 1st ed. Baltimore: Lippincott Williams and Wilkins; 2003. 595–606.

[45] Waylett-Rendall J. Interventions to improve personal skills and abilities, sensory reeducation. In: Crepeau EB, Cohn ES, Schell BAB, editors. Willard and Spackman's Occupational Therapy. 1st ed. Baltimore: Lippincott Williams & Wilkins; 2003.579–580.

[46] Giles GM. Learning perspectives, cognitive therapy. In: Crepeau EB, Cohn ES, Schell BAB, editors. Willard & Spackman's Occupational Therapy. 1st ed. Baltimore: Lippincott Williams and Wilkins; 2003.259–260.

[47] Bernardo-Filho M, Barbosa ML, da Cunha Sá-Caputo D, de Oliveira Guedes E, Pacheco Carvalho de Lima R. The relevance of the procedures related to physiotherapy in interventions in patients with prostate cancer: short review with practice approach. Int J Biomed Sci. 2014; 10 (2): 73–84.

[48] Tamminga SJ, De Boer AGEM, Verbeek JHAM, Frings-Dresen MHW. Return-to-work interventions integrated into cancer care: a systematic review. Occup Environ Med. 2010; 67 (9): 639–648. DOI:10.1136/oem.2009.050070

[49] Klemm P, Bunnell D, Cullen M, Soneji R, Gibbons P, Holecek A. Online cancer support groups: a review of the research literature. Comp Inform Nurs. 2003; 21 (3): 136–142. DOI: 10.1097/00024665-200305000-00010

[50] Prochnau C, Liu L, Boman, J. (2003). Personal–professional connections in palliative care occupational therapy. Am J Occup Ther. 2003; 57 (2): 196–204.

[51] Kealey P, McIntyre, I. An evaluation of the domiciliary occupational therapy service in palliative cancer care in a community trust: a patient and carers perspective. Eur J Cancer Care. 2005; 14(3): 232–243.